The COVID-19 Pandemic and Older Adults

T0256395

The COVID-19 pandemic has disrupted life globally through virus-related mortality and morbidity and the social and economic impacts of actions taken to stop the virus' spread. It became evident early on during the pandemic that older adults are especially vulnerable to morbidity and mortality from COVID-19, and the adverse consequences of strategies taken to mitigate its effects. While no more likely to become infected than younger populations, the risk for hospitalization and death rises considerably with age. Residents of long-term care facilities have been among the hardest hit. The pandemic has brought many facets of ageism to the fore. Community stay-at-home messages, lockdowns, social distancing requirements, and visitation restrictions contributed to a concomitant epidemic in social isolation and loneliness. Economic and social impacts have been dramatic; so too has been the disproportionate hardship experienced by members of racial and ethnic minority communities.

This book reports original empirical research and perspectives on the ramifications of the COVID-19 pandemic for the older adult population, and draws lessons for policy, research, and practice. Key issues pertaining to the impact of COVID-19 on older adults and their families, caregivers, and communities are highlighted. Four main areas are examined: personal experiences with COVID-19; long-term care system impacts; end-of-life care; and technology and innovation.

The chapters in this book were originally published as a special issue of the *Journal of Aging & Social Policy.*

Edward Alan Miller is Professor and Chair, Department of Gerontology, and Fellow, Gerontology Institute, at the John W. McCormack Graduate School of Policy & Global Studies, University of Massachusetts Boston, and Adjunct Professor of Health Services, Policy & Practice at the School of Public Health, Brown University. His research focuses on understanding the determinants and effects of public policies and practices affecting older adults in need of long-term services and support. He is author/co-author/editor/co-editor of more than 134 journal articles, 21 book chapters, and 6 books. He is the Editor-in-Chief of the *Journal of Aging & Social Policy*, and Fellow within the Gerontological Society of America.

The COVID-19 Pandemic and Older Adults

Experiences, Impacts, and Innovations

Edited by
Edward Alan Miller

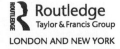

Routledge
Taylor & Francis Group

LONDON AND NEW YORK

First published 2022
by Routledge
4 Park Square, Milton Park, Abingdon, Oxon OX14 4RN

and by Routledge
605 Third Avenue, New York, NY 10158

Routledge is an imprint of the Taylor & Francis Group, an informa business

Chapters 1–4 and 6–18 © 2022 Taylor & Francis
Chapter 5 © 2021 Gabriella Nilsson, Lisa Ekstam, Anna Axmon, and Janicke Andersson.
Originally published as Open Access.

British Library Cataloguing in Publication Data
A catalogue record for this book is available from the British Library

ISBN: 978-1-032-22636-1 (hbk)
ISBN: 978-1-032-22637-8 (pbk)
ISBN: 978-1-003-27346-2 (ebk)

DOI: 10.4324/9781003273462

Typeset in Minion Pro
by Newgen Publishing UK

Publisher's Note
The publisher accepts responsibility for any inconsistencies that may have arisen during the conversion of this book from journal articles to book chapters, namely the inclusion of journal terminology.

Disclaimer
Every effort has been made to contact copyright holders for their permission to reprint material in this book. The publishers would be grateful to hear from any copyright holder who is not here acknowledged and will undertake to rectify any errors or omissions in future editions of this book.

Contents

Citation Information   viii
Notes on Contributors   xi

Introduction

1   Shining a Spotlight: The Ramifications of the COVID-19
    Pandemic for Older Adults   3
    Edward Alan Miller

Personal Experiences

2   Coronavirus-Related Anxiety, Social Isolation, and Loneliness in
    Older Adults in Northern California during the Stay-at-Home Order   21
    Laura Gaeta and Christopher R. Brydges

3   Pandemic Place: Assessing Domains of the Person-Place Fit
    Measure for Older Adults (PPFM-OA) during COVID-19   33
    Joyce Weil

4   The Impact of Stigmatization on Social Avoidance and Fear of
    Disclosure among Older People: Implications for Social Policy
    Preparedness in a Public Health Crisis   43
    Jiannan Li, Chulan Huang, Bocong Yuan, and Haixuan Liang

5   Old Overnight: Experiences of Age-Based Recommendations in
    Response to the COVID-19 Pandemic in Sweden   60
    Gabriella Nilsson, Lisa Ekstam, Anna Axmon, and Janicke Andersson

6   Living Through the COVID-19 Pandemic: Community-Dwelling
    Older Adults' Experiences   81
    Bo Xie, Kristina Shiroma, Atami Sagna De Main, Nathan W Davis,
    Karen Fingerman, and Valerie Danesh

7   "We Are Saving Their Bodies and Destroying Their Souls.":
    Family Caregivers' Experiences of Formal Care Setting Visitation
    Restrictions during the COVID-19 Pandemic   99
    *Whitney A. Nash, Lesley M. Harris, Kimberly E. Heller, and Brandon
    D. Mitchell*

Long-Term Care System Impacts

8   Prevalence of COVID-19 in Ohio Nursing Homes: What's Quality
    Got to Do with It?   117
    John Bowblis and Robert Applebaum

9   The Impact of COVID-19 on Nursing Homes in Italy: The Case of
    Lombardy   134
    Marco Arlotti and Costanzo Ranci

10 COVID-19 and Long-Term Care Policy for Older People in Japan   147
    Margarita Estévez-Abe and Hiroo Ide

11 The Impact of COVID-19 on Social Isolation in Long-term Care
    Homes: Perspectives of Policies and Strategies from Six Countries 162
    *Charlene H. Chu, Jing Wang, Chie Fukui, Sandra Staudacher, Patrick
    A. Wachholz, and Bei Wu*

12 COVID-19 Pandemic and Resilience of the Transnational Home-
    Based Elder Care System between Poland and Germany   177
    *Magdalena Nowicka, Susanne Bartig, Theresa Schwass, and Kamil
    Matuszczyk*

End-of-Life Care

13 Rethinking the Role of Advance Care Planning in the Context of
    Infectious Disease   199
    Sara Moorman, Kathrin Boerner, and Deborah Carr

14 Palliative Care for Older Adults with Multimorbidity in the Time
    of COVID 19   206
    Victoria D. Powell and Maria J. Silveira

Technology and Innovation

15 Cross-Border Medical Services for Hong Kong's Older Adults in
    Mainland China: The Implications of COVID-19 for the Future of
    Telemedicine   217
    Genghua Huang, Yin Ma, and Zhaiwen Peng

16 Telephone-Based Emotional Support for Older Adults during the
    COVID-19 Pandemic   230
    Liora Bar-Tur, Michal Inbal-Jacobson, Sharon Brik-Deshen,
    Yael Zilbershlag, Sigal Pearl Naim, and Yitzhak Brick

17 Technology Recommendations to Support Person-Centered Care
    in Long-Term Care Homes during the COVID-19 Pandemic and
    Beyond   247
    Charlene H. Chu, Charlene Ronquillo, Shehroz Khan, Lillian Hung,
    and Veronique Boscart

18 Redesigning Memory Care in the COVID-19 Era: Interdisciplinary
    Spatial Design Interventions to Minimize Social Isolation in
    Older Adults   263
    Farhana Ferdous

    Index   278

Citation Information

The chapters in this book were originally published in the *Journal of Aging & Social Policy*, volume 33, issue 4–5 (2021). When citing this material, please use the original page numbering for each article, as follows:

Chapter 1

Shining a Spotlight: The Ramifications of the COVID-19 Pandemic for Older Adults
Edward Alan Miller
Journal of Aging & Social Policy, volume 33, issue 4–5 (2021), pp. 305–319

Chapter 2

Coronavirus-Related Anxiety, Social Isolation, and Loneliness in Older Adults in Northern California during the Stay-at-Home Order
Laura Gaeta and Christopher R. Brydges
Journal of Aging & Social Policy, volume 33, issue 4–5 (2021), pp. 320–331

Chapter 3

Pandemic Place: Assessing Domains of the Person-Place Fit Measure for Older Adults (PPFM-OA) during COVID-19
Joyce Weil
Journal of Aging & Social Policy, volume 33, issue 4–5 (2021), pp. 332–341

Chapter 4

The Impact of Stigmatization on Social Avoidance and Fear of Disclosure among Older People: Implications for Social Policy Preparedness in a Public Health Crisis
Jiannan Li, Chulan Huang, Bocong Yuan, and Haixuan Liang
Journal of Aging & Social Policy, volume 33, issue 4–5 (2021), pp. 342–358

Chapter 5

Old Overnight: Experiences of Age-Based Recommendations in Response to the COVID-19 Pandemic in Sweden
Gabriella Nilsson, Lisa Ekstam, Anna Axmon, and Janicke Andersson
Journal of Aging & Social Policy, volume 33, issue 4–5 (2021), pp. 359–379

Chapter 6
Living Through the COVID-19 Pandemic: Community-Dwelling Older Adults'
Experiences
Bo Xie, Kristina Shiroma, Atami Sagna De Main, Nathan W Davis, Karen
Fingerman, and Valerie Danesh
Journal of Aging & Social Policy, volume 33, issue 4–5 (2021), pp. 380–397

Chapter 7
"We Are Saving Their Bodies and Destroying Their Souls.": Family Caregivers'
Experiences of Formal Care Setting Visitation Restrictions during the COVID-
19 Pandemic
Whitney A. Nash, Lesley M. Harris, Kimberly E. Heller, and Brandon
D. Mitchell
Journal of Aging & Social Policy, volume 33, issue 4–5 (2021), pp. 398–413

Chapter 8
Prevalence of COVID-19 in Ohio Nursing Homes: What's Quality Got to Do
with It?
John Bowblis and Robert Applebaum
Journal of Aging & Social Policy, volume 33, issue 4–5 (2021), pp. 414–430

Chapter 9
The Impact of COVID-19 on Nursing Homes in Italy: The Case of Lombardy
Marco Arlotti and Costanzo Ranci
Journal of Aging & Social Policy, volume 33, issue 4–5 (2021), pp. 431–443

Chapter 10
COVID-19 and Long-Term Care Policy for Older People in Japan
Margarita Estévez-Abe and Hiroo Ide
Journal of Aging & Social Policy, volume 33, issue 4–5 (2021), pp. 444–458

Chapter 11
The Impact of COVID-19 on Social Isolation in Long-term Care Homes:
Perspectives of Policies and Strategies from Six Countries
Charlene H. Chu, Jing Wang, Chie Fukui, Sandra Staudacher, Patrick
A. Wachholz, and Bei Wu
Journal of Aging & Social Policy, volume 33, issue 4–5 (2021), pp. 459–473

Chapter 12
COVID-19 Pandemic and Resilience of the Transnational Home-Based Elder
Care System between Poland and Germany
Magdalena Nowicka, Susanne Bartig, Theresa Schwass, and Kamil
Matuszczyk
Journal of Aging & Social Policy, volume 33, issue 4–5 (2021), pp. 474–492

Chapter 13

Rethinking the Role of Advance Care Planning in the Context of Infectious Disease
Sara Moorman, Kathrin Boerner, and Deborah Carr
Journal of Aging & Social Policy, volume 33, issue 4–5 (2021), pp. 493–499

Chapter 14

Palliative Care for Older Adults with Multimorbidity in the Time of COVID 19
Victoria D. Powell and Maria J. Silveira
Journal of Aging & Social Policy, volume 33, issue 4–5 (2021), pp. 500–508

Chapter 15

Cross-Border Medical Services for Hong Kong's Older Adults in Mainland China: The Implications of COVID-19 for the Future of Telemedicine
Genghua Huang, Yin Ma, and Zhaiwen Peng
Journal of Aging & Social Policy, volume 33, issue 4–5 (2021), pp. 509–521

Chapter 16

Telephone-Based Emotional Support for Older Adults during the COVID-19 Pandemic
Liora Bar-Tur, Michal Inbal-Jacobson, Sharon Brik-Deshen, Yael Zilbershlag, Sigal Pearl Naim, and Yitzhak Brick
Journal of Aging & Social Policy, volume 33, issue 4–5 (2021), pp. 522–538

Chapter 17

Technology Recommendations to Support Person-Centered Care in Long-Term Care Homes during the COVID-19 Pandemic and Beyond
Charlene H. Chu, Charlene Ronquillo, Shehroz Khan, Lillian Hung, and Veronique Boscart
Journal of Aging & Social Policy, volume 33, issue 4–5 (2021), pp. 539–554

Chapter 18

Redesigning Memory Care in the COVID-19 Era: Interdisciplinary Spatial Design Interventions to Minimize Social Isolation in Older Adults
Farhana Ferdous
Journal of Aging & Social Policy, volume 33, issue 4–5 (2021), pp. 555–569

For any permission-related enquiries please visit:
www.tandfonline.com/page/help/permissions

Notes on Contributors

Janicke Andersson, Associate Professor, School of Health and Welfare, Halmstad University, Halmstad, Sweden.

Robert Applebaum, Professor of Gerontology and Director of the Ohio Long-Term Care Research Project, Scripps Gerontology Center, Miami University, Oxford, Ohio, USA.

Marco Arlotti, Lecturer in Economic Sociology, Department of Architecture and Urban Studies, DASTU Politecnico Di Milano, Milano, Italy.

Anna Axmon, Associate Professor, EPI@LUND (Epidemiology, Population Studies, and Infrastructures at Lund University), Department of Occupational and Environmental Medicine, Lund University, Lund, Sweden.

Susanne Bartig, Department Integration, DeZIM-Institut, Berlin, Germany.

Liora Bar-Tur, Department of Clinical Geropsychology, Faculty of Social & Community Sciences, Ruppin Academic Center, Emek Hefer, Israel.

Kathrin Boerner, Associate Professor, Department of Gerontology, John W. McCormack Graduate School of Policy and Global Studies, University of Massachusetts Boston, Boston, Massachusetts, USA.

Veronique Boscart, Affiliate Scientist, KITE, Toronto Rehabilitation Institution, Toronto, Ontario, Canada.

Executive Dean, School of Health & Life Sciences, Conestoga College Institute of Technology and Advanced Learning, Kitchener, Ontario, Canada.

John Bowblis, Professor, Department of Economics, Farmer School of Business, Miami University, Oxford, Ohio, USA; Research Fellow, Scripps Gerontology Center, Miami University, Oxford, Ohio, USA.

Yitzhak Brick, Department of Gerontology, University of Haifa, Haifa, Israel.

Sharon Brik-Deshen, Israel Gerontological Society, Israel.

Christopher R. Brydges, Principal Statistician, West Coast Metabolomics Center, University of California, Davis, California, USA.

Deborah Carr, Professor and Chair, Department of Sociology, Boston University, Boston, Massachusetts, USA.

Charlene H. Chu, Assistant Professor, Lawrence S. Bloomberg Faculty of Nursing, University of Toronto, Toronto, Ontario, Canada; Assistant Professor (cross-appointed), Institute for Life Course and Aging, University of Toronto, Toronto, Ontario, Canada; Affiliate Scientist, KITE, Toronto Rehabilitation Institution, Toronto, Ontario, Canada.

Valerie Danesh, School of Nursing, The University of Texas at Austin, Austin, Texas, USA.

Nathan W Davis, School of Information, The University of Texas at Austin, Austin, Texas, USA.

Atami Sagna De Main, School of Nursing, The University of Texas at Austin, Austin, Texas, USA.

Lisa Ekstam, Associate Professor, Department of Arts and Cultural Sciences, Lund University, Lund, Sweden.

Margarita Estèvez-Abe, Associate Professor of Political Science, Maxwell School of Citizenship and Public Affairs, Syracuse University, Syracuse, New York, USA.

Farhana Ferdous, Assistant Professor, Department of Architecture, Howard University, Washington DC, USA.

Karen Fingerman, Department of Human Development and Family Sciences, The University of Texas at Austin, Austin, Texas, USA.

Chie Fukui, Assistant Professor, Department of Gerontological Home-Care & Long-term Care Nursing, School of Health Sciences & Nursing, Graduate School of Medicine, The University of Tokyo, Tokyo, Japan.

Laura Gaeta, Assistant Professor, Department of Communication Sciences and Disorders, College of Health and Human Services, California State University, Sacramento, Sacramento, California, USA.

Lesley M. Harris, Associate Professor, Kent School of Social Work, University of Louisville, Louisville, KY, USA.

Kimberly E. Heller, Graduate Student, School of Nursing, University of Louisville, Louisville, KY, USA.

Chulan Huang, Undergraduate, School of Tourism Management, Sun Yat-sen University, Guangzhou, Guangdong, China.

Genghua Huang, Lingnan University, Tuen Mun, Hong Kong.

Lillian Hung, Assistant Professor, School of Nursing, University of British of Columbia, Vancouver, British Columbia, Canada.

Hiroo Ide, Project Associate Professor, Institute for Future Initiatives, The University of Tokyo, Tokyo, Japan.

Michal Inbal-Jacobson, Department of Gerontology, University of Haifa, Haifa, Israel.

Shehroz Khan, Affiliate Scientist, KITE, Toronto Rehabilitation Institution, Toronto, Ontario, Canada.

Jiannan Li, Research Associate Professor, Institute of Advanced Studies in Humanities and Social Sciences, Beijing Normal University, Zhuhai, China.

Haixuan Liang, Undergraduate, School of Tourism Management, Sun Yat-sen University, Guangzhou, Guangdong, China.

Yin Ma, Research Professor, Lanzhou University, Lanzhou, Gansu, China.

Kamil Matuszczyk, Faculty of Political Science and International Studies, Centre of Migration Research, Uniwersytet Warszawski, Warsaw, Poland.

Edward Alan Miller, Professor and Chair, Department of Gerontology, and Fellow, Gerontology Institute, John W. McCormack Graduate School of Policy and Global Studies, University of Massachusetts, Boston, Massachusetts, USA Adjunct Professor of Health Services, Policy and Practice, Brown University, Providence, Rhode Island, USA.

Brandon D. Mitchell, PhD Student, Kent School of Social Work, University of Louisville, Louisville, KY, USA.

Sara Moorman, Associate Professor, Department of Sociology, Boston College, Chestnut Hill, Massachusetts, USA.

Sigal Pearl Naim, Department of Human Services, Max Stern Yezreel Academic College, Yezreel Valley, Israel.

Whitney A. Nash, Professor, School of Nursing, University of Louisville, Louisville, Kentucky, USA.

Gabriella Nilsson, Associate Professor, Department of Arts and Cultural Sciences, Lund University, Lund, Sweden.

Magdalena Nowicka, Department Integration, DeZIM-Institut, Berlin, Germany.

Victoria D. Powell, Palliative Care Program, Division of Geriatric and Palliative Medicine, University of Michigan School of Medicine, Ann Arbor, Michigan, USA; Geriatric Research Education and Clinical Center, Ann Arbor Veterans Administration Medical Center, Ann Arbor, Michigan, USA.

Zhaiwen Peng, Assistant Professor, Center for Chinese Public Administration Research, Sun Yat-sen University, Guangzhou, China.

Costanzo Ranci, Professor in Economic Sociology, Department of Architecture and Urban Studies, DASTU Politecnico Di Milano, Milano, Italy.

Charlene Ronquillo, Scientist, School of Nursing, University of British Columbia Okanagan, Kelowna, BC, Canada.

Theresa Schwass, Department Integration, DeZIM-Institut, Berlin, Germany.

Kristina Shiroma, School of Information, The University of Texas at Austin, Austin, Texas, USA.

Maria J. Silveira, Palliative Care Program, Division of Geriatric and Palliative Medicine, University of Michigan School of Medicine, Ann Arbor, Michigan, USA; Geriatric Research Education and Clinical Center, Ann Arbor Veterans Administration Medical Center, Ann Arbor, Michigan, USA.

Sandra Staudacher, Postdoc, Department of Public Health, University of Basel, Basel, Switzerland.

Patrick A. Wachholz, Collaborating Professor, Departamento de Clínica Médica, Faculdade de Medicina de Botucatu - Universidade Estadual Paulista (UNESP), Ourinhos, Brazil.

Jing Wang, Assistant Professor, School of Nursing, Fudan University, Shanghai, China.

Joyce Weil, Associate Professor, Gerontology Program, University of Northern Colorado, Greeley, Colorado, USA.

Bei Wu, Professor, Rory Meyers College of Nursing, New York University, New York, New York, USA.

Bo Xie, School of Nursing, The University of Texas at Austin, Austin, Texas, USA; School of Information, The University of Texas at Austin, Austin, Texas, USA.

Bocong Yuan, Associate Professor, School of Tourism Management, Sun Yat-sen University Guangzhou, Guangdong, China.

Yael Zilbershlag, Department of Occupational Therapy, Faculty of Health Allied Professions, Ono Academic College, Kiryat Ono, Israel.

Introduction

Shining a Spotlight: The Ramifications of the COVID-19 Pandemic for Older Adults

Edward Alan Miller

ABSTRACT

The COVID-19 pandemic has disrupted life globally through virus-related mortality and morbidity and the social and economic impacts of actions taken to stop the virus' spread. It became evident early in the pandemic that COVID-19 and the strategies adopted to mitigate its effects would have a disproportionate impact on older adults. This special issue of the *Journal of Aging & Social Policy* reports original empirical research and perspectives on the ramifications of the COVID-19 pandemic for this population. This introductory essay highlights key issues pertaining to the impact of COVID-19 on older adults and their families, caregivers, and communities. The prevalence and susceptibility of COVID-19 infection in the older adult population is discussed, including the devastating consequences of the pandemic for residents and staff of long-term care facilities. This is followed by a brief examination of ageism and social isolation brought to the fore during the pandemic, as well as the adverse effects of the pandemic for the economy and racial and ethnic minority populations. It concludes with an overview of issue content.

Introduction

Severe acute respiratory syndrome coronavirus 2 (SARS-CoV-2), the virus that causes coronavirus disease 2019 (COVID-19) infection, has disrupted life globally through virus-related mortality and morbidity and the social and economic impacts of actions taken to stop the virus' spread. As of August 16, 2021, COVID-19 infections exceeded 207 million worldwide, with nearly 4.5 million reported deaths (World Health Organization [WHO], 2021). Vaccines became available late last year; currently, 31.7% of the global population has received one vaccine dose with 23.7% being fully vaccinated (Our World in Data, 2021). Thus, although 4.76 billion vaccine doses have been administered and the rates of COVID-19 infections and deaths declined through the spring, pandemic-related disruptions continue as large segments of the population have yet to be vaccinated, especially in low-income countries.

The United States is less than 5% of the global population (U.S. Census Bureau, 2021), but leads the world in number of cases (36.4 million, 17.6%) and deaths (615,747, 14.1%) from COVID-19 (WHO, 2021). The U.S. is currently in its fourth wave of infections driven by the emergence of the highly contagious Delta variant. COVID-19 cases and deaths have risen in large part because a high proportion of the population remains unvaccinated even though eligible. By mid-August 2021, 50.44% of the U.S. population had been totally vaccinated with an additional 9.03% partially so (Our World in Data, 2021). There is considerable variation across states, however, ranging from lows of fully vaccinated adults of around 45% in Alabama, Mississippi, and West Virginia to highs of 75% and greater in Maine, Massachusetts, Connecticut, and Vermont (*The New York Times*, 2021b).

The recent increase in COVID-19 cases and deaths has occurred in the context of continued opposition among segments of the public to preventive measures such as mask wearing and social distancing, and reluctance on the part of some elected officials to reinstate previous virus mitigation require-ments or to adopt new ones (e.g., "vaccine passports"). Executive and legisla-tion actions taken in some conservative states with Republican leadership explicitly preclude the adoption or enforcement of such measures (Abbasi, 2021; Drees, 2021). Indeed, it is official policy in states such as Florida, Texas, and Arizona to punish local communities and school districts that opt to adopt virus mitigation measures in defiance of such statewide bans (Mabus, 2021; Vestal, 2021).

The politicization of basic vaccination and public health measures in the U.S. is reflected in recent polls. Republicans constitute a much higher propor-tion than Democrats of adults to report being unvaccinated (51% v. 23%), that they are definitely not getting the vaccine (58% v. 15%), and never wearing masks, including in grocery stores (55% v. 18%) and at work (57% v. 32%) (Kirzinger, Sparks et al., 2021). Republicans are also much more likely to oppose the federal government recommending that employers require employees to get vaccinated (67% v. 24%). Comparable partisan breakdowns are reflected in parents' responses to similar questions about children's vacci-nation status and school vaccine and mask wearing policies (Hamel et al., 2021).

This special double issue of the *Journal of Aging & Social Policy*, "The COVID-19 Pandemic and Older Adults: Experiences, Impacts, and Innovations," reports original empirical research and perspectives stemming from the COVID-19 pandemic to draw lessons for policy, research, and practice. This introductory essay highlights key issues pertaining to the impact of COVID-19 on older adults and their families, caregivers, and communities. The prevalence and susceptibility of COVID-19 infection in the older adult population is discussed, including the disproportionate impact on residents and staff of long-term care facilities. This is followed by a review of ageism and social isolation brought to the fore during the pandemic, as well as the adverse effects of the pandemic for the economy. The disproportionate hardship based on racial and ethnic minority status is noted as well. It concludes with an overview of issue content.

Health effects and older adults

It became evident early during the pandemic that older adults were especially vulnerable to the morbidity and mortality effects of COVID-19. While no more likely to become infected than younger populations, Centers for Disease Control and Prevention [CDC] (2021b) data indicate that the risk for hospitalization and death rises considerably with age. Compared with 18- to 29-year-olds, the rate of hospitalization is six, nine, and 15 times higher among people aged 65 to 74, 75 to 84, and 85 years and older, respectively. Compared to the younger age group, the rate of death is 95, 230, and 600 times higher among people aged 65 to 74, 75 to 84, and 85 years and older. Thus, although adults aged 65 years and older represent about 16.6% of the population in the U.S. (U.S. Census Bureau, 2021), 79.4% of all COVID-19 deaths (482,727) have occurred in this age group (CDC, 2021c).

Not all older adults are equally susceptible to adverse outcomes stemming from the virus. Those at greatest risk tend to be found among frailer adults at more advanced ages who are more likely to demonstrate high viral shedding, delayed prognosis due to atypical disease presentation and limited testing, and difficulties quarantining, particularly in congregate living settings (Smorenberg et al., 2021). Respiratory, cardiovascular, cerebrovascular, and diabetes co-morbidities; reductions in physiological reserve (increased frailty); and compromised immune responses contribute to increased risk as well.

Residents of long-term care facilities have been among the hardest hit by the pandemic. In U.S. nursing homes, there have been 664,815 confirmed COVID-19 infections and 133,631 deaths, accounting for less than 2% of cases nationally but more than 20% of fatalities (Centers for Medicare and Medicaid Services [CMS], 2021; WHO, 2021). At 597,087 and 1,994, respectively, cases and deaths among nursing home staff have been comparatively high as well (CMS, 2021). Looking at congregate living settings more broadly, it has been estimated that even though only 4% of all cases were among residents and staff in nursing homes, assisted living facilities, memory care facilities, retirement and senior communities, and rehabilitation facilities, these individuals represented 31% of all COVID-19 deaths (*The New York Times*, 2021a). Comparably high proportions of COVID-19 deaths among care home residents have also been reported internationally (Comas-Herrera et al., 2021).

By spring 2021, cases and deaths in long-term care facilities from COVID-19 had reached all-time lows, mainly due to widespread vaccination of residents and staff (Chidambaram & Garfield, 2021). Nationally, 82.4% of residents and 60.0% of staff have been vaccinated per facility (CMS, 2021), consistent with national figures for the proportion of fully vaccinated people ages 65+ (81%) and 18+ (62%) more generally (*The New York Times*, 2021b); however, vaccination rates among nursing facility staff lag behind front line health care workers in hospitals and other settings (Kirzinger, Kearney et al., 2021). Vaccine hesitancy among staff, combined with breakthrough infections among vaccinated residents in wake of the Delta variant, suggests potential reversal in progress made as infections and deaths again begin to rise. Increasing numbers of nursing home operators are thus requiring staff to be vaccinated (Paulin, 2021); so too are a growing chorus of states mandating vaccination among all long-term care workers (Connecticut, Washington), nursing home workers (Massachusetts), workers in group settings (Illinois, Maryland), and health care workers more generally (California, New Jersey, New York) (Kamp, 2021). The Biden Administration recently announced that it plans to withhold Medicare and Medicaid funding from nursing facilities that do not fully vaccinate their employees (Z. Miller, 2021).

Social effects and older adults

The disproportionate impact of the COVID-19 pandemic on older adults brought many facets of ageism to the fore (Ehnia & Wahl, 2020; Previtali et al., 2020). At the extreme, this revealed ageism has been reflected in rhetoric and decisions that devalue the lives of older adults relative to other age groups in triage and resource allocation decisions. More commonly, though, it has been reflected in policy discussions and choices based on chronological age. Treating older adults as uniformly susceptible and vulnerable to the virus compromises older adults' autonomy, reinforces age stereotypes, ignores intra-group differences, and fails to ground interventions in individual capacities, risk levels, and needs.

Community stay-at-home messages, lockdowns, social distancing requirements, and visitation restrictions in long-term care facilities contributed to a concomitant epidemic in social isolation and loneliness among older adults during the COVID-19 pandemic. This reflects the exacerbation of already high burdens of social isolation among older adults before the pandemic, especially among certain subgroups, including the oldest old, unmarried, and residents of long-term care facilities (Donovan & Blazer, 2020; Simard & Volicer, 2020). Social isolation and loneliness have a range of adverse effects. These include declines in mental health and physical functioning, increased psychological distress and behavioral problems, and heightened mortality risk, especially among people with cognitive impairment (Gorenko et al., 2021). Recognition of the risks posed by limited social interaction spurred increased use of information and communication technologies during the pandemic to maintain connections between older adults and their families and friends, on the part of both long-term care facilities and community-based providers and older adults themselves (Kakulla, 2021; Veiga-Siejo et al., 2021). Physical and cognitive limitations, cost, availability, knowledge, awareness, experience, comfort, attitude, and aptitude may serve as impediments to successful usage, however.

Economic effects and older adults

Economic and social impacts stemming from the COVID-19 pandemic and the local, regional, and national government actions taken to mitigate the spread of the virus have been dramatic. The pandemic resulted in the deepest global recession since the end of World War II with the global economy contracting by 3.5% in 2020 (Yeyati & Filippini, 2021). In the U.S., 2.4 million women and 1.8 million men left the labor force between February 2020 and February 2021, reductions of 3.1% and 2.1%, respectively (Kochhst & Bennett, 2021). During the peak of the pandemic, the unemployment rate topped out at 14.8%, a level not seen since data collection started in 1948, while the labor force participation rate bottomed out at 60.2%, a level not witnessed since the early 1970s (Falk et al., 2021). As of May 2021, the unemployment and labor force participation rates have both recovered, reaching 5.8% and 61.6%, respectively, but still remain below immediate pre-pandemic levels (3.5%, 63.4%).

Critically, nursing homes, assisted living facilities, and home and community-based services providers continue to struggle to recruit and retain sufficient direct care staff despite the improved economic outlook (Brown, 2021; Kaiser Family Foundation, 2021). These chronic shortages, driven by low pay, lack of career advancement, high turnover, and work environment factors, were severely exacerbated by the pandemic (Tyler et al., 2021; Xu et al., 2020). This was due, in part, to the high risk of infection stemming from the nature of the work and insufficient personal protective equipment. It was also due to increased professional demands posed by the need to isolate care recipients and implement infection control protocols and to reduced informal support provided by relatives due to visitor bans and stay at home orders. Increased personal demands stemming, perhaps most notably, from school and day care closures contributed to staff retention challenges as well.

Federal and state officials recognize the severity of the workforce issue. State officials report plans to increase provider payment rates and support workforce recruitment using enhanced federal funding for Medicaid home and community-based services under the American Rescue Plan Act of 2021 (Watts et al., 2021). The Nursing Home Improvement and Accountability

Act recently introduced in the Senate includes a range of provisions to bolster staffing, including minimum staffing requirements, temporary resources to enhance wages and support staff recruitment and retention, and RN availability 24 hours per day (rather than the current 8 hours). It is possible that implementation of vaccine mandates could promote resignations among some workers. Recent case study evidence, however, suggests that the adverse impact of vaccine mandates for retention may be minimal in the context of strong support and communication on the part of nursing home leadership (Ritter et al., 2021).

Racial and ethnic disparities and older adults

Adverse health effects stemming from the pandemic have not been uniformly distributed. Native American, Hispanic/Latino, and Black/African American communities have suffered disproportionate hardship. The CDC (2021a) reports that, compared to white, Non-Hispanic individuals, the age-adjusted risk of infection, hospitalization, and death from COVID-19 is higher among Native Americans (1.7, 3.4, and 2.4 times, respectively), Black or African Americans (1.1, 2.8, and 2.0 times), and Hispanic or Latino persons (1.9, 2.8 and 2.3 times). Reductions in projected life expectancy at birth and age 65 stemming from COVID-19 are projected across all racial and ethnic groups, but are greater among Black and Latino populations, thereby widening the gap in life expectancy between Blacks and whites (from 3.6 years to 5.0 years) and narrowing the advantage in life expectancy Latinos have traditionally had over whites (known as the "Latino or Hispanic epidemiological paradox," from 3 years to <1 year) (Andrasfaya & Goldman, 2021). Black and Hispanic persons are less likely than whites to have received the vaccine, though the gap has narrowed over time (Ndugga & Hill, 2021).

Economic disparities are similarly evident with Blacks and Hispanics experiencing higher peaks of unemployment and greater troughs in labor force participation during the pandemic (Falk et al., 2021). Black and Hispanic women constitute less than one-third of the female labor force in the U.S., for example, but 46% of the women who left the labor force between February 2020 and February 2021 (Kochhst & Bennett, 2021). Vulnerabilities steeped in structural racism and the social determinants of health place racial and ethnic minority older adults at particularly high risk for poor heath, economic, and social outcomes. These vulnerabilities relate to the higher prevalence of co-morbid conditions; housing/residential segregation; income, education, and wealth disparities; unequal health care access and quality; occupational segregation (e.g., employment in high-risk occupations in health care and other industries); and chronic resource deficits and stresses accumulated over the life course (Garcia et al., 2021; Shippee et al., 2020).

Issue content

The 17 articles included in this issue were submitted to the Journal between April 2020 and April 2021. Contributions to the current issue are divided between original empirical research (seven) and commentaries/perspectives (ten). Four general areas are addressed: (1) personal experiences with COVID-19 (Gaeta & Brydges; Weil; Li, Huang, Yuan, & Liang; Nilsson, Ekstam, Axmon, & Andersson; Xie, Shiroma, De Main, Davis, Fingerman, & Danesh; Nash, Harris, Heller, & Mitchell); (2) long-term care system impacts (Bowblis & Applebaum; Arlotti & Ranci; Estévez-Abe & Ide; Chu, Wang, Fukui, Staudacher-Preite, Wachholz, & Wu; Nowicka, Bartig, Schwass, & Matuszczyk); (3) end-of-life care (Moorman, Boerner, & Carr; Powell & Silveria); and (4) technology and innovation (Huang, Ma, & Peng; Bar-Tur, Inbal-Jacobson, Brick-Deshen, Zilbershlag, & Naim; Chu, Ronquillo, Khan, & Hung; Ferdous).

Assessing personal experiences with COVID-19

Six articles focus on personal experiences during the COVID-19 pandemic, primarily in relation to community-dwelling older adults but also with respect to family caregivers in formal care settings. These articles stress the adverse effects of the pandemic on psychosocial outcomes, including social isolation, loneliness, anxiety, person-place fit, stigmatization, and reactions to age-based policy making and pandemic-imposed visitation restrictions.

Gaeta & Brydges report the results of a survey of 514 older adults in Northern California during the stay-at-home order. The results document comparatively high levels of loneliness and social isolation with the former (but not the latter) related to anxiety about COVID-19. The need to safely increase social interaction with older adults during the pandemic is thus highlighted.

Weil argues for broadly exploring COVID-19-era changes on older adults to assess the range of impact more fully beyond the health and biomedical changes most frequently highlighted in the literature. The importance of place-based identity and person-place fit is demonstrated across five domains assessed in the Person-Place Fit Measure for Older Adults: primary or basic needs/necessities, neighborhood changes and moving, identity and place attachment, community value, and services and resources. The author concludes that assessing the changing relationship between older adults and place can inform the development of policies to mitigate the adverse effects of the pandemic on this population.

Li, Huang, Yuan, & Liang report the results of a three-wave survey of 429 older adults with epicenter travel experience to Hubei, China at the start of the COVID-19 pandemic. Results reveal positive associations between perceived stigmatization and fear of disclosure and social avoidance, mediated, in part, by stress. Based on these results, the authors recommend that public health efforts to control and limit the virus should include de-stigmatization measures and psychological supports for older adults in quarantine.

Nilsson, Ekstam, Axmon, & Andersson analyzed 851 responses to a web-based qualitative survey to assess the impact on older adults of the abrupt adoption of age-based quarantine recommendations in Sweden that contrasted with the active aging ideal and values such as individuality, self-determination, and quality. Six ways in which respondents related to the age-based recommendations were identified based on varying degrees of acceptance and resistance. The authors conclude that age-based policy making can be a problematic governing principle that may be deemed less legitimate and lead to negative self-image and poorer health among those targeted when social responsibility has otherwise become more individualized.

Xie, Shiroma, De Main, Davis, Fingerman, & Danesh conducted phone interviews with 200 older adults in Central Texas to assess the impact of the COVID-19 pandemic on community-dwelling older adults' lived experiences. The results reveal the complexity of the pandemic's impact, with a range of positive, mixed, and negative experiences being reported. The authors point to the need to attend to the long-term consequences of the pandemic for older adults' mental health and recommend that policies and interventions leverage older adults' effective coping and resilience while attending to the negative effects on certain subgroups.

In contrast to the other studies in this section, Nash, Harris, Heller, & Mitchell focus on elucidating the experiences of 512 family caregivers recruited from an international caregiving social media site during the COVID-19 pandemic due to the implementation of visitation restrictions in formal care settings (i.e., assisted living facilities and nursing homes). When asked to describe the feelings around reduced visitation the most common words used expressed a range of negative emotions (sadness, trauma, anger, frustration, helplessness, anxiety); major themes included isolation, rapid decline, inhumane care, and lack of oversight. The authors urge that policies be developed that address the mental, emotional, and physical needs of both family caregivers and care recipients.

Elucidating the impact of COVID-19 on long-term care systems

Five articles address the impact of the COVID-19 pandemic on long-term care, mainly with respect to nursing homes, and, in one case, home care. Three articles focus on system impacts in specific countries – the U.S. (Ohio), Italy (Lombardy), and Japan; a fourth reports the results of a cross-national comparison of six nations; a fifth reports on the implications of COVID-19 on the flow of workers between countries (in this case, from Poland to Germany).

Bowblis and Applebaum examine the relationship between COVID-19 cases and quality in 921 Ohio nursing homes using state data on COVID-19 prevalence and the federal Nursing Home Compare system and Payroll-based Journal data. Results reveal no differences in the susceptibility to any COVID-19 cases or especially high caseloads across poor- and high-quality nursing homes after accounting for other factors, including urban location. The authors conclude that community prevalence and the nature of nursing home care itself is a larger driver of COVID-19 infections in nursing homes than the quality of care provided in specific facilities.

Focusing on the Lombardy region, Arlotti and Ranci analyze the root causes of high mortality rates in Italian nursing homes during the first wave of the COVID-19 pandemic. They conclude that the negative outcomes experienced derived from financial and management challenges stemming from policy legacies in the way of inadequate investment on the part of the regional and national governments in residential institutions within the health care system. The authors argue that increased government attention needs to be paid to addressing structural weaknesses within the residential care sector that created the conditions for the severe impact of COVID-19 in nursing homes, even within Lombardy, the wealthiest region in Italy.

Estévez-Abe and Ide sought to explain why, in contrast to the United States and European countries, Japan experienced relatively low levels of virus transmission and deaths in nursing homes due to the COVID-19 pandemic. The authors argue that the primary factor explaining this difference was the decision to lockdown long-term care facilities several weeks earlier than their counterparts in Europe and the U.S. The authors explain that Japan was able to move quickly due to the presence of effective communication between long-term care facilities and hierarchically organized government agencies charged exclusively with overseeing elder care within the country and a well-established routine protocol for preventing and controlling communicable diseases in long-term care facilities.

Chu, Wang, Fukui, Staudacher-Preite, Wachholz, & Wu recognize the exacerbation of social isolation in long-term care homes stemming from well-meaning policies to mitigate the spread of COVID-19 by restricting visits to these facilities. The authors thus identify common characteristics of policies enacted in Brazil, Canada, China, Japan, Switzerland, and the U.S. during the pandemic to inform recommendations to mitigate social isolation. Proposed actions would promote person-centered care and prioritize residents' social and psychological well-being by, for example, using information technologies to connect residents to family and friends, maintaining/supporting safe resident interactions, and providing for increased monitoring and resident support to identify and minimize the negative effects of visitation restrictions.

The increased risk COVID-19 poses to older adults in long-term institutional care further heightens the importance of home-based care; consequently, Nowicka, Bartig, Schwass, & Matuszczyk conducted 28 stakeholder interviews to gauge the resilience of a transnational elder care system characterized by Germany's reliance on migrant caregivers from Poland following travel restrictions imposed because of the pandemic. Results highlight the mobilization of adaptative capacities to deliver services with fewer resources, but limitations in the system's ability to provide the same level and quality of care under the circumstances. The authors recommend greater formalization and legalization of the transnational labor system and better assurances for the qualification and payment of workers.

Examining the role of end-of-life care in COVID-19

Two articles address issues critical to end-of-life care: advanced care planning and palliative care. Moorman, Boerner, & Carr reflect on barriers to advanced care planning in the context of infectious diseases such as COVID-19 where the process from illness to death occurs quickly. Heightened interpersonal and sociostructural barriers to advanced care planning stemming from social isolation and racial and socioeconomic inequalities are noted; so too are impediments posed by health system overload and orientation of advanced care planning around death from chronic illness. The authors conclude that these factors need to be accounted for in efforts to increase the rate of advanced care planning due to the expected resurgence of death from infectious disease in forthcoming decades.

Powell & Silveria highlight the role of palliative care in supporting older adults with multimorbidity during COVID-19. In outpatient settings, telehealth has increased the accessibility of palliative care providers, though barriers to use among some older adults remain depending on the ability to navigate the technology and to access family assistance in using it. In inpatient settings, palliative care consult teams have provided relief in the context of restrictive hospital visitation policies and limited access to post-acute care by playing a larger role in communicating with families and in emotionally supporting front-line colleagues.

Proposing technologies and innovations in the wake of COVID-19

Four articles recommend broader adoption of technologies and innovations as a result of social distancing, lock-down, visitation, and travel restrictions and guidelines adopted due to the COVID-19 pandemic. Two focus on improving communication between community-dwelling older adults and clinicians; one on adopting communication and social technologies to improve person-centered care in institutional settings; and another on applying spatial redesign strategies to improve memory care in residential care settings.

Huang, Ma, & Peng highlight the challenges of providing cross-border services and supports to Hong Kong citizens electing to live in mainland China during the COVID-19 pandemic. These older adults would otherwise return to Hong Kong for needed medical services but are prevented from doing so due to stringent immigration controls. The authors discuss remedial measures taken by governmental and non-governmental organizations to meet the need for prescription medications and suggest accelerating the role of telemedicine in addressing continuing gaps in treatment and follow-up.

Bar-Tur, Inbal-Jacobson, Brick-Deshen, Zilbershlag, & Naim describe a telephone-based emotional care program developed and implemented by gerontologists in Israel to provide emotional care to older adults in the face of increased social isolation stemming from lockdowns during the COVID-19 pandemic. They report that the intervention provides an effective and efficient strategy for supporting older adults and their families and assisting caregiving agencies. The authors recommend that online and telephone-based solutions such as this one be adopted widely in the post-pandemic world to better reach older adults at risk for social isolation and loneliness who might otherwise not receive emotional support.

Chu, Ronquillo, Khan, & Hung observe that long-term care homes often lack the capacity to take advantage of technologies used to keep residents connected with the outside world during the COVID-19 pandemic. To enable these connections and better support person-centered care, the authors point to the urgent need for the government and facilities to prioritize upgrading the current antiquated technological infrastructure. Recommendations include stable and reliable wi-fi access and usable software and hardware and technologies that support clinical decision making, social engagement, and environmental control.

Finally, Ferdous observes that older adults in memory care facilities are especially vulnerable to the adverse effects of social isolation and loneliness resulting from social distancing guidelines adopted during the COVID-19 pandemic. Though largely missing from current discussions, one potential avenue for mitigating this harm is through the adoption of evidence-based spatial redesign. Drawing from multiple disciplines, the author thus identifies eight themes to inform the development and implementation of evidence-based spatial redesign interventions and strategies in memory care facilities.

Conclusion

The content for this special issue stems from a call for papers whereby authors were invited to submit balanced, thoughtful, and analytical contributions on the effects of and response to COVID-19 across the range of issues affecting older adults. All submissions were subject to the Journal's usual double blind peer review process. The editorial team would thus like to thank those individuals who generously agreed to devote their time to conducting these reviews. Of course, the Journal's managing editor, Elizabeth Simpson; International Editor, Michael K. Gusmano; and the staff at Taylor and Francis, Inc., Jessica Ingle, Debraj Chattaraj, and Alyse Taggart, among others, proved instrumental in producing this issue as well.

This special issue complements the first special issue on COVID-19, "Older Adults and COVID-19: Implications for Aging Policy and Practice," published July 2020 (Volume 32, Issue 4–5; see, E. A. Miller, 2020, for an overview). The first special issue consisted of contributions from leading scholars invited to address the myriad ways in which the COVID-19 pandemic had affected older adults and their families, caregivers, and communities early on during the pandemic, and to propose policies and strategies to mitigate the pandemic's effects and draw lessons for aging policy and practice going forward. Given the volume of COVID-19-related submissions currently under review and still coming into the Journal weekly, we anticipate a third special issue next year.

Key points

- The health, social, and economic effects of the COVID-19 pandemic has disrupted life globally.
- The COVID-19 pandemic and strategies to mitigate its effects have had a disproportionate impact on older adults.
- Key issues pertaining to the impact of COVID-19 on older adults and their families, caregivers, and communities are highlighted.
- Other content in the special issue reports original empirical research and perspectives to draw lessons from the COVID-19 pandemic for policy, research, and practice.
- Four main areas are examined: Personal experiences with COVID-19; long-term care system impacts; end-of-life care; and technology and innovation.

References

Abbasi, E. (2021, August 2). *State by state face mask mandates*. LeadingAge. https://leadingage.org/regulation/state-state-face-mask-mandates

Andrasfaya, T., & Goldman, N. (2021). Reductions in 2020 US life expectancy due to COVID-19 and the disproportionate impact on the Black and Latino populations. *Proceedings from the National Academy of Sciences of the United States of America*, 118(5), 1–6. https://doi.org/10.1073/pnas.2014746118

Brown, D. (2021, June 24). 94% of all nursing home still facing staffing shortages, new survey shows. *McKnights Long-Term Care News*. https://www.mcknights.com/news/94-of-all-nursing-homes-still-facing-staffing-shortages-new-survey-shows/

Center for Disease Control and Prevention. (2021a, July 16). *Risk for COVID-19 infection, hospitalization, and death by race/ethnicity*. https://www.cdc.gov/coronavirus/2019-ncov/covid-data/investigations-discovery/hospitalization-death-by-race-ethnicity.html

Centers for Disease Control and Prevention. (2021b, July 19). *Risk for COVID-19 infection, hospitalization, and death by age group*. https://www.cdc.gov/coronavirus/2019-ncov/covid-data/investigations-discovery/hospitalization-death-by-age.html

Centers for Disease Control and Prevention. (2021c, August 11). *COVID-19 mortality overview: Provisional death counts for COVID-19*. https://www.cdc.gov/nchs/nvss/vsrr/covid_weekly/index.htm#SexAndAge

Centers for Medicare and Medicaid Services. (2021, August 1). *COVID-19 nursing home data*. https://data.cms.gov/stories/s/COVID-19-Nursing-Home-Data/bkwz-xpvg/

Chidambaram, P., & Garfield, R. (2021, August 2). *COVID-19 cases and deaths in long-term care facilities through June 2021*. Kaiser Family Foundation. https://www.kff.org/coronavirus-covid-19/issue-brief/covid-19-cases-and-deaths-in-long-term-care-facilities-through-june-2021/

Comas-Herrera, A., Zalakaín, J., Lemmon, E., Henderson, D., Litwin, C., Hsu, A. T., Schmidt, A. E., Arling, G., Kruse, F., & Fernández, J.-L. (2021, February 1). *Mortality associated with COVID-19 in care homes: International evidence*. International Long-Term Care Policy Network. https://ltccovid.org/wp-content/uploads/2021/02/LTC_COVID_19_international_report_January-1-February-.pdf

Donovan, N. J., & Blazer, D. (2020). Social isolation and loneliness in older adults: Review and commentary of a national academies report. *American Journal of Geriatric Psychiatry*, 28 (12), 1233–1244. https://doi.org/10.1016%2Fj.jagp.2020.08.005

Drees, J. (2021, July 3). *Vaccine passports: 50 states with bands, limitations & green lights*. Becker's Health IT. https://www.beckershospitalreview.com/digital-transformation/vaccine-passports-10-states-with-bans-limitations-green-lights.html

Ehnia, H.-J., & Wahl, H.-W. (2020). Six propositions against ageism in the COVID-19 pandemic. *Journal of Aging & Social Policy*, 32(4–5), 515–525. https://doi.org/10.1080/08959420.2020.1770032

Falk, G., Nicchitta, I. A., Romero, P. D., Nyof, E. C., & Carter, R. A. (2021, June 15). *Unemployment rates during the COVID-19 pandemic*. Congressional Research Service. https://fas.org/sgp/crs/misc/R46554.pdf

Garcia, M. A., Homan, P. A., Garcia, C., & Brown, T. H. (2021). The color of COVID-19: Structural racism and the disproportionate impact of the pandemic on older Black and Latinx adults. *Journal of Gerontology: Social Sciences*, 76(3), e75–e80. https://doi.org/10.1093/geronb/gbaa114

Gorenko, J. A., Moran, C., Flynn, M., Dobson, K., & Konnert, C. (2021). Social isolation and psychological distress among older adults related to COVID-19: A narrative review of remotely-delivered interventions and recommendations. *Journal of Applied Gerontology*, 40(1), 1–13. https://doi.org/10.1177/0733464820958550

Hamel, L., Lopes, L., Kearney, A., Krizinger, A., Sparks, G., Stokes, M., & Brodie, M. (2021, August 11). *KFF COVID-19 vaccine monitor: Parents and the pandemic*. Kaiser Family Foundation. https://www.kff.org/coronavirus-covid-19/poll-finding/kff-covid-19-vaccine-monitor-parents-and-the-pandemic/

Kaiser Family Foundation. (2021, August 10). *Direct care workforce shortages worsened in many states during the pandemic, hampering providers of home and community-based services.* https://www.kff.org/coronavirus-covid-19/press-release/direct-care-workforce-shortages-have-worsened-in-many-states-during-the-pandemic-hampering-providers-of-home-and-community-based-services/

Kakulla, B. (2021, April). *Personal tech and the pandemic: Older adults are upgrading for a better online experience.* AARP. https://www.aarp.org/research/topics/technology/info-2021/2021-technology-trends-older-americans.html-CMP=RDRCT-PRI-TECH-040721/?cmp=RDRCT-907b618d-20210416

Kamp, J. (2021, August 6). COVID-19 vaccine mandates are on the rise for nursing home workers. *The Wall Street Journal.* https://www.wsj.com/articles/covid-19-vaccine-mandates-are-on-the-rise-for-nursing-home-workers-11628254164

Kirzinger, A., Kearney, A., Hamel, L., & Brodie, M. (2021, April 6). *KFF/The Washington Post frontline health care workers survey.* Kaiser Family Foundation. https://www.kff.org/report-section/kff-washington-post-frontline-health-care-workers-survey-vaccine-intentions/

Kirzinger, A., Sparks, G., Hamel, L., Lopes, L., Kearney, A., Stokes, M., & Brodie, M. (2021, August 4). *KFF-COVID-19 vaccine monitor: July 2021.* Kaiser Family Foundation. https://www.kff.org/coronavirus-covid-19/poll-finding/kff-covid-19-vaccine-monitor-july-2021/

Kochhst, R., & Bennett, J. (2021, April 14). *U.S. labor market inches back from the COVID-19 shock, but recovery is far from complete.* Pew Research Center. https://www.pewresearch.org/fact-tank/2021/04/14/u-s-labor-market-inches-back-from-the-covid-19-shock-but-recovery-is-far-from-complete/

Mabus, K. (2021, July 27). Mask mandates by states: As COVID cases spike, see what the rules are where you live. *USA Today.* https://www.usatoday.com/story/news/nation/2021/07/27/mask-requirements-state/8087357002/

Miller, E. A. (2020). Protecting and improving the lives older adults in the COVID-19 era. *Journal of Aging & Social Policy, 32*(4–5), 297–309. https://doi.org/10.1080/08959420.2020.1780104

Miller, Z. (2021, August 18). Biden to require COVID vaccines for nursing home staff. *AP.* https://apnews.com/article/business-health-coronavirus-pandemic-nursing-homes-2e6189cd41068b1e0f643ee7e4bfbb92

Ndugga, N., & Hill, L. (2021, August 4). *Latest data on COVID-19 vaccinations by race/ethnicity.* The Kaiser Family Foundation. https://www.kff.org/coronavirus-covid-19/issue-brief/latest-data-on-covid-19-vaccinations-race-ethnicity/

Nearly one-third of U.S. coronavirus deaths are linked to nursing homes. (2021a, June 1). *The New York Times.* https://www.nytimes.com/interactive/2020/us/coronavirus-nursing-homes.html

Our World in Data. (2021, August 17). *Coronavirus (COVID-19) vaccinations.* University of Oxford. https://ourworldindata.org/covid-vaccinations

Paulin, E. (2021, May 27). *More nursing homes are requiring staff COVID-19 vaccinations.* AARP. https://www.aarp.org/caregiving/health/info-2021/nursing-homes-covid-vaccine-mandate.html

Previtali, F., Allen, L. D., & Varlamova, M. (2020). Not only virus spread: The diffusion of ageism during the outbreak of COVID-19. *Journal of Aging & Social Policy, 32*(4–5), 506–514. https://doi.org/10.1080/08959420.2020.1772002

Ritter, A. Z., Kelley, J., Kent, R. M., Howard, P., Theil, R., Cavanaugh, P., Hollingsworth, J., Duffey, J. S., Schuler, M., & Nayor, M. D. (2021). Implementation of a coronavirus disease 2019 vaccination condition of employment in a community nursing home. *Journal of the American Medical Director Association.* 1-5.[Epub Ahead of Print]. https://doi.org/10.1016/j.jamda.2021.07.035

See how vaccinations are going in your county and state. (2021b, August 16). *The New York Times*. https://www.nytimes.com/interactive/2020/us/covid-19-vaccine-doses.html

Shippee, T. P., Akosionu, O., Ng, W., Woodhouse, M., Duan, Y., Thao, M. S., & Bowblis, J. R. (2020). COVID-19 pandemic: Exacerbating racial/ethnic disparities in long-term services and supports. *Journal of Aging & Social Policy, 32*(4–5), 323–333. https://doi.org/10.1080/08959420.2020.1772004

Simard, J., & Volicer, L. (2020). Loneliness and isolation in long-term care and the COVID-19 pandemic. *Journal of the American Medical Directors Association, 21*(7), 966–968. https://doi.org/10.1016%2Fj.jamda.2020.05.006

Smorenberg, A., Petters, E. J. G., Van Daele, P. L. A., Nossent, E. J., & Muller, M. (2021). How does SARS-CoV-2 targets the elderly patients? A review on potential mechanisms increasing disease severity. *European Journal of Internal Medicine, 83*, 1–5. https://doi.org/10.1016/j.ejim.2020.11.024

Tyler, D., Hunger, M., Mulmule, N., & Porter, K. (2021, May 31). *COVID-19 intensifies home care workforce challenges*. Office of the Assistant Secretary for Programming and Evaluation. https://aspe.hhs.gov/sites/default/files/private/aspe-files/265686/homecarecovid.pdf

U.S. Census Bureau. (2021, May 5). *Older Americans month: 2021*. https://www.census.gov/newsroom/stories/older-americans-month.html

U.S. Census Bureau. (2021, August 17). *U.S. and world population clock*. https://www.census.gov/popclock/

Veiga-Siejo, R., Miranda-Duro, M., & Veiga-Seijo, S. (2021). Strategies and actions to enable meaningful family connections in nursing homes during the COVID-19. *Clinical Gerontologist*, 1–11. [Epub Ahead of Print]. https://doi.org/10.1080/07317115.2021.1937424

Vestal, C. (2021, August 10). 10 states have school mask mandates while 8 forbid them. *Stateline*. PEW. https://www.pewtrusts.org/en/research-and-analysis/blogs/stateline/2021/08/10/10-states-have-school-mask-mandates-while-8-forbid-them

Watts, M. O., Musumeci, M., & Ammula, M. (2021, August 10). *State Medicaid home & community-based services (HCBS) programs respond to COVID-19: Early findings from a 50-state survey*. Kaiser Family Foundation. https://www.kff.org/coronavirus-covid-19/issue-brief/state-medicaid-home-community-based-services-hcbs-programs-respond-to-covid-19-early-findings-from-a-50-state-survey/

World Health Organization. (2021, August 17). *WHO coronavirus (COVID-19) dashboard*. https://covid19.who.int/

Xu, H., Intrator, O., & Bowblis, J. R. (2020). Shortages of staff in nursing homes during the COVID-19 pandemic: What are the driving factors?. *Journal of the American Directors Association, 21*(10), 1371–1377. https://doi.org/10.1016/j.jamda.2020.08.002

Yeyati, L., & Filippini, F. (2021, June). *Social and economic impact of COVID-19*. The Brookings Institution. https://www.brookings.edu/wp-content/uploads/2021/06/Social-and-economic-impact-COVID.pdf

Personal Experiences

Coronavirus-Related Anxiety, Social Isolation, and Loneliness in Older Adults in Northern California during the Stay-at-Home Order

Laura Gaeta ⓘ and Christopher R. Brydges

ABSTRACT

This study aimed to determine the prevalence of and associations between anxiety, social isolation, and loneliness in a sample of older adults in Northern California during the stay-at-home order enacted during the COVID-19 pandemic. 514 older adults completed a 24-item survey. Perceived isolation and loneliness were reported in 56.4% and 36.0% of participants, respectively. Loneliness was found to be associated with both social isolation and COVID-19-related anxiety; however, social isolation and coronavirus-related anxiety were unrelated. Healthcare providers, social service providers, and families are encouraged to maintain or increase contact with older adults during the COVID-19 pandemic.

Introduction

Social isolation and loneliness are important issues and concerns for community-dwelling older adults because of their effects on overall health. Both loneliness and isolation have been shown to negatively affect one's health (Coyle & Dugan, 2012), including increased risk of stroke and coronary heart disease (Valtorta et al., 2016), and increased likelihood of mortality (Holt-Lunstad et al., 2015). These documented negative sequelae are important for healthcare professionals, public health professionals, and community service providers to be aware of in order to identify older adults at risk of social isolation and loneliness and/or take action to reduce prevalence rates in this population.

Although commonly discussed alongside each other, the two constructs are distinct: Social isolation often refers to whether an individual is a member of a social network (e.g., through living with another person and/or participating in social activities). Conversely, loneliness refers to a perceived state of isolation, in that a person is not receiving the quality and/or quantity of social interactions they require (Cacioppo et al., 2014). Prevalence rates of social isolation and loneliness in older adults are commonly reported to be around 20–25% during daily life (e.g.,

Fokkema et al., 2012; Theeke, 2009; Victor & Yang, 2012), although a recent study found that social isolation and loneliness prevalence estimates were as low as 7.3% and 11.4%, respectively, in a national sample of Canadian adults aged 65 years and older (Menec et al., 2019), and 3% in English adults aged 65 years and older (Office for National Statistics, 2018).

In 2019, a novel coronavirus, COVID-19, emerged from Wuhan, China. The typical clinical presentation of COVID-19 was largely respiratory and varied in severity. Human-to-human transmission among those with COVID-19 and those without in close proximity was the primary form of spread. Because most with COVID-19 experience mild symptoms, transmission can affect more people (Vetter et al., 2020). In response to the growing number of cases of the virus, public health measures (similar to those taken during the 1918–1920 Spanish influenza; Bootsma & Ferguson, 2007) were implemented to slow the rate at which COVID-19 was spreading. Examples of these measures included washing hands frequently, avoiding touching the face and nose with one's hands, and practicing social distancing (World Health Organization, 2020). Social distancing occurred in the community (e.g., cancellation and/or closure of schools, places of worship, non-essential businesses and events) and at the individual level (e.g., maintaining six feet of physical distance between people and limiting close contact with other people) as it is effective in mitigating pandemic influenza (Glass et al., 2006).

Prior to the COVID-19 outbreak, loneliness was a major public health concern among older Americans (Gerst-Emerson & Jaywardhana, 2015). The potential implications of the COVID-19-related stay-at-home order and measures of social distancing, particularly for the older adult population who were already vulnerable, must be given attention. Given the increased risk of adverse consequences associated with social isolation (Morrow-Howell et al., 2020), it is necessary to investigate the prevalence of and risk factors associated with feelings of social isolation and loneliness during the COVID-19 pandemic. However, given the unusual circumstances of the current study (namely, the stay-at-home order), no formal hypotheses were specified. Rather, the current study tested two research questions: First, to estimate the prevalence of feelings of loneliness and feelings of social isolation in a sample of older adults during the COVID-19 pandemic. Second, to investigate associations between objective measures of loneliness, isolation, and COVID-19-related anxiety during the stay-at-home order (i.e., a novel and unusual context). As past research has not occurred during mass quarantine/self-isolation, it is unknown whether these constructs are associated with each other.

Methods

The study was reviewed and approved by the Institutional Review Board at California State University, Sacramento (IRB-19-20-259).

Participants

Participants were 551 adults who were members of an organization for older adults interested in lifelong learning in Northern California. This organization, which is composed of more than 1900 members, provides over 200 seminars and forums on a range of topics on the California State University, Sacramento campus each year. Thirty-seven participants did not complete the survey and were excluded from all analyses. As such, the final sample size was 514.

Measures

Participants completed a total of 24 survey items regarding demographic information, loneliness, isolation, and COVID-19-related anxiety (see Supplemental Materials for complete list of items). To measure loneliness and COVID-19-related anxiety, the short-form UCLA Loneliness Scale (ULS-6; Neto, 2014) and the Coronavirus Anxiety Scale (CAS; Lee, 2020) were administered, respectively. These measures have been previously validated and achieved Cronbach's α of 0.74 and 0.80 in the current study. Isolation was measured by asking participants about their marital status, household size, and whether they use social media. Additionally, participants were asked questions pertaining to feelings of isolation/loneliness, change in loneliness, frequency of in-person interactions, and change in that frequency were considered subjective measures. The survey was created in Qualtrics and took approximately five minutes to complete. The survey was sent to prospective participants via e-mail on May 28 2020, approximately two months after the March 19, 2020, stay-at-home order was enacted throughout California, and 74 days after recommendations for people aged 65 and older to stay at home. The organization of which the participants were members had also suspended its programs for 80 days.

Statistical analyses

All analyses were conducted using R 4.0.0 (R Core Team, 2020), and confirmatory factor analysis (CFA) was conducted and visualized using the lavaan 0.6.-6 (Rosseel, 2012) and semPlot 1.1.2 (Epskamp, 2015) packages. CFA was conducted to investigate associations between factors of loneliness (measured by the ULS-6), isolation (measured by marital status, household size, and social media use), and COVID-19-related anxiety (measured by the CAS). The ULS-6 and CAS were coded in accordance with the original papers describing the measures (Lee, 2020; Neto, 2014) such that a higher score indicated greater loneliness and greater COVID-19-related anxiety, respectively. For the CFA, marital status was recoded to give "married" a value of 0, and all other responses ("widowed", "never married", and "divorced or separated") a value of 1. Social media use was coded so that a "yes" response, where participants indicate they do use social media, was assigned a value of 0, and a "no" response was assigned a value of 1. Household size was multiplied by −1. In short, a higher score for each item entered into the CFA was associated with worse symptoms.

The inter-factor correlations were of key interest. In order to evaluate the associations between the loneliness, isolation, and COVID-19-related anxiety factors for dimensional distinctness. The full three-factor model, where the loneliness, isolation, and COVID-19-related anxiety factors were free to correlate, was compared to an independent three-factor model (where the inter-factor correlations were constrained to 0), a one-factor model (where all survey items loaded onto a single factor), and a series of two-factor models where two factors were merged into one and then correlated with the third (e. g., a loneliness and isolation factor is correlated with the COVID-19-related anxiety factor). Additionally, the factors were considered to be distinct if the 95% upper-bound correlation confidence intervals (CIs) did not intersect with 1.0. Following the guidelines summarized by Scheizer (2010), the CFA model was considered to have acceptable fit based on the following criteria: Comparative Fit Index (CFI) $\geq$ 0.90; Tucker-Lewis Index (TLI) $\geq$ 0.90; standardized root mean residual (SRMR) $\leq$ 0.10; and the root mean square error of approximation (RMSEA) $\leq$ 0.08. The 90% CIs of the RMSEA were also reported. The Bayesian Information Criterion (BIC) was also used for model comparison. A smaller BIC value indicates a better fitting model. For thoroughness, the model chi-square statistics were also included, although this statistic is considered to be overly sensitive with large sample sizes (Scheizer, 2010). All models were tested using maximum likelihood estimation, although standard errors and confidence intervals were estimated via bias-corrected bootstrapping with 2000 replications to help ensure robustness to any deviations from normality.

Results

Prevalence of isolation and loneliness

Descriptive statistics of all items are presented in Table 1. Over half (56.4%) of participants reported feeling isolated as a result of the COVID-19 outbreak, and more than one third (36.0%) reported feeling lonely. Additionally, just over half of participants (50.1%) reported an increase in loneliness since the COVID-19 outbreak. Over half (54.5%) of participants reported having daily in-person interactions before the stay-at-home order, and 88.1% reported a decrease in their in-person interactions. Nearly half (40.9%) of participants

Table 1. Descriptive statistics of survey items (n = 514).

Survey Item	Responses
1. What is your age? (in years)	M = 73.25 years, SD = 6.56, range = 57–93
2. What is your gender?	387 females; 127 males
3. What is your race/ethnicity?	471 White; 14 Asian; 11 Mixed; 5 Black or African American; 2 Native Hawaiian or Pacific Islander; 1 American Indian or Alaska Native; 0 Hispanic; 10 Other
4. What is your marital status?	275 married; 129 divorced or separated; 83 widowed; 27 never married
5. During this COVID-19 outbreak, have you felt isolated?	290 yes; 224 no
6. During this COVID-19 outbreak, have you felt lonely?	185 yes; 329 no
7. Indicate how often the statement below is descriptive of you: I lack companionship.	108 never; 168 rarely; 181 sometimes; 57 often
8. Indicate how often the statement below is descriptive of you: I feel part of a group of friends.	9 never; 42 rarely; 188 sometimes; 275 often
9. Indicate how often the statement below is descriptive of you: I feel left out.	80 never; 261 rarely; 148 sometimes; 25 often
10. Indicate how often the statement below is descriptive of you: I feel isolated from others.	80 never; 156 rarely; 219 sometimes; 59 often
11. Indicate how often the statement below is descriptive of you: I am unhappy being so withdrawn.	147 never; 184 rarely; 153 sometimes; 30 often
12. Indicate how often the statement below is descriptive of you: People are around me but not with me.	110 never; 191 rarely; 154 sometimes; 59 often
13. During the COVID-19 outbreak and stay-at-home order, how have your feelings of loneliness changed?	75 a lot more; 183 slightly more; 210 unchanged; 34 slightly less; 12 a lot less
14. How many people live in your household, including yourself?	210 one person; 262 two people; 31 three people; 4 four people; 7 five or more people
15. Are you connected to others (e.g., family, friends) through social media like Facebook?	399 yes; 115 no
16. During the COVID-19 outbreak, how frequently do you interact with others (e.g., phone call, video call, Skype, messaging, in person)?	280 daily; 136 4–6 times a week; 79 2–3 times a week; 19 once a week or less
17. Compared to before the COVID-19 outbreak, how often did you have in-person interactions?	280 daily; 126 4–6 times a week; 73 2–3 times a week; 19 once a week; 16 less than once a week
18. Since the stay-at-home order, how has the frequency of your in-person interactions changed?	291 much lower; 113 moderately lower; 49 slightly lower; 40 about the same; 6 slightly higher; 9 moderately higher; 6 much higher
19. How often have you experienced the following activities over the last 2 weeks? I felt dizzy, lightheaded, or faint, when I read or listened to news about the coronavirus.	474 not at all; 27 rare, less than a day or two; 9 several days; 2 more than seven days; 2 nearly every day over the last two weeks
20. How often have you experienced the following activities over the last 2 weeks? I had trouble falling or staying asleep because I was thinking about the coronavirus.	345 not at all; 119 rare, less than a day or two; 35 several days; 9 more than seven days; 6 nearly every day over the last two weeks
21. How often have you experienced the following activities over the last 2 weeks? I felt paralyzed or frozen when I thought about or was exposed to information about the coronavirus.	425 not at all; 67 rare, less than a day or two; 18 several days; 1 more than seven days; 3 nearly every day over the last two weeks
22. How often have you experienced the following activities over the last 2 weeks? I lost interest in eating when I thought about or was exposed to information about the coronavirus.	471 not at all; 33 rare, less than a day or two; 9 several days; 0 more than seven days; 1 nearly every day over the last two weeks
23. How often have you experienced the following activities over the last 2 weeks? I felt nauseous or had stomach problems when I thought about or was exposed to information about the coronavirus.	455 not at all; 42 rare, less than a day or two; 14 several days; 1 more than seven days; 2 nearly every day over the last two weeks
24. Optional: If you would like to share your experiences with social activities during the COVID-19 outbreak, please share them below.	Open-ended responses entered in a text box.

reported living alone, and the majority reported using some form of social media.

Associations between loneliness, isolation, and COVID-19-related anxiety

Correlations between items entered into the CFA are presented in Table 2. The full three-factor model provided acceptable or close to acceptable model fit (see Table 3 for model fit statistics), and provided a better fit of the data than the next best fitting model (three independent factors), $\Delta\chi^2$ (3) = 62.388, p < .001, ΔBIC = −43.662. Figure 1 presents the full three-factor CFA model.

Upon examination of the inter-factor correlations, it was noted that the correlation between the isolation and anxiety factors was very low (r = .020, 95% CI = −.081 – .143). Removal of this correlation did not significantly worsen model fit in comparison to the full three-factor model, $\Delta\chi^2$ (1) = 0.126, p = .723, and the BIC also decreased, ΔBIC = −6.116. Therefore, it was implied that the loneliness factor was associated with isolation (r = .319, 95% CI = .191-.453) and with COVID-19-related anxiety (r = .303, 95% CI = .173-.433), but that the isolation and COVID-19-related anxiety factors were independent. The final model fit statistics were close to acceptable or acceptable, CFI = 0.890, TLI = 0.867, RMSEA = 0.071 (90% CI = 0.062– 0.080), SRMR =0.058, χ^2 (75) = 267.795, BIC = 12,796.354. Lastly, it should be noted that the loading of social media use on to the isolation factor was non-significant. However, as removing it made no difference to the outcome of any analysis, it was kept in all models.

Discussion

The current study aimed to estimate the prevalence of feelings of loneliness and feelings of social isolation and to investigate associations between objective measures of loneliness, isolation, as well as COVID-19-related anxiety during the stay-at-home order (i.e., a novel and unusual context). The findings of this survey reveal that over half of the older adults in the study sample felt isolated. Given that estimates of isolation and loneliness in older adults commonly report prevalence rates of 25% or lower during daily life (Fokkema et al., 2012; Menec et al., 2019; Theeke, 2009; Victor & Yang, 2012), the value observed in the current study is markedly higher. This difference may be attributed to the higher engagement that the participants likely had as a result of belonging to a lifelong learning organization. Perhaps surprisingly, this value was not as high for feelings of loneliness; that is, more participants feel isolated than lonely during the COVID-19 outbreak (although loneliness prevalence in the current study was still higher than 25%).

Additionally, CFA models found that loneliness was significantly associated with both isolation and COVID-19-related anxiety. However, isolation and

Table 2. Correlations between measures of loneliness, isolation, and COVID-19-related Anxiety (n = 514).

Measure	1	2	3	4	5	6	7	8	9	10	11	12	13
1. ULS 1	-												
2. ULS 2	.25***	-											
3. ULS 3	.36***	.24***	-										
4. ULS 4	.46***	.25***	.43***	-									
5. ULS 5	.36***	.21***	.42***	.52***	-								
6. ULS 6	.31***	.16***	.32***	.32***	.27***	-							
7. Marital status	.49***	.03	.07	.09*	.10*	.07	-						
8. Household size	.36***	.00	.10*	.10*	.10*	.08	.58***	-					
9. Social media use	.08	.16***	.08	.05	.02	-.06	.08	.05	-				
10. CAS 1	.08	.04	.10*	.13**	.12**	.11*	-.02	-.01	.03	-			
11. CAS 2	.13**	.09*	.14**	.25***	.25***	.12**	.05	.05	.03	.28***	-		
12. CAS 3	.10*	.03	.10*	.18***	.20***	.10*	-.03	-.03	-.02	.50***	.35***	-	
13. CAS 4	.13**	.07	.05	.15***	.18***	.08	.04	.04	.07	.52***	.48***	.44***	-
14. CAS 5	.09*	.03	.12**	.16***	.16***	.14**	-.01	-.01	-.02	.53***	.44***	.48***	.57***

* $p < .05$. ** $p < .01$. *** $p < .001$.

Table 3. Fit indices for the full confirmatory factor analysis model and reduced models of loneliness, isolation, and COVID-19-related anxiety (n = 514).

Model	CFI	TLI	RMSEA (90% CI)	SRMR	χ^2	df	BIC
Full three-factor	0.890	0.865	0.071 (0.062-0.081)	0.058	267.669	74	12802.470
Independent three-factor	0.856	0.830	0.080 (0.071-0.089)	0.101	330.057	77	12846.132
One-factor	0.483	0.389	0.151 (0.143-0.160)	0.135	985.380	77	13501.455
Two-factor (Loneliness = Isolation)	0.788	0.743	0.098 (0.089-0.106)	0.077	448.325	76	12970.642
Two-factor (Loneliness = Anxiety)	0.600	0.521	0.134 (0.126-0.143)	0.124	779.345	76	13301.662
Two-factor (Isolation = Anxiety)	0.755	0.707	0.105 (0.096-0.114)	0.093	506.456	76	13028.774

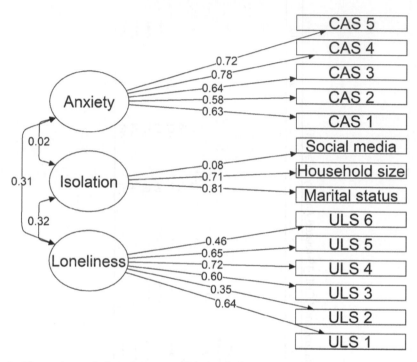

Figure 1. The estimated three-factor model. Single-headed arrows have standardised factor loadings next to them. Double-headed arrows have inter-factor correlations next to them. All factor loadings are significant to $p < .05$ except for the social media use loading.

COVID-19-related anxiety were not associated. Specifically, the CFA models found that loneliness and isolation are related, yet distinct, constructs. Isolation, in this case, refers more to the physical aspect. Aspects of loneliness may include not seeing family and friends often, wishing for more friends, feeling lonely the majority of the time, and having no friends nearby; whereas social isolation may include living alone, never visiting anyone, having no contact with neighbors, being alone for nine or more hours a day, and never leaving the house (Wenger & Burholt, 2004). These manifestations are of particular relevance to the current study and situation, in which participants are likely falling under the description of social isolation. The stay-at-home order has affected social interactions by reducing the number of people who can gather in a group, maintaining about six feet between people, and limiting trips and travel to only essential places, such as to medical appointments or grocery stores. Given that loneliness commonly refers to a perceived state of isolation (Cacioppo et al., 2014), it appears that those who perceive themselves to be isolated also worry the most about COVID-19. Prior to the COVID-19 outbreak, the majority of participants reported daily in-person interactions. With the stay-at-home order, however, opportunities to have in-person interactions and meetings have decreased, causing a large proportion of participants to notice a marked change. This may be resulting in increased anxiety with regards to COVID-19 (although it should be noted that this study is purely correlational and that the direction of associations between constructs cannot be determined).

With the aforementioned risks and effects of social isolation in mind, healthcare professionals and social service providers need to be aware of this finding. Older adults may already be at risk for loneliness, but the stay-at-home orders associated with COVID-19 have increased their vulnerability to isolation (see Office for National Statistics, 2018, however, for data showing that self-reported loneliness is more prevalent in young than older adults), and worry about the COVID-19 pandemic. To address this potential issue, it is important to maintain or increase contact (i.e., not in-person interactions) with older adults' social networks through social media, phone calls, and video-based calls (Ouslander, 2020). Additionally, providers should encourage older adults to quickly reestablish in-person interactions and social activities once the COVID-19 pandemic has ended; doing so could potentially alleviate any lingering feelings of isolation and/or loneliness from the stay-at-home order. Interventions that are focused on social connectedness can be effective for alleviating feelings of loneliness (Masi et al., 2011). To address isolation, interventions that provide opportunities for social support and activity, particularly in group formats, may be beneficial (Dickens et al., 2011). However, these approaches are highly dependent on the characteristics and needs of individuals (Fakoya et al., 2020). Recommendations specific to feelings resulting from the COVID-19 pandemic would likely require additional research and consideration of related health risks for how to best tailor the interventions for older adults, keeping in mind that feelings of loneliness vary between individuals.

Limitations and future research

Although this study provides estimates of prevalence of feelings of loneliness and isolation in a sample of older adults, as well as investigating associations between loneliness, isolation, and COVID-19-related anxiety, there are some limitations that should be noted. First, this sample was not nationally representative, as the sample was based in Northern California. As well as potential variation in demographic factors, stay-at-home orders varied by county and state, so experiences of those in other regions or states are likely different. Given the racial/ethnic and socio-economic disparities in COVID-19-related outcomes (Hooper et al., 2020; Van Lancker & Parolin, 2020), it could be the case that COVID-19-related anxiety may also vary substantially between demographic groups. Second, the participants were members of a lifelong learning program, so they were likely social and active participants who may have been more affected than other community-dwelling older adults because the program's classes were suspended during the pandemic. Older adults who are not as active, not community-dwelling, or who have smaller social networks may experience greater loneliness and/or isolation as a result of the stay-at-home order. On the other hand, those who are not as socially active as the participants in this study may feel no change in their perceived isolation. Third, the study design was cross-sectional, so it is possible that these feelings and the other variables of interest may change during the stay-at-home order. This survey captured the experiences of the participants about two months after the stay-at-home orders were enacted. In addition to differences in location, respondents may have different answers if this survey had been administered at other time points, such as after one month or three months. Future research could potentially follow up with older adults repeatedly during this period to see if feelings of loneliness and isolation change, and could also investigate the moderating effects of personality, as it could be a factor for determining one's risk for isolation.

Conclusion

In conclusion, this study demonstrates that feelings of isolation and loneliness appear to be higher than usual as a result of the COVID-19 pandemic and the resulting stay-at-home orders, and that loneliness (but not isolation) is associated with anxiety about COVID-19. Although the research is relatively exploratory, it suggests that older adults who report feeling lonely appear to be most at risk for being anxious about the COVID-19 pandemic. Reducing isolation – both objective and perceived – is important within the context of this pandemic. Families and friends should place greater emphasis on connecting with older adults in their social networks, and providers should follow up with their patients to ensure that they are participating in activities that address their social needs.

Key points:

- Older adults are thought to be at increased risk of loneliness and social isolation.
- A survey about loneliness during the coronavirus pandemic was sent to older adults.
- The majority of respondents felt lonelier during the stay-at-home order.

- Loneliness, but not isolation, is related to COVID-19-related anxiety.
- Safely increasing social interactions may alleviate feelings of loneliness.

Disclosure statement

Laura Gaeta is a seminar co-leader in the Renaissance Society (volunteer position).

Funding

There was no funding for this study.

ORCID

Laura Gaeta Ph.D ⓘ http://orcid.org/0000-0001-5493-9636

References

Bootsma, M. C. J., & Ferguson, N. M. (2007). The effect of public health measures on the 1918 influenza pandemic in U.S. cities. *Proceedings of the National Academy of Sciences*, *104*(18), 7588–7593. https://doi.org/10.1073/pnas.0611071104

Cacioppo, S., Capitanio, J. P., & Cacioppo, J. T. (2014). Toward a neurology of loneliness. *Psychological Bulletin*, *140*(6), 1464–1504. https://doi.org/10.1037/a0037618

Coyle, C. E., & Dugan, E. (2012). Social isolation, loneliness and health among older adults. *Journal of Aging & Health*, *24*(8), 1346–1363. https://doi.org/10.1177/0898264312460275

Dickens, A. P., Richards, S. H., Greaves, C. J., & Campbell, J. L. (2011). Interventions targeting social isolation in older people: A systematic review. *BMC Public Health*, *11*(1), 647. https://doi.org/10.1186/1471-2458-11-647

Epskamp, S. (2015). Semplot: Unified visualizations of structural equation models. *Structural Equation Modeling: A Multidisciplinary Journal*, *22*(3), 474–483. https://doi.org/10.1080/10705511.2014.937847

Fakoya, O. A., McCorry, N. K., & Donnelly, M. (2020). Loneliness and social isolation interventions for older adults: A scoping review of the evidence. *BMC Public Health*, *20* (1), 129. https://doi.org/10.1186/s12889-020-8251-6

Fokkema, T., De Jong Gierveld, J., & Dykstra, P. A. (2012). Cross-national differences in older adult loneliness. *The Journal of Psychology*, *146*(1-2), 201–228. https://doi.org/10.1080/00223980.2011.631612

Gerst-Emerson, K., & Jaywardhana, J. (2015). Loneliness as a public health issue: The impact of loneliness on health care utilization among older adults. *American Journal of Public Health*, *105*(5), 1013–1019. https://doi.org/10.2105/AJPH.2014.302427

Glass, R. J., Glass, L. M., Beyeler, W. E., & Min, H. J. (2006). Targeted social distancing designs for pandemic influenza. *Emerging Infectious Diseases*, *12*(11), 1671–1681. https://doi.org/10.3201/eid1211.060255

Holt-Lunstad, J., Smith, T. B., Baker, M., Harris, T., & Stephenson, D. (2015). Loneliness and social isolation as risk factors for mortality: A meta-analytic review. *Perspectives on Psychological Science*, *10*(2), 227–237. https://doi.org/10.1177/1745691614568352

Hooper, M. W., Nápoles, A. M., & Pérez-Stable, E. J. (2020). COVID-19 and racial/ethnic disparities. *Journal of the American Medical Association 323*(24), 2466–2467. https://doi.org/10.1001/jama.2020.8598

Lee, S. A. (2020). Coronavirus Anxiety Scale: A brief mental health screener for COVID-19 related anxiety. *Death Studies, 44*(7), 393–401. https://doi.org/10.1080/07481187.2020.1748481

Masi, C. M., Chen, H. Y., Hawkley, L. C., & Cacioppo, J. T. (2011). A meta-analysis of interventions to reduce loneliness. *Personality and Social Psychology Review, 15*(3), 219–266. https://doi.org/10.1177/1088868310377394

Menec, V. H., Newall, N. E., Mackenzie, C. S., Shooshtari, S., & Nowicki, S. (2019). Examining individual and geographic factors associated with social isolation and loneliness using Canadian longitudinal study on aging (CLSA) data. *PLoS ONE, 14*(2), e0211143. https://doi.org/10.1371/journal.pone.0211143

Morrow-Howell, N., Galucia, N., & Swinford, E. (2020). Recovering from the COVID-19 pandemic: A focus on older adults. *Journal of Aging and Society 32(4-5),* 526–535. https://doi.org/10.1080/08959420.2020.1759758

Neto, F. (2014). Psychometric analysis of the short-form UCLA Loneliness Scale (ULS-6) in older adults. *European Journal of Ageing,* 11, 313-319. https://doi.org/10.1007/s10433-014-0312-1

Office for National Statistics. (2018) *Analysis of characteristics and circumstances associated with loneliness in England using the community life survey, 2016 to 2017.* Retrieved April 12, 2020, from https://www.ons.gov.uk/peoplepopulationandcommunity/wellbeing/articles/lonelinesswhatcharacteristicsandcircumstancesareassociatedwithfeelinglonely/2018-04-10

Ouslander, J. G. (2020). Coronavirus-19 in geriatrics and long-term care: An update. *Journal of the American Geriatrics Society, 68*(5), 918–921. https://doi.org/10.1111/jgs.16464

R Core Team. (2020). *R: A language and environment for statistical computing (Version 4.0.0) [Computer Software].* https://www.R-project.org/

Rosseel, Y. (2012). Lavaan: An R package for structural equation modeling and more. *Journal of Statistical Software, 48*(2), 1–36. https://doi.org/10.18637/jss.v048.i02

Scheizer, K. (2010). Some guidelines concerning the modeling of traits and abilities in test construction. *European Journal of Psychological Assessment, 26*(1), 1–2. https://doi.org/10.1027/1015-5759/a000001

Theeke, L. A. (2009). Predictors of loneliness in U.S. adults over age sixty-five. *Archives of Psychiatric Nursing, 23*(5), 387–396. https://doi.org/10.1016/j.apnu.2008.11.002

Valtorta, N. K., Kanaan, M., Gilbody, S., Ronzi, S., & Hanratty, B. (2016). Loneliness and social isolation as risk factors for coronary disease and stroke: Systematic review and meta-analysis of longitudinal observational studies. *Heart, 102*(13), 1009–1016. https://doi.org/10.1136/heartjnl-2015-308790

Van Lancker, W., & Parolin, Z. (2020). COVID-19, school closures, and child poverty: A social crisis in the making. *The Lancet Public Health, 5*(5), e243–e244. https://doi.org/10.1016/S2468-2667(20)30084-0

Vetter, P., Eckerle, I., & Kaiser, L. (2020). Covid-19: A puzzle with many missing pieces. *BMJ, 368*(8235), m627. https://doi.org/10.1136/bmj.m627

Victor, C. R., & Yang, K. (2012). The prevalence of loneliness among adults: A case study of the United Kingdom. *The Journal of Psychology, 146*(1–2), 85–104. https://doi.org/10.1080/00223980.2011.613875

Wenger, G. C., & Burholt, V. (2004). Changes in levels of social isolation and loneliness among older people in a rural area: A twenty–year longitudinal study. *Canadian Journal of Aging/la Revue Canadienne Du Vieillissement, 23*(2), 115–127. https://doi.org/10.1353/cja.2004.0028

World Health Organization. (2020) *Coronavirus disease (COVID-19) advice for the public website.* Retrieved April 3, 2020, from https://www.who.int/emergencies/diseases/novel-coronavirus-2019/advice-for-public

Pandemic Place: Assessing Domains of the Person-Place Fit Measure for Older Adults (PPFM-OA) during COVID-19

Joyce Weil (iD)

ABSTRACT

Place-based identity and person-place fit are called into question during a pandemic, such as COVID-19, when older adults' relationship to place may be in flux. Both academic and gray literature detail drastic changes in the way many aspects of place will be affected by a pandemic. While the dominant discourse focuses on medical and health changes, this brief report uses the Person-Place Fit Measure for Older Adults (PPFM-OA) and its broader, five subscale place domains (Primary or Basic Needs/Necessities; Neighborhood Changes and Moving; Identity and Place Attachment; Community Value; and Services and Resources) as a way to assess the pandemic's impact on the daily lives of older adults from their own points of view.

Introduction

During the COVID-19 pandemic, initial research has tended toward a medical or health-based focus. This is particularly true for older adults – leaving other aspects of their lives to fade into the background. Medical practitioners report increased mortality rates and find those 65 years or older "accounting for 45% of hospitalizations, 53% of ICU admissions, and 80% of deaths" (Le Couteur et al., 2020, p. 2). Skilled-care facilities express concern about liability related to resident coronavirus deaths (Runyeon, 2020). Early on the Associated Press (AP) kept a tally of deaths in skilled-care facilities (11,000 as of April 23, 2020) because, it states, no federal agencies have done so (Condon et al., 2020). By May 2020, researchers suggest coronavirus-related deaths in skilled care account for a "staggering one-third of the more than 80,000 deaths due to COVID-19 in the U.S. (Behrens & Naylor, 2020). Community-dwelling older adults, who outnumber those in skilled care, are also targeted as high risk (Cohen & Tavares, 2020). During this period larger gerontological and sociology-of-aging-and-the-lifecourse communities have called for placing the virus in a broader, social, non-medical context to humanize the impact of the disease. For example, researchers have developed strategies that focus on the dignity of older adults during the pandemic (Ehni & Wahl, 2020). Articles call for the restoration of human rights of older adults instead of promoting negative age-based policies and divisions (Previtali et al., 2020).

The Secretary-General of the United Nations issued policy briefs (United Nations, 2020a, 2020b) calling for a "response to COVID-19 [that] must respect the rights and dignity of older people" (Guterres, 2020, video). One priority is the meaningful inclusion of older adults in "the socio-economic and humanitarian response to COVID-19" (p. 4). Policies developed must authentically include older adults and their needs because "the voices, perspectives, and expertise of older persons in identifying problems and solutions are sometimes not sufficiently incorporated in policy-making" (p. 15).

Ayalon et al. (2020) ask that gerontological researchers "contribute to more balanced discourse about COVID-19" (2020, p. 2). Viewed biomedically, older adults are cited as being most at-risk, yet socially they face increased ageism. Some observers have even called this a "parallel outbreak of ageism" (Ayalon et al., 2020, p. 1). This labeling occurs at many levels, for example, the "BoomerRemover" hashtag on social media, present in 780,000 posts by mid-March 2020 (Aronson, 2020a, 2020b; Ehni & Wahl, 2020; Godfrey, 2020; Schmich, 2020; Sparks, 2020). The hashtag has been attributed to Millennials who used the term to show they are not at risk of COVID-19 infection because they falsely believe it kills only older adults. Some posts have characterized the hashtag as a joking reaction, while others have used the hashtag when trying to "help" older adults by offering patronizing advice (such as "remember to wash your hands"). Aronson (2020a, 2020b) further explains how the construction of older adults during the COVID-19 pandemic is not balanced in the discourse. She highlights the paradox of targeting older adults as those with the highest rate of infection yet having the population almost absent from peer-reviewed medical journals.

Social policies are impacted by the negative framing of COVID-19 as a disease only of the old. Examples include the triaging of care for those 80 years of age and older, making decisions as to who gets an ICU bed by age (Le Couteur et al., 2020), or countries acting slowly in creating policies to contain COVID-19 because they feel the virus is a risk solely to the old (Aronson, 2020a, 2020b). Resurfacing, too, are more familiar stereotypes, such as older adults being a drain on the healthcare system and on such federal programs as Social Security, Medicare, and Medicaid. Legal groups are challenging ageism in states' health and medical policies targeting older adults, abuses of civil rights, and diminution of the rights of skilled-care residents (Justice in Action, 2020).

Adhering to a solely biomedical assessment of the effects of the pandemic can become regressive. Little discussed are the non-medical markers of quality of life during COVID-19–especially when it comes to the meaning and aspects of place – particularly when sheltering-in-place. Framing the pandemic in a biomedical view without including a broader view embracing societal, policy, and human rights concerns limits our understanding of the lived experience of older adults as they remain in pandemic place. The remaining sections of this brief focus on: the role and meaning of place for older adults; the need to broadly measure person-place fit from older adults' own assessments using the Person-Place Fit Measure for Older Adults (PPFM-OA; Weil, 2017); how each of the PPFM-OA's subscales can be used to assess the impact of pandemic place/COVID-19 upon place; and the way accurate place assessments can be used to inform policy.

Why older adults' relationship to place matters

Gerontological literature has long valued the relationship of person and place for older adults. While building upon the framework created by early models of person-environment fit (such as Lawton & Nahemow, 1973), more recent models have broadened to include an expanded sense of place, acknowledging those who are stuck in place (Torres-Gil & Hofland, 2012), the value of "being in place" (Rowles, 2019), and what constitutes the "right place" for the individual (Golant, 2015). Researchers have focused on having older adults self-define the meaning and relationship place holds for them (Wiles et al., 2012) and how understanding place can inform policy-making (Greenfield, 2012).

While place-based research has been expanding the concept of place, the work of the author of this manuscript has concentrated on bringing a deeper understanding of older adults' agency in assessing place, the way place-fit evolves over time, and the complexity and nuance of how older adults attach meaning to place. For example, aging in place has moved beyond being defined as one's longstanding home in a community setting; the term should be embraced across the continuum of care as older adults' need and choice of place may change (Weil & Smith, 2016). The relationship of place that an older adult chooses to live and how that place suits their needs continues evolve – as virtual place, co-housed place, and people and policies that support person-place fit (see Weil, 2020). Place has grown to include an understanding of what it means to live in a rural place, to live in places that are undergoing rapid gentrification, and global or transnational places. Place work acknowledges that older adults can affect and be affected differently by place. Namely, intersectional characteristics of older person, such as social class, race, ethnicity gender, sexual orientation, health status, and geographic setting, influence how well a place matches an older adult's needs, as do changes in the society in which they live (Mitra & Weil, 2014; Weil, 2014). The person-place fit, or older adult's relationship to place, is seen as dynamic, fluid, and influenced by both individual and societal phenomena.

Person-Place Fit Measure for Older Adults (PPFM-OA)

The Person-Place Fit Measure for Older Adults (PPFM-OA) was created to incorporate broader domains of place often missing from traditional assessments of how well an environment meets the needs of an older adult. The full, self-assessment based, 44-item measure has five subscales: Primary or Basic Needs/Necessities, Neighborhood Changes and Moving, Identity and Place Attachment, Community Value, Services and Resources. Each subscale contains Likert-style items that an older adult can rate with their level of agreement/disagreement. The online administration of the PPFM-OA allows for utility during COV1D-19 sequestering and in a COVID-19 and post-COVID -19 context, thus challenging assumptions about how older adults are assessed. As a 10–15 minute online tool, the PPFM-OA can easily transition into virtual administration for use in the current COVID-19 and post-COVID-19 new-normal – much like the case of telemedicine. (For a full description of the measure see, Weil, 2019).

In this research report, the PPFM-OA serves as an example of how showing the effect of a pandemic upon place attachment and the meaning of place can make the lived experience of older adults visible. This increased visibility can broaden the view of a pandemic that was initially seen through a lens of medical surveillance.

Primary or basic needs and necessities

This subscale comprises items related to basic needs, those at the base of Maslow's Hierarchy of Needs. Items asked about health (overall and in relation to being able to live in the community, and healthcare suited to current needs) and general safety (in one's home and community both during the day and at night). Also explored are basic concerns about finances (and affording current rent or mortgage payments), housing being adequate for one's needs, and the individual being able to care for their own home. Having neighbors rated as good, a social network (having a spouse/partner around), and not wanting to move from the neighborhood are parts of this subscale. Items in this subscale can track discourse about healthcare changes and access that have changed drastically during COVID-19.

During the pandemic, there is a focus on assessing the impact of COVID-19 on older adults' financial security and safety. For example, older adults who are financially insecure are reported to fare even less well during COVID-19 (Annelies, 2020). While more affluent older adults may manage well, the National Council on Aging predicts "the COVID-19 pandemic will push between 1.4 and 2.1 million more older Americans into poverty, and older adults with the least wealth will be the hardest hit" (p. 1).

Personal safety and community safety have also been frequent news topics during the pandemic. News stories cover financial scams targeted at older adults (e.g., phone calls asking for investments to find a cure or soliciting funding for medication or treatment). Though financial changes are currently reported, the PPFM-OA can quantify the extent to which they are experienced and rated as satisfactory/dissatisfactory by older persons.

Social networks and social isolation in a pandemic also fill the literature. Older adults sheltering-in-place in Spain and watching the news coped with low self-efficacy and the feeling of being a burden to others. These factors contributed to increased levels of distress (Losada-Baltar et al., 2020). In the U.S., literature reports social isolation is increasing (Golant in McElwee, 2020). Armitage and Nellums (2020) suggest that, because many older adults socialize outside, isolation is a severe public-health and mental-health threat. Items such as older persons seeing their neighbors as good and having a readily available social network while rating their neighborhood's "feel" are parts of this subscale.

Community value

An assessment of community value is measured by older adults' feeling of being accepted in their own communities and being heard. It includes an evaluation of the community as one that "advocate[s] for older persons" and "is a good one for older people." Such thoughts can evaluate if this resurgence of negative labeling impacts older adults' own assessment of the value/lack of value of the community in which they live and its acceptance of them.

Identity and place attachment

Place attachment and identity refer to place being an integral part of how older adults define or see themselves. The subdomain is measured by older adults feeling they have a history with the place they live and wanting to remain in that place until they die. It assesses whether older people live in their community by choice and if the natural environment keeps the individual there.

During COVID-19, emphasis is given to how the nature of place is changing as a society; we are "navigating the uncharted" (Fauci et al., 2020). News reports suggest familiar and favored places may lack access to vital resources – food, transportation, and other necessities. As Golant (in McElwee, 2020) suggests, maintaining the same quality of life for those aging in place pre- and post-COVID-19 may be a "serious challenge … as they are [without resources] … 'trapped in place'" (para. 2). Items asking directly about the self-rated identity-place relationship can show the variation in the ways the pandemic may impact the meaning and attachment to place for older adults.

Services and resources

Health resources for older adults are scarce during COVID-19, with access to mental-health services even rarer. As in the case of China during its initial outbreak, if mental-health services were available, they were often in person and could not be traveled to owing to sequestering (Yang et al., 2020). National organizations are creating toolkits and websites to address older adults' increased demand for information about where to find resources – from food, housing, and transportation to health care and medication (Annelies, 2020; Hartford Foundation, 2020). For example, the National Council on Aging (NCOA, 2020a, 2020b) has established a guide for the "most urgently needed" COVID-19 Resources for Older Adults & Caregivers, and the Hartford Foundation has developed a frequently updated website, "Coronavirus Disease (COVID-19) Resources for Older Adults, Family Caregivers, and Health Care Providers." The Hartford Foundation's website offers links to federal organizations (such as the CDC or Administration for Community Living), national organizations (such as the Alzheimer's Association or AARP), and news stories and articles. The website has sections dedicated to information for health professionals and long-term care providers. Using a measure can assess, via older persons' views, both the lack of resources and the way that more newly created resources in response to COVID-19 may have filled the gap.

Neighborhood changes and consideration of moving

Kuwahara et al. (2020) draw attention to the specific ways COVID-19 may affect community-dwelling older adults. It is possible the pandemic will add stress to the neighborhood-based social connections older adults may have. Any strained networks or relationships, possibly aiding in alleviating pandemic effects, may also be weakened or made more vulnerable to negative change. In many ways, neighborhood-feeling can capture many ways that a place works or does not work for the older adult. Assessment of satisfaction with multiple neighborhood-based markers can allow for the impact of COVID-19 sequestering on neighborhood to be evaluated.

Summary

As researchers, we need to explore the impact that the COVID-19-era changes reported in the academic and gray literature have on the daily lives of older adults. Measures that work across multiple domains – in this case, of place (like the PPFM-OA) – are useful to gauge change from older persons' point of view. The assessment of place includes many crucial areas of change from the pandemic, beyond medical ones, and can aid in assessing the full range of the pandemic's impact on the lives of older adults.

The pandemic and its related scapegoating of older adults are reported to have likely long-lasting ramifications on levels of community acceptance, being heard, and being advocated for as older persons. Yes, older adults are more likely to struggle to access resources and be at greater risk from severe illness (CDC, 2020), but questions can capture if older adults perceive risk from heath rationing or feel they are not being prioritized in treatment order due to their less-likely chances of survival (Emanuel et al., 2020; Orecchio-Egresitz, 2020). While local news stations run reports about changes in Medicare, Medicaid, and Social Security and about scarcity of face-to-face coordination of care (Siegel, 2020), this aspect of the measure includes older adults' assessment of this scarcity in their own local place.

Implications for policy

Understanding Person-Place Fit and the changing relationship between older adults and place during the COVID-19 pandemic can influence policies at a community-based and national level. Each of the subscales of the PPFM-OA (Primary or Basic Needs/Necessities, Neighborhood Changes and Moving, Identity and Place Attachment, Community Value, Services and Resources) has direct implications for policy. Information learned from the Primary-needs subscale can influence community-based policies about food and nutrition, access to healthcare and long-term care, poverty, and financial security. For example, this evaluation of how well primary needs are met can inform housing policy in terms of supportive housing and rent assistance. At the federal level, this indicator can influence Medicare, Medicaid, and Social Security as age-based policies.

Data gathered from the two subscales of Neighborhood Changes and Moving and Services and Resources are directly tied to policy at both the community and national levels, as well. Older adults' assessment of their current situation on these two scales can direct local services and resources that are ultimately provided by the Older Americans Act at the federal level. These services and resources include nutrition sites, transportation, community-based information and referral services, recreation and leisure, and legal assistance often provided in senior center settings. Policy makers can use the Community Value and Identity and Place Attachment subscales to create or improve policies addressing social isolation, mental health, and the status of older adults in a community. Broader measures of place expand, beyond the health experiences of those in acute medical care, the ability to capture the pandemic's full impact on the daily lives of older adults and incorporate that information in guiding policy.

Disclosure statement

No potential conflict of interest was reported by the author.

ORCID

Joyce Weil Ph.D., MPH, C.P.G. (iD) http://orcid.org/0000-0002-1573-6534

References

Annelies, G. (2020 March 16). *For millions of low-income seniors, coronavirus is a food- security issue.* Brookings Institute. https://www.brookings.edu/blog/the-avenue/2020/03/16/for-millions-of-low-income-seniors-coronavirus-is-a-food-security-issue/

Armitage, R., & Nellums, L. B. (2020). COVID-19 and the consequences of isolating the elderly. *The Lancet Public Health, 5*(5), e256. https://doi.org/10.1016/S2468-2667(20)30061-X

Aronson, L. (2020a, March 28). Ageism is making the pandemic worse: The disregard for the elderly that's woven into American culture is hurting everyone. *The New York Times.* https://www.theatlantic.com/culture/archive/2020/03/americas-ageism-crisis-is-helping-the-coronavirus/608905/

Aronson, L. (2020b, March 22). Covid-19 kills only old people. *The New York Times.* https://www.nytimes.com/2020/03/22/opinion/coronavirus-elderly.html

Ayalon, L., Chasteen, A., Diehl, M., Levy, B., Neupert, S. D., Rothermund, K., & Wahl, H. W. (2020). Aging in times of the COVID-19 pandemic: Avoiding ageism and fostering inter-generational solidarity. *The Journals of Gerontology: Series B, gbaa051*(2020), 1–4. https://doi.org/10.1093/geronb/gbaa051

Behrens, L. L., & Naylor, M. D. (2020). "We are alone in this battle": A framework for a coordinated response to COVID-19 in nursing homes. *Journal of Aging & Social Policy, 32*(4–5), 1–7. https://doi.org/10.1080/08959420.2020.1773190

CDC. (2020, April 11). *COVID-19, people who need extra protection: Older adults.* U.S. Department of Health & Human Services. https://www.cdc.gov/coronavirus/2019-ncov/need-extra-precautions/older-adults.html

Cohen, M. A., & Tavares, J. (2020). Who are the most at-risk older adults in the COVID-19 era? It's not just those in nursing homes. *Journal of Aging & Social Policy, 32*(4–5), 1–7. https://doi.org/10.1080/08959420.2020.1764310

Condon, B., Sedensky, M., & Mustian, J. (2020, April 24). 11,000 deaths: Ravaged nursing homes plead for more testing. *The Associated Press.* https://apnews.com/e34b42d996968cf9fa0ef85697418b01

Ehni, H. J., & Wahl, H. W. (2020). Six propositions against ageism in the COVID-19 pandemic. *Journal of Aging & Social Policy, 32*(4–5), 1–11. https://doi.org/10.1080/08959420.2020.1770032

Emanuel, E. J., Persad, G., Upshur, R., Thome, B., Parker, M., Glickman, A., & Phillips, J. P. (2020). Fair allocation of scarce medical resources in the time of COVID-10. *The New England Journal of Medicine, 382*(21), 2049–2055. https://doi.org/10.1056/NEJMsb2005114

Fauci, A. S., Lane, H. C., & Redfield, R. R. (2020). COVID-19 — Navigating the uncharted. *The New England Journal of Medicine, 382*(13), 1268–1269. https://doi.org/10.1056/NEJMe2002387

Godfrey, A. (2020 March 29). Millennials' shocking new term for coronavirus - 'Boomer Remover'. *7News*. Retrieved April 11, 2020, from https://7news.com.au/lifestyle/health-wellbeing/millennials-shocking-new-term-for-coronavirus-boomer-remover-c-770457

Golant, S. M. (2015). *Aging in the right place*. Health Professions Press.

Greenfield, E. A. (2012). Using ecological frameworks to advance a field of research, practice, and policy on aging-in-place initiatives. *The Gerontologist, 52*(1), 1–12. https://doi.org/10.1093/geront/gnr108

Guterres, A. (2020, May 1). *UN secretary general on the launch of the policy brief on older persons* (video). United Nations. Retrieved May 30, 2020, from https://www.youtube.com/watch? time_continue=13&v=YOua9Y1D5mM&feature=emb_logo

Hartford Foundation. (2020, April 9). *Coronavirus disease (COVID-19) resources for older adults, family caregivers and health care providers*. The John A. Hartford Foundation. https://www.johnahartford.org/dissemination-center/view/coronavirus-disease-covid-19-resources-for-older-adults-family- caregivers-and-health-care-providers

Justice in Action. (2020). *From DC: COVID-19 updates*. Retrieved April 24, 2020, from.

Kuwahara, K., Kuroda, A., & Fukuda, Y. (2020). COVID-19: Active measures to support community-dwelling older adults. *Travel Medicine and Infectious Disease, 36*(2020), 101638. https://doi.org/10.1016/j.tmaid.2020.101638

Lawton, M., & Nahemow, L. (1973). *The psychology of adult development and aging*. APA.

Le Couteur, D. G., Anderson, R. M., & Newman, A. B. (2020). COVID-19 through the lens of gerontology. *The Journals of Gerontology: Series A*. https://doi.org/10.1093/gerona/glaa077

Losada-Baltar, A., Jiménez-Gonzalo, L., Gallego-Alberto, L., Pedroso-Chaparro, M. D. S., Fernandes-Pires, J., & Márquez-González, M. (2020). "We're staying at home": Association of self-perceptions of aging, personal and family resources and loneliness with psychological distress during the lock-down period of COVID-19. *The Journals of Gerontology: Series B, gbaa048*. https://doi.org/10.1093/geronb/gbaa048

McElwee, C. (2020, March 23). America's seniors and COVID-19 (Interview with StephenGolant). *City Talk*. Retrieved April 11, 2020, from https://www.city-journal.org/americas-seniors-and-covid-19

Mitra, D., & Weil, J. (Eds.). (2014). *Race and the lifecourse: Readings from the intersection of race, ethnicity, and age*. Palgrave.

NCOA. (2020a, March 18). *4 Coronavirus scams to avoid*. Author. Retrieved April 11, 2020, from https://www.ncoa.org/blog/4-coronavirus-scams-to-avoid/

NCOA. (2020b). *Economic insecurity for older adults in the presence of the COVID-19 pandemic.NCOA issue brief*. Cohen, M., Tavares, J., Silberman, S, & Popham, P. National Council on Aging.

Orecchio-Egresitz, H. (2020, March 10). *Faced with tough choices, Italy is prioritizing young COVID-19 patients over the elderly. That likely 'would not fly' in the US*. Business Insider. Retrieved April 11, 2020, from https://www.businessinsider.com/prioritizing-covid-19-patients-based-age-likely-wont-fly-us-2020-3

Previtali, F., Allen, L. D., & Varlamova, M. (2020). Not only virus spread: The diffusion of ageism during the outbreak of COVID-19. *Journal of Aging & Social Policy, 32*(4–5), 1–9. https://doi.org/10.1080/08959420.2020.1772002

Rowles, G. (2019). Being in place identity and attachment in later life. In M. W. Skinner, G. J. Andrews, & M. P. Cutchin (Eds.), *Geographical gerontology: Perspectives, concepts, approaches* (pp. 203–215). Routledge.

Runyeon, F. (2020, April 17). NY immunity law shields nursing homes as virus toll soars. *Law360*. Retrieved April 20, 2020, from https://www.law360.com/articles/1264434

Schmich, M. (2020, March 24). Column: COVID-19 as the 'Boomer Remover'? Let's talk about that. *Chicago Tribune*. Retrieved April 11, 2020, from, https://www.chicagotribune.com/

columns/mary-schmich/ct-met-schmich-coronavirus-boomer-remover-20200324-mk3f7sut6bdj5fuuvrgvixd5su-story.html

Siegel, S. (2020, March 20). COVID-19's impact multiplies for seniors and vulnerable adults. *National Law Review*. Retrieved April 11, 2020, from https://www.natlawreview.com/article/covid-19-s-impact-multiplies-seniors-and-vulnerable-adults

Sparks, H. (2020, March 19). Morbid 'boomer remover' coronavirus meme only makes millennials seem more awful. *New York Post*. Retrieved May 30, 2020, from https://nypost.com/2020/03/19/morbid-boomer-remover-coronavirus-meme-only-makes-millennials-seem-more-awful/

Torres-Gil, F., & Hofland, H. (2012). Vulnerable populations. In D.-C. Cisneros & Hickie (Eds.), *Independent for life* (pp. 221–232). University of Texas Press.

United Nations. (2020a, May). *Policy brief: The impact of COVID-19 on older persons*. Author. Retrieved May 30, 2020, from https://www.un.org/development/desa/ageing/wp-content/uploads/sites/24/2020/05/COVID-Older-persons.pdf

United Nations. (2020b, April). *Issue brief: Older persons and COVID-19: A defining moment for informed, inclusive and targeted response*. Author. https://www.un.org/development/desa/ageing/wp-content/uploads/sites/24/2020/04/POLICY-BRIEF-ON-COVID19-AND-OLDER-PERSONS.pdf

Weil, J. (2014). *The new neighborhood senior center: Redefining social and service roles for the baby boom generation*. Rutgers University Press.

Weil, J. (2017). Aging in rural communities: Older persons' narratives of relocating in place to maintain rural identity. *Online Journal of Rural Research & Policy, 12*(1), 1–28. https://doi.org/10.4148/1936-0487.1076

Weil, J. (2019). Developing the person–place fit measure for older adults: Broadening place domains. *The Gerontologist, gnz112*, 1–11. https://doi.org/10.1093/geront/gnz112

Weil, J. (2020). Is the place the thing?: The role of place in later life. *Journal of Women & Aging, 32*(1), 1–2. https://doi-org.unco.idm.oclc.org/10.1080/08952841.2019.1681890

Weil, J., & Smith, E. (2016). Revaluating aging in place: From traditional definitions to the continuum of care. *Working with Older People, 20*(4), 223–230. https://doi.org/10.1108/WWOP-08-2016-0020

Wiles, J. L., Leibing, A., Guberman, N., Reeve, J., & Allen, R. E. (2012). The meaning of "aging in place" to older people. *The Gerontologist, 52*(3), 357–366. https://doi.org/10.1093/geront/gnr098

Yang, Y., Li, W., Zhang, Q., Zhang, L., Cheung, T., & Xiang, Y. T. (2020). Mental health services for older adults in China during the COVID-19 outbreak. *The Lancet Psychiatry, 7*(4), e19. https://doi.org/10.1016/S2215-0366(20)30079-1

The Impact of Stigmatization on Social Avoidance and Fear of Disclosure among Older People: Implications for Social Policy Preparedness in a Public Health Crisis

Jiannan Li (iD), Chulan Huang, Bocong Yuan (iD),
and Haixuan Liang,

ABSTRACT

This study examined whether older people with epicenter travel experiences in the event of the novel coronavirus disease epidemic suffered from stigmatization, which in turn affected subsequent behavior, including fear of disclosure and social avoidance. A three-wave survey was conducted using a time-lagged design of older people who had travel experiences in Hubei, China on the eve of the outbreak. Results reveal positive associations between stigmatization and stress, social avoidance, and fear of disclosure, in addition to positive associations between stress and social avoidance and fear of disclosure. Findings thus suggest that the effects of stigmatization on social avoidance and fear of disclosure is mediated, in part, by stress. De-stigmatization and psychological supports should be prioritized for epidemic prevention and control among older people in quarantine.

Since the outbreak of novel coronavirus disease in China, people who have had epicenter travel have been subject to ongoing stigmatization (Kanmodi & Kanmodi, 2020). Unnecessary stigmatization may cause travelers who might not be infected to potentially lose jobs, friends, and family connections. In China, people who have been to the epicenter – Hubei province – during or before the outbreak of the pandemic were quarantined and underwent rigorous detection of virus nucleic acid testing. It is reported that these people experienced rejection, isolation, prejudice, and discrimination even after quarantine (Hardinges, 2020; Lin, 2020; Zhai & Du, 2020), whether they were infected or not. Individuals tend to cope with the fear of getting an infection by blaming a new disease outbreak on someone or some group of people outside of their own social sphere; those who are blamed may experience stigmatization as a result (McCauley et al., 2013). Such experiences more frequently happen to older people in the context of COVID-19 as they are considered to have higher likelihood of getting infected.

Stigmatization can lead to negative consequences, as evidenced by prior infectious disease emergencies (Cheung, 2015; Maunder et al., 2003; Person et al., 2004). For example, in 1994 when Yersinia pestis infection had been identified publicly, half a million people who fled Surat, India were turned away from other communities and cities. Goods, flights, and passengers from this city were also rejected by other countries, resulting in billion-dollar losses and a major decline in the Bombay Stock Exchange (McCauley et al., 2013). Similarly, in April 2009 when a novel strain of human influenza (H1N1) first appeared in some Mexican pig farms and spread rapidly around the world, Latino immigrants were rejected and products from Mexico were shunned across many countries (McCauley et al., 2013).

Similar phenomena of stigmatization exist in almost every infectious disease emergency. Previous research on disease-related stigmatization devotes much attention to patients as the stigmatized group, but little to the group of people in healthy conditions but suffering epidemic-related stigmatization. The investigation of this latter group can help extend and generalize relevant research findings into a new population. Further, older people with epicenter travel experience could be more vulnerable to the effects of stigmatization and at a much higher risk of getting infected. As such, this study focuses on older people with epicenter travel experience in the event of the novel coronavirus disease epidemic in order to examine the effect of stigmatization on subsequent behavior. The exploration of the internal, individual psychological mechanisms in the field of stigmatization research remains insufficient. This study helps to fill this gap by considering stress as a potential mediator explaining subsequent behavior among older adults experiencing stigmatization during COVID-19.

This study proposes that novel coronavirus disease-related stigmatization could expose older people who had epicenter travel experiences to increased stress resulting from prejudice and discrimination. In order to relieve this stress, it posited that these individuals engage in socially avoidant or withdrawal responses (social avoidance), and an unwillingness to disclose personal information (fear of disclosure). Understanding the behavioral tendencies and the related psychological mechanisms of uninfected older people with epicenter travel experiences could inform public health interventions during the pandemic.

The relationship between stigmatization and social avoidance and fear of disclosure

Stigmatization is defined as the process of social relations through which specific groups are labeled as undesirable and dangerous and are thus treated as an "outsider" or "other" (Goffman, 2009). It is generally regarded as a kind of interpersonal rejection (Smart Richman & Leary, 2009). Stigmatization stems from fears that are often suffered by people in times of uncertainty, like the current novel coronavirus disease pandemic (McCauley et al., 2013). Individuals with a concealable stigma have the fear that someone will discover their stigma and reject, ridicule, or discriminate against them accordingly (Jones, 1984; Link & Phelan, 2001; Pachankis, 2007; Stutterheim et al., 2011). In response, it is more likely for individuals such as these to experience cognitive and affective reactions, such as self-consciousness, vigilance, shame, and guilt (Pachankis, 2007). To avoid further interpersonal rejection and its accompanying hurt, these individuals, in turn, develop socially avoidant or withdrawal responses (Smart Richman & Leary, 2009).

Stigmatization is also the most prevalent reason reported for concealing one's condition (Adebiyi & Ajuwon, 2015; Akani & Erhabor, 2006; Anakwa et al., 2020; Kumar et al., 2006; Stutterheim et al., 2011; Toth & Dewa, 2014; Vanable et al., 2006; Wright, 2015, April). Virus carriers who experience a higher level of perceived infectious disease-related stigma are found to have a greater level of disclosure concerns, and accordingly, are less likely to disclose their positive testing status (Anakwa et al., 2020). As such, people who have epicenter travel experience in the event of the pandemic may have fear of disclosure and be inclined to keep their conditions concealed when perceiving the potential suffering of stigmatization. Hence, it is conceivable that the perceived stigmatization for one with epicenter travel experience during the novel coronavirus disease pandemic, may lead to the subsequent behavior of fear of disclosure as well as social avoidance.

The relationship between stigmatization and stress

Stress, as a kind of internal arousal, emanates from discrepancies between external conditions and individual characteristics including needs, values, perceptions, resources, and skills (Aneshensel, 1992). Stress is defined as the experience of unpleasant and negative emotions, such as anger, anxiety, tension, frustration, or depression (Kyriacou, 2001). Any event and condition that causes changes or requires an individual to adapt to new situations or life circumstances are defined as stressors (Meyer, 2003). As a kind of interpersonal rejection, stigmatization can destroy one's original sense of belonging in groups he or she is a part of, leading them to adapt to this new situation to assuage their mental discomfort. Accordingly, stigmatization can be viewed as a type of stressor.

Individuals who test positive for potential stigmatizing conditions face a host of psychological and social stressors caused by challenging social situations, stemming from prejudice, discrimination, confidentiality, and disclosure (Miller & Kaiser, 2001; Miller & Major, 2000; Pakenham et al., 1994, 1996; Pakenham & Rinaldis, 2002). This suggests that people who have epicenter travel experience during COVID-19 may perceive stigmatization as a type of stressor that leads to heightened psychological stress within them, based on others' stereotypical or prejudicial attitudes.

The mediating role of stress

The transactional model of stress and coping proposed by Lazarus and Folkman (1984) provides a theoretical framework for understanding the mediation mechanism proposed in this study. The transactional model asserts that individuals make cognitive appraisals of potentially stressful situations. If a situation is appraised as being stressful, the individual will seek to prevent and/or minimize the stress by implementing coping strategies that match the specific situation faced. Coping strategies include cognitive, affective, and behavioral responses to manage stressful events.

Avoidance coping is one primary coping strategy (Nicholls & Polman, 2007). It focuses on taking actions to remove oneself from a stressful situation. Social avoidance may manifest as living without companionship, having low levels of social contact and little social support, feeling separate from others, being an outsider, being isolated, and suffering loneliness (Hawthorne, 2006). This physical or social withdrawal acts as an avoidance strategy to disengage from and cope with stress (Miller & Kaiser, 2001).

It has been found that individuals suffering from stigmatization practice social avoidance to avoid the stress brought on by stigmatization (Courtwright, 2013). This suggests that psychological stress resulting from stigmatization perceived by older adults with epicenter travel experience may evoke social avoidance in the context of COVID-19. As such, we propose that stress plays a mediating role in the relationship between stigmatization and social avoidance in the present study.

Non-disclosure serves as a way of coping with stress by avoiding potentially stressful encounters with others. The perceptions of stress are found to strongly influence the process of disclosure (Murphy et al., 1999). Prior studies show that PLHIV (people living with HIV) who report experiencing higher levels of HIV-related emotional stress also report greater levels of HIV status disclosure concerns. Disclosure of HIV-status is a difficult emotional task, creating opportunities for both support and rejection (Anakwa et al., 2020); thus, not being open about their HIV serostatus often serves as a way of managing the stress of their own internalized stigma (Hult et al., 2012). Recent research has shown that HIV-related stress such as fear of divorce and intimate partner violence can weaken the resolve to disclose among HIV-positive women (Anakwa et al., 2020).

The experience with PLHIV suggests that the psychological stress caused by perceived stigmatization could, in turn, trigger a fear of disclosure among older adults with epicenter travel experience during COVID-19. Therefore, we propose that stigmatization perceived by people with epicenter travel experience may trigger fear of disclosure stemming from resulting psychological stress, leading to stress playing a mediating role in the relationship between stigmatization and fear of disclosure in the present investigation.

Method

Sample and procedure

A convenience sampling method was used to collect data from 429 respondents willing to participate in this survey. The sample consisted of uninfected individuals aged 60 years and above who had travel experience in Hubei around the novel coronavirus disease outbreak and were put in quarantine at home for 14 days upon returning to the city of Guangzhou. It is worth noting that the quarantine required by the local government not only affected those infected with COVID-19, but any individual who had traveled to Hubei during the outbreak.

Community workers in charge of the delivery of food and goods to households of quarantined people were invited to assist in the implementation of the survey. These individuals were asked to send an invitation letter to those who had traveled to Hubei Province and been under quarantine at home since their return to Guangzhou. Participants completed the questionnaire online. The QR (two-dimension) code link to the questionnaire was printed at the bottom of the invitation letter. Respondents scanned the QR code with a smartphone to complete the questionnaire. Participants completed an online consent form, informing them that the survey would only be used for academic research and that answers and personal information would be kept confidential. Because the completed questionnaires were submitted online, answers were not available to the community workers who recruited them.

A time-lagged design was used to reduce common method bias, which leads to bias in estimate and results from predictors and outcome variables rated by the same person in the same measurement context at the same time points (Podsakoff et al., 2003). Since the cross-sectional data generally share the same method of collection (that is, collected from the same person at the same points), the observed covariance between predictors and outcome variables may include covariance caused by the same method of collection (Podsakoff et al., 2003). Consistent with common practice, an effective way to avoid common method bias is to collect the data at different time points. Three-wave surveys with a three-day interval between each time point were conducted. Respondents were asked to report demographic information (i.e., age, gender, education, in Wave 1), and to complete measures of "stigmatization" (Wave 1), "perceived stress" (Wave 2), "social avoidance" (Waive 3) and "fear of disclosure" (Wave 3), and to report "how many days you have experienced in the quarantine?" (Wave 3). The three-day interval was adopted considering the period of quarantine was 14 days and a long-time interval between waves may cause high sample loss rate.

Of the 429 individuals who agreed to participate, 353 completed the three-wave survey (valid response rate = 82.28%). Of those who responded, 230 (65.20%) were male, 83.90% were aged 60–70 years, 75.10% had a middle school education or below, and all were no less than seven days in quarantine when they completed the third wave of the questionnaire. This study was approved by the Institutional Review Board at Sun Yat-sen University, in compliance with the World Medical Association Declaration of Helsinki.

Measures

Measures of variables were translated from English to Chinese through the translation-back translation procedure (supplemental Appendix available upon request).

Stigmatization was measured by a 17-item scale adapted from Visser et al.'s (2008). The items were tailored to reflect stigma of epicenter travel experiences (e.g., "My neighbors would not like me living next door if they knew I had traveled in Hubei").

Perceived stress was measured using a 10-item scale developed by Cohen et al. (1983) (e.g., "Around events and situations that occurred recently, you felt difficulties were piling up so high that you could not overcome them").

Social avoidance was measured using a 14-item scale adapted from Razian et al. (2017). The items were tailored to reflect the extent to which participants had concerns about interpersonal interactions upon finishing quarantine (e.g., "I tend to withdraw from people when finishing quarantine shortly thereafter").

Fear of disclosure was measured using a 8-item scale adapted from Chaudoir and Quinn (2010). The items were tailored to reflect the extent to which participants had concerns about disclosing their epicenter travel experiences to others (e.g., "Sometimes I am unable to confide my travel experience in Hubei even in someone who is close to me").

Respondents rated items on the stigmatization, social avoidance, and feature of disclosure scales from 1 = *strongly disagree* to 7 = *strongly agree*. Individual items on the stress scale were rated from 1 = *never* to 5 = *very often*.

Control variables

Gender, age, education, and the time participants had spent in quarantine served as controls. Gender was coded as 1 = *male* and 0 = *female*. Education was coded as 1 = *primary school or below*, 2 = *middle school*, 3 = *high school or technical school*, 4 = *college or above*. Age was measured by the year of age. The time that participants had spent in quarantine was measured by the number of days.

Confirmatory factor analyses

Consistent with common practice in studies that use scales, confirmatory factor analysis (CFA) was conducted to test whether participants' scores on the scales used in this study had good convergent and discriminant validity. Good convergent validity meant that each indicator on the scale sufficiently reflected the meaning of the scale. Good discriminant validity indicated that unrelated items across scales were indeed unrelated. Results of convergent validity was be determined by the statistical significance of standard factor loadings of indicators on the same scale, while results of discriminant validity could be obtained by the comparison of measurement models across scales

The comparison of measurement models was conducted by comparing the model fit of a baseline measurement model with that of alternative measurement models. In this study, the baseline model was the hypothesized four-factor model (i.e., *stigmatization, stress, social avoidance, and fear of disclosure*). One of the alternative models was the three-factor model specified by combining variables measured at the same time point (i.e., *social avoidance and fear of disclosure*, at Time 3) into one factor and the other was the one-factor model specified by combining self-report measures (i.e., *stigmatization, stress, social avoidance, and fear of disclosure*) into one factor.

The criterion of model comparison was the model fit indices, including p-value of $\Delta\chi^2/\Delta df$, rroot-mean-squareerror of approximation (RMSEA), standardized residual mean root (SRMR), comparative fit index (CFI), and Tucker Lewis index (TLI) (Bollen, 1989). If the fit indices of alternative models were worse than those of the baseline model, it demonstrated that all factors in the baseline model were distinctive, combining any factor with others into one would harm the fit between model and data. The following cutoff scores were used to conclude a relatively good fit between the hypothesized model and the observed data: P-value of $\Delta\chi^2/\Delta df$ less than 0.05 (Hou et al., 2004); a value close to 0.1 for RMSEA (Browne & Cudeck, 1993; Steiger, 1990); a value close to 0.08 for SRMR (Hu & Bentler, 1999); and CFI and TLI values larger than 0.90 (Wang et al., 2011).

As shown in Table 1, the hypothesized four-factor model (i.e., stigmatization, stress, social avoidance, and fear of disclosure) was shown to fit the data well, χ^2 (293, $N = 353$) = 944.691, RMSEA = .079, SRMR = .040, CFI = .930, TLI = .922. The three-factor model exhibited significantly worse fit than the four-factor model, as the p-value of $\Delta\chi^2$ (4, $N = 353$) was below .01, RMSEA = .121, SRMR = .139, CFI = .834, and TLI = .819. The one-factor model also fit the data significantly worse than the four-factor model, as the p-value of $\Delta\chi^2$ (9, $N = 353$) was below .01, RMSEA = .228, SRMR = .252,

Table 1. Comparison of measurement models.

Model	Description	χ^2	df	$\Delta\chi^2$	RMSEA	SRMR	CFI	TLI
The baseline four-factor model	SG, SS, SA, FD.	944.691	293		0.079 [0.074, 0.085]	0.040	0.930	0.922
The three-factor model	SA and FD were combined into one factor.	1835.830	297	891.139**	0.121 [0.116, 0.127]	0.139	0.834	0.819
The one-factor model	SG, SS, SA, and FD were combined into one factor.	5832.607	302	4887.916**	0.228 [0.223, 0.233]	0.252	0.405	0.359

SG = stigmatization; SS = stress; SA = social avoidance; FD = fear of disclosure. RMSEA = root mean square error of approximation; SRMR = standardized residual mean root; CFI = comparative fit index; TLI = non-normed fit index (NNFI). 90% confidence interval estimate is in brackets.
* $p < .05$, ** $p < .01$.

CFI = .405, and TLI = .359. Results of the comparison of measurement models indicated that the discriminant validity of variables was acceptable.

Moreover, the significant standard factor loadings (i.e., t-value of factor loading ≥ 1.96) showed that all the indicators corresponded well to their respective scales. Accordingly, the convergent validity of variables was adequate. Together these results of CFA indicate that the regression results accurately reflected the theoretical relationship among the scales used and not statistical relationships resulting from measurement bias.

Analytic strategy

This study followed the steps outlined by Baron and Kenny (1986) for assessing potential mediation. The requisite steps were simultaneously estimated using structural equation modeling (SEM), as follows.

$$SA, \ FD = \ b_{01} + \ b_{11}Control + \ b_{21}SG + \varepsilon_1 \tag{1}$$

$$SS = \ b_{02} + \ b_{12}Control + \ b_{22}SG. + \varepsilon_2 \tag{2}$$

$$SA, \ FD = \ b_{03} + \ b_{13}Control + \ b_{23}SG. + \ b_{33}SS. + \varepsilon_3 \tag{3}$$

where SA = social avoidance, FD = fear of disclosure, SG = stigmatization, SS = stress, $Control$ = control variables; b_{01}, b_{02}, b_{03} = intercept terms, b_{11}, b_{12}, b_{13} = slope of control variables, b_{21}, b_{22}, b_{23} = slope of SG, b_{33} = slope of $SS; \varepsilon_1, \varepsilon_2, \varepsilon_3,$ = residuals.

In Equation (1), dependent variables (SA, FD) were regressed on the independent variable (SG). The coefficient b_{21} was an estimate of the total or unadjusted effect of the independent variable (SG) on the dependent variables (SA, FD). In Equation (2), the mediation variable (SS) was regressed on the independent variable (SG). The coefficient b_{22} was an estimate of the effect of the independent variable (SG) on the mediation variable (SS). In Equation (3), the dependent variables (SA, FD) were regressed on the independent variable

(SG) and mediation variable (SS). The coefficient b_{23} was an estimate of the direct effect of the independent variable (SG) on dependent variables (SA, FD) considering the mediation variable (SS), and the coefficient b_{33} in Equation (3) was an estimate of the effect of the mediation variable (SS) on dependent variables (SA, FD).

Substituting Equation (2) into Equation (3) yielded Equation (4) as following.

$$SA,\ FD = b_{03} + b_{02}b_{33} + (b_{13} + b_{12}b_{33})Control + b_{23}SG + b_{22}b_{33}SG + \varepsilon_4$$

$$(4)$$

In Equation (4), the product of the two parameters $b_{22}b_{33}$ was an estimate of the mediation effect of the independent variable (SG) on the dependent variables (SA, FD) through the mediation variable (SS), which was equivalent to b_{21}- b_{23}. The bias-corrected bootstrapping approach was used to estimate confidence intervals (CI) of the hypothesized mediation relationships ($b_{22}b_{33}$) to determine their significance (Preacher & Hayes, 2008).

Hierarchical regression was conducted in this study. According to common practice, only control variables were entered in regression analysis in Step 1, then controls and independent variables were both included in regression analysis in Step 2 (for Equations (1) & (2)). Additionally, for Equation (3), Step 3 included controls, independent, and mediation variables.

The item parceling method was used to address the problem of estimation bias resulting from excessive items of a scale (Bandalos, 2002; Nasser-Abu Alhija & Wisenbaker, 2006). Accordingly, 17 items of stigmatization scale and 14 items of social avoidance scale were parceled into four items in a sequential packing manner, respectively. The hypothesized relationships and confirmatory factor analysis were estimated with Mplus 7.0 (Muthén & Muthén, 2012) and the reliability test and descriptive statistical analysis were conducted with SPSS16.0.

Results

Means, standard deviations, and bivariate correlations of variables are shown in Table 2. The positive relationships between stigmatization and social avoidance/fear of disclosure ($r = .214$ and $.210$, $p < .01$, respectively), between stigmatization and stress ($r = .267$, $p < .01$), and between stress and social avoidance/fear of disclosure ($r = .196$ and $.215$, $p < .01$, respectively) provided preliminary support for the hypothesized relationships.

Table 3 shows the results of the hierarchical multiple regression analyses. Stigmatization was shown to significantly and positively predict social avoidance/fear of disclosure ($b = .116$ and $.143$, $p < .01$ in Step 2, regression 2 & 3) and stress ($b = .228$, $p < .01$ in Step 2, regression 1) and stress was shown to

Table 2. Means, standard deviations, and bivariate correlations among variables.

Variable	M	SD	1	2	3	4	5	6	7	8
1.Gender	.652	.477	–							
2.Age	66.963	3.095	.001	–						
3.Education	2.034	.885	−.053	−.121*	–					
4.Days	9.127	1.586	.029	−.031	.009	–				
5. Stigmatization	5.260	.924	.045	−.064	.061	−.034	(.975)			
6. Stress	4.463	.764	−.119*	−.014	.066	.121*	.267**	(.968)		
7. Social avoidance	5.169	.496	−.050	.054	.078	−.032	.214**	.196**	(.900)	
8. Fear of disclosure	5.281	.644	−.023	−.096	.063	.054	.210**	.215**	.337**	(.930)

n = 353. Gender is coded as 1 for males and 0 for females. Education is coded as 1 = primary school or below, 2 = middle school, 3 = high school or technical school, 4 = college or above. Internal consistency coefficients, Cronbach's alphas are reported in the parentheses on the diagonal. * p < .05, ** p < .01.

Table 3. Regression results.

	Regression 1. *Mediator: Stress*		
Variable	Step1		Step2
Controls			
Gender	−0.192** (0.072)		−0.214** (0.067)
Age	−0.001 (0.013)		0.003 (0.013)
Education	0.050 (0.047)		0.037 (0.047)
Days	0.059** (0.022)		0.064** (0.020)
Independent variable			
Stigmatization			0.228** (0.043)
	Regression 2. *Dependent variable: Social avoidance*		
Variable	Step1	Step2	Step3
Controls			
Gender	−0.046 (0.054)	−0.057 (0.053)	−0.037 (0.055)
Age	0.010 (0.009)	0.012 (0.008)	0.012 (0.008)
Education	0.047 (0.031)	0.040 (0.030)	0.036 (0.030)
Days	−0.009 (0.015)	−0.007 (0.015)	−0.013 (0.015)
Independent variable			
Stigmatization		0.116** (0.027)	0.094** (0.027)
Mediator			
Stress			0.095** (0.032)
	Regression 3. *Dependent variable: Fear of disclosure*		
Variable	Step1	Step2	Step3
Controls			
Gender	−0.029 (0.073)	−0.043 (0.071)	−0.013 (0.072)
Age	−0.018 (0.011)	−0.016 (0.011)	−0.016 (0.011)
Education	0.037 (0.037)	0.028 (0.037)	0.023 (0.036)
Days	0.021 (0.021)	0.024 (0.020)	0.015 (0.021)
Independent variable			
Stigmatization		0.143** (0.032)	0.112** (0.033)
Mediator			
Stress			0.138** (0.039)

n = 353. Value are unstandardized regression coefficients; standard error estimates are in parentheses. The regression models involved were simultaneously estimated. The model fit indices were shown with RMSEA and SRMR were close to 0, CFI and TLI were close to 1. * p < .05, ** p < .01.

significantly and positively predict social avoidance/fear of disclosure (b = .095 and .138, p < .01 in Step 3, regression 2 & 3).

With 2,000 bootstrap replications, the results showed that the indirect effects of stigmatization on social avoidance/fear of disclosure through stress were significant and positive (indirect effect = .022 and .031, 95% bias-corrected bootstrap CI [.008, .040] and [.015, .058], respectively).

Discussion

The empirical results support the hypotheses of the present study. Psychological stress generated within older people who traveled to Hubei on the eve of the novel coronavirus disease outbreak was found to be a mediating mechanism between experienced stigmatization and the behavioral tendency toward social avoidance and fear of disclosure. These findings indicate that the experience of stigmatization among an uninfected group of older people can be detrimental to the epidemic control efforts of public health authorities by, for example, preventing others from having knowledge of the dynamics of their physical conditions. Use of social media technologies can be a feasible and effective way for governments to help people develop scientific under-standing of the novel coronavirus disease and to quell unnecessary fear impeding public health efforts. Social media can also be helpful for older people in quarantine to access psychological care through online psychological aids to relieve the negative effects of epidemic-related stigmatization.

Prioritizing de-stigmatization is necessary for epidemic prevention and control

The stigmatization of epicenter travel experience could encourage people to conceal their past travel to high-risk areas. Although epicenter travel does not necessarily imply infection, stigmatization forces ambient social pressure upon people. This stigmatization may cause people to suffer from prejudice, dis-crimination, and loss of employment and friends. Thus, people with epicenter travel experience have a strong motivation to hide their past travel status in order to avoid adverse social consequences.

Intentional concealment of epicenter travel could also bring additional risks to infectious disease prevention and control. At the present time, a growing number of asymptomatic carriers of novel coronavirus and close contacts have been identified. Communities, social institutions, and government depart-ments thus need to use social media technologies to facilitate education and publicity activities on de-stigmatization of epicenter travel experience in order to eliminate misunderstanding of this experience. The relief of stigmatization could lead people to disclose their status more readily and could facilitate tracking and treatment of potentially infected people as a result.

De-Stigmatization is particularly important for older people as a susceptible population in the practice of epidemic prevention and control

It is known that older people are more vulnerable to this public health crisis because they have a higher likelihood of getting infected and dying once infected. This risk, combined with stigmatization, acts as a barrier to disclo-sure and places older people at higher of adverse outcomes, both due to the health effects of COVID-19 itself and due to the social isolation resulting from measures adopted to control it. Required, therefore, are the use of social media technologies to promote health communication for de-stigmatization that emphasize the experience of older people. The focus of these de-stigmatization measures should be on reducing unnecessary concerns about epicenter travel among the public and finding an appropriate manner to treat older people with this travel experience.

Urgent need to care for the psychological health of older people in quarantine

Older people who suffer from stigmatization can experience high levels of psychological distress, which in turn leads to social avoidance and fear of disclosure. It is known that older people are particularly vulnerable to adverse psychological health outcomes (e.g., Goulia et al., 2012; Kim, 2003). The compulsory request for quarantine for "once been to epicenter" travelers can further strengthen these negative psychological responses. Loneliness is one of the main psychological health concerns among older people, since an increasing number of older adults are living alone. In the wake of compulsory quarantine during the public health crisis, the psychological health status of older people resulting from stigmatization could be even worse. Although we know that older people suffer from great stress in the quarantine, it is not clear whether this stress would recede when the quarantine is over. Thus, it is necessary to adopt early psychological intervention during the quarantine, viewed, perhaps as "psychological first aid" (McNally et al., 2003). Feasible tactics include guidance for older people in quarantine on how to get strong social support from families and friends and how to improve their psychological reserves through the provision of information about common psychological dynamics. Feasible tactics also include instructions on how to access psychological services and education about what stress reactions are normal and expected. These practices can be facilitated by using social media technologies and could help buffer older people against great stress in quarantine.

Limitations

This study is not free from limitations. The outbreak of infectious disease can last for months or even years. Since the epidemiologic picture is dynamic, the perception of stigmatization, level of psychological stress, and subsequent behaviors can also vary over time. Hence, future research is needed to depict the dynamic features of this process in different stages of the novel coronavirus disease emergency.

Moreover, the present study used a time-lagged design in which data were collected at different time points to avoid the common method bias,; however, self-report measures of variables in this study might still suffer from this problem. Hence, future research should collect data from different sources (multiple-source data) to avoid common method bias and achieve adequate discriminate validity.

Finally, limited by human, material, and financial resources as well as other factors, the present study adopted a convenience sampling method to collect data rather than random sampling. Due to the convenience sample, the study may not represent the population of interest and the findings of this study may not apply to the full population. Future research should use additional samples to investigate the validity and transportability of our findings.

Conclusion

This study finds that novel coronavirus disease-related stigmatization could lead to the behavioral tendency toward social avoidance and fear of disclosure among older people who had epicenter travel experiences. Psychological stress generated within older people played a mediating role between experienced stigmatization and these behavioral tendencies. De-stigmatization and psychological supports should thus be prioritized for epidemic prevention and control among older people in quarantine.

Key points

- Stigmatization promotes social avoidance and fear of disclosure among older adults
- The effects of stigmatization on older adults is mediated by stress
- De-stigmatization should be prioritized for epidemic prevention and control among older people
- Caring for the psychological health of older population in quarantine is urgently needed

Acknowledgments

We sincerely thank all respondents participating in this study and community workers who provided us with help in the survey process.

Disclosure statement

This study was approved by institutional review board of Sun Yat-sen University. This study was conducted in compliance with the WMA declaration of Helsinki. Informed consent was obtained online from participants.

Funding

This study receives support from the National Social Science Fund of China (Grant No. 20CTY017); National Office for Philosophy and Social Sciences [20CTY017].

ORCID

Jiannan Li (iD) http://orcid.org/0000-0001-5981-6731
Bocong Yuan (iD) http://orcid.org/0000-0002-6918-5483

References

Adebiyi, I., & Ajuwon, A. J. (2015). Sexual behaviour and serostatus disclosure among persons living with HIV in Ibadan, Nigeria. *African Journal of Biomedical Research, 18* (2), 69–80. https://www.ajol.info/index.php/ajbr/article/view/118466

Akani, C. I., & Erhabor, O. (2006). Rate, pattern and barriers of HIV serostatus disclosure in a resource-limited setting in the Niger delta of Nigeria. *Tropical Doctor, 36*(2), 87–89. https://doi.org/10.1258/004947506776593378

Anakwa, N. O., Teye-Kwadjo, E., & Kretchy, I. A. (2020). Effect of HIV-related stigma and HIV-related stress on HIV disclosure concerns: A study of HIV-positive persons on antiretroviral therapy at two urban hospitals in Ghana. *Applied Research in Quality of Life*, 1–16. https://link.springer.com/article/10.1007/s11482-020-09813-6

Aneshensel, C. S. (1992). Social stress: Theory and research. *Annual Review of Sociology, 18*(1), 15–38. https://doi.org/10.1146/annurev.so.18.080192.000311

Bandalos, D. L. (2002). The effects of item parceling on goodness-of-fit and parameter estimate bias in structural equation modeling. *Structural Equation Modeling, 9*(1), 78–102. https://doi.org/10.1207/S15328007SEM0901_5

Baron, R. M., & Kenny, D. A. (1986). The moderator-mediator variable distinction in social psychological research: Conceptual, strategic, and statistical considerations. *Journal of Personality and Social Psychology, 51*(6), 1173–1182. https://doi.org/10.1037/0022-3514.51.6.1173

Bollen, K. A. (1989). A new incremental fit index for general structural equation models. *Sociological Methods & Research, 17*(3), 303–316. https://doi.org/10.1177/0049124189017003004

Browne, M. W., & Cudeck, R. (1993). Alternative ways of assessing model fit. In K. A. Bollen & J. S. Long (Eds.), *Testing structural equation models* (pp. 136–162). Sage.

Chaudoir, S. R., & Quinn, D. M. (2010). Revealing concealable stigmatized identities: The impact of disclosure motivations and positive first-disclosure experiences on fear of disclosure and well-being. *Journal of Social Issues, 66*(3), 570–584. https://doi.org/10.1111/j.1540-4560.2010.01663.x

Cheung, E. Y. (2015). An outbreak of fear, rumours and stigma: Psychosocial support for the Ebola Virus disease outbreak in West Africa. *Intervention, 13*(1), 70–76. https://doi.org/10.1097/WTF.0000000000000079

Cohen, S., Kamarck, T., & Mermelstein, R. (1983). A global measure of perceived stress. *Journal of Health and Social Behavior, 24*(4), 385–396. https://doi.org/10.2307/2136404

Courtwright, A. (2013). Stigmatization and public health ethics. *Bioethics, 27*(2), 74–80. https://doi.org/10.1111/j.1467-8519.2011.01904.x

Goffman, E. (2009). *Stigma: Notes on the management of spoiled identity*. Simon and Schuster.

Goulia, P., Papadimitriou, I., Machado, M. O., Mantas, C., Pappa, C., Tsianos, E., ... Hyphantis, T. (2012). Does psychological distress vary between younger and older adults in health and disease. *Journal of Psychosomatic Research*, *72*(2), 120–128. https://doi.org/10.1016/j.jpsychores.2011.11.011

Hardinges, N. (2020, February 6). *British-Chinese people tell of 'discrimination' and hate as fears rise over coronavirus*. Leading Britain's Conversation. https://www.lbc.co.uk/news/british-chinese-people-discrimination-coronavirus/

Hawthorne, G. (2006). Measuring social isolation in older adults: Development and initial validation of the friendship scale. *Social Indicators Research*, *77*(3), 521–548. https://doi.org/10.1007/s11205-005-7746-y

Hou, J. T., Wen, Z. L., & Cheng, Z. J. (2004). *Structural equation models and its applications*. Educational Science Press.

Hu, L. T., & Bentler, P. M. (1999). Cutoff criteria for fit indexes in covariance structure analysis: Conventional criteria versus new alternatives. *Structural Equation Modeling*, *6*(1), 1–55. https://doi.org/10.1080/10705519909540118

Hult, J. R., Wrubel, J., Bränström, R., Acree, M., & Moskowitz, J. T. (2012). Disclosure and nondisclosure among people newly diagnosed with HIV: An analysis from a stress and coping perspective. *AIDS Patient Care and STDs*, *26*(3), 181–190. https://doi.org/10.1089/apc.2011.0282

Jones, E. E. (1984). *Social stigma: The psychology of parked relationships*. WH Freeman.

Kanmodi, K., & Kanmodi, P. (2020). COVID-19 stigmatization: A devil and a deep blue sea. *Population Medicine*, *2*(5), 10. https://doi.org/10.18332/popmed/121098

Kim, H. R. (2003). Health status among community elderly in Korea. *Journal of Korean Academy of Nursing*, *33*(5), 544–552. https://doi.org/10.4040/jkan.2003.33.5.544

Kumar, A., Waterman, I., Kumari, G., & Carter, A. O. (2006). Prevalence and correlates of HIV serostatus disclosure: A prospective study among HIV-infected postparturient women in Barbados. *AIDS Patient Care & STDs*, *20*(10), 724–730. https://doi.org/10.1089/apc.2006.20.724

Kyriacou, C. (2001). Teacher stress: Directions for future research. *Educational Review*, *53*(1), 27–35. https://doi.org/10.1080/00131910120033628

Lazarus, R. S., & Folkman, S. (1984). *Stress, appraisal and coping*. Springer.

Lin, C. Y. (2020). Social reaction toward the 2019 novel coronavirus (COVID-19). *Social Health and Behavior*, *3*(1), 1. https://doi.org/10.4103/SHB.SHB_11_20

Link, B. G., & Phelan, J. C. (2001). Conceptualizing stigma. *Annual Review of Sociology*, *27*(1), 363–385. https://doi.org/10.1146/annurev.soc.27.1.363

Maunder, R., Hunter, J., Vincent, L., Bennett, J., Peladeau, N., Leszcz, M., ... Mazzulli, T. (2003). The immediate psychological and occupational impact of the 2003 SARS outbreak in a teaching hospital. *CMAJ*, *168*(10), 1245–1251. https://www.ncbi.nlm.nih.gov/pmc/articles/PMC154178/

McCauley, M., Minsky, S., & Viswanath, K. (2013). The H1N1 pandemic: Media frames, stigmatization and coping. *BMC Public Health*, *13*(1), 1116. https://doi.org/10.1186/1471-2458-13-1116

McNally, R. J., Bryant, R. A., & Ehlers, A. (2003). Does early psychological intervention promote recovery from posttraumatic stress. *Psychological Science in the Public Interest*, *4*(2), 45–79. https://doi.org/10.1111/1529-1006.01421

Meyer, I. H. (2003). Prejudice, social stress, and mental health in lesbian, gay, and bisexual populations: Conceptual issues and research evidence. *Psychological Bulletin*, *129*(5), 674. https://doi.org/10.1037/0033-2909.129.5.674

Miller, C. T., & Kaiser, C. R. (2001). A theoretical perspective on coping with stigma. *Journal of Social Issues*, *57*(1), 73–92. https://doi.org/10.1111/0022-4537.00202

Miller, C. T., & Major, B. (2000). Coping with stigma and prejudice. In T. F. Heatherton, R. E. Kleck, M. R. Hebl, & J. G. Hull (Eds.), The social psychology of stigma (p. 243–272). GuilfordPress. https://psycnet.apa.org/record/2000-05051-009

Murphy, L. M. B., Koranyi, K., Crim, L., & Whited, S. (1999). Disclosure, stress, and psychological adjustment among mothers affected by HIV. AIDS Patient Care and STDs, 13(2), 111–118. https://doi.org/10.1089/apc.1999.13.111

Muthén, L. K., & Muthén, B. O. (2012). Mplus user's guide (7th ed.). Author

Nasser-Abu Alhija, F., & Wisenbaker, J. (2006). A Monte Carlo study investigating the impact of item parceling strategies on parameter estimates and their standard errors in CFA. Structural Equation Modeling, 13(2), 204–228. https://doi.org/10.1207/s15328007sem1302_3

Nicholls, A. R., & Polman, R. C. J. (2007). Coping in sport: A systematic review. Journal of Sports Sciences, 25(1), 11–31.

Pachankis, J. E. (2007). The psychological implications of concealing a stigma: A cognitive-affective-behavioral model. Psychological Bulletin, 133(2), 328. https://doi.org/10.1037/0033-2909.133.2.328

Pakenham, K., & Rinaldis, M. (2002). Development of the HIV/AIDS stress scale. Psychology and Health, 17(2), 203–219. https://doi.org/10.1080/08870440290013680

Pakenham, K. I., Dadds, M. R., & Terry, D. J. (1994). Relationship between adjustment to HIV and both social support and coping. Journal of Consulting and Clinical Psychology, 62(6), 1194. https://doi.org/10.1037/0022-006X.62.6.1194

Pakenham, K. I., Dadds, M. R., & Terry, D. J. (1996). Adaptive demands along the HIV disease continuum. Social Science & Medicine, 42(2), 245–256. https://doi.org/10.1016/0277-9536(95)00099-2

Person, B., Sy, F., Holton, K., Govert, B., & Liang, A. (2004). Fear and stigma: The epidemic within the SARS outbreak. Emerging Infectious Diseases, 10(2), 358. https://doi.org/10.3201/eid1002.030750

Podsakoff, P. M., MacKenzie, S. B., Lee, J. Y., & Podsakoff, N. P. (2003). Common method biases in behavioral research: A critical review of the literature and recommended remedies. Journal of Applied Psychology, 88(5), 879–903. https://doi.org/10.1037/0021-9010.88.5.879

Preacher, K. J., & Hayes, A. F. (2008). Asymptotic and resampling strategies for assessing and comparing indirect effects in multiple mediator models. Behavior Research Methods, 40(3), 879–891. https://doi.org/10.3758/BRM.40.3.879

Razian, S., Fathi Ashtiani, A., & Bozorgmehr, A. (2017). Psychometric properties of the Persian version of social avoidance and distress scale (SADS). International Journal of Behavioral Sciences, 11(2), 82–85. http://www.behavsci.ir/article_67977_3c0f6a309065cdc51c02a1380aa087a1.pdf

Smart Richman, L., & Leary, M. R. (2009). Reactions to discrimination, stigmatization, ostracism, and other forms of interpersonal rejection: A multimotive model. Psychological Review, 116(2), 365. https://doi.org/10.1037/a0015250

Steiger, J. H. (1990). Structural model evaluation and modification: An interval estimation approach. Multivariate Behavioral Research, 25(2), 173–180. https://doi.org/10.1207/s15327906mbr2502_4

Stutterheim, S. E., Shiripinda, I., Bos, A. E., Pryor, J. B., De Bruin, M., Nellen, J. F., ... Schaalma, H. P. (2011). HIV status disclosure among HIV-positive African and Afro-Caribbean people in the Netherlands. AIDS Care, 23(2), 195–205. https://doi.org/10.1080/09540121.2010.498873

Toth, K. E., & Dewa, C. S. (2014). Employee decision-making about disclosure of a mental disorder at work. Journal of Occupational Rehabilitation, 24(4), 732–746. https://doi.org/10.1007/s10926-014-9504-y

Vanable, P. A., Carey, M. P., Blair, D. C., & Littlewood, R. A. (2006). Impact of HIV-related stigma on health behaviors and psychological adjustment among HIV-positive men and women. *AIDS and Behavior*, *10*(5), 473–482. https://doi.org/10.1007/s10461-006-9099-1

Visser, M. J., Kershaw, T., Makin, J. D., & Forsyth, B. W. (2008). Development of parallel scales to measure HIV-related stigma. *AIDS and Behavior*, *12*(5), 759–771. https://doi.org/10.1007/s10461-008-9363-7

Wang, J. C., Wang, X. Q., & Jiang, B. F. (2011). *Structural equation models: Methods and applications*. Higher Education Press.

Wright, R. S. (2015, April). Influence of quality of life and reason for non-disclosure on HIV stress among urban HIV-infected African American men. In UWM undergraduate research symposium. Symposium conducted at 2015 NCUR, University of Wisconsin-Milwaukee, Wisconsin, USA.

Zhai, Y., & Du, X. (2020). Mental health care for international Chinese students affected by the COVID-19 outbreak. *The Lancet Psychiatry*, *7*(4), e22. https://doi.org/10.1016/S2215-0366(20)30089-4

Old Overnight: Experiences of Age-Based Recommendations in Response to the COVID-19 Pandemic in Sweden

Gabriella Nilsson ⓘ, Lisa Ekstam ⓘ, Anna Axmon ⓘ, and Janicke Andersson ⓘ

ABSTRACT

The Swedish response to the COVID-19 pandemic included age-based recommendations of voluntary quarantine specifically for those 70 years of age or older. This paper investigates the experiences of a sudden change of policy in the form of an age restriction that trumped the contemporary active aging ideal. A web-based qualitative survey was conducted in April 2020. Through manual coding of a total of 851 responses, six different ways of relating to the age-based recommendations were identified. The results show that age is not an unproblematic governing principle. Instead, in addition to protecting a vulnerable group, the age-based recommendation meant deprivation of previously assigned individual responsibility and, consequently, autonomy. It is shown how respondents handled this tension through varying degrees of compliance and resistance. Findings highlight the importance of continuously tracking the long-term consequences of age-based policy to avoid negative self-image and poorer health among older adults.

Introduction

On March 11, 2020, the World Health Organization (WHO) declared the COVID-19 outbreak to be a pandemic. Countries were urged to take all necessary measures to slow the spread of the virus and to prevent their healthcare systems from being overwhelmed with seriously ill patients. In Sweden, the Public Health Agency, with national responsibility for public health, issued recommendations specifically targeting the 70 and older age group. At a press conference on March 16, state epidemiologist Anders Tegnell emphasized that "people over 70 need help limiting their contact with other people ... Now is the time to try to isolate them as much as possible" (Press Conference, 2020). Aside from the call for the entire Swedish population to increase hand hygiene and to stay home at the first signs or symptoms of illness, Swedes 70 years of age or older were the only group given specific recommendations. The argument for this recommendation was susceptibility to the virus: "High age is the main risk factor. This is shown in available studies on the outbreak of COVID-19. Therefore, those who are 70 years or older are in a risk group" (the Public Health Agency, 2020). Among the general population in Sweden as well as in the media, the recommendation was interpreted and discussed as a call for voluntary quarantine or isolation.

Persons who were between the ages of 70 and 80 in the spring of 2020 are members of the so-called baby-boom generation of Swedes, born in the 1940s. In Sweden, this is a generation of retirees often described according to what makes them distinct from previous generations – they are perceived to be healthier and more active with a better financial situation than the generations before them (Age Cap, 2020; Nilsson, 2011). Whether or not this characterization holds true at the individual level, baby boomers have retired at a time when the ideal of active aging has come to dominate the aging discourse. Active aging is the view that the negative aspects of aging can be countered through an active lifestyle (FUTURAGE, 2011). This view combined with the normative concept "successful aging" (Rowe & Kahn, 1997) makes it the duty of older people to demonstrate a high degree of activity in order to show that they are not being a burden on society (Blaakilde, 2007; Katz, 2000). In other words, many belonging to the group of people targeted by the Public Health Agency in their response to the COVID-19 pandemic were accustomed to seeing themselves as anything but old and vulnerable (see also Meisner, 2021).

Studies have shown a correlation between the health of older people and the internalization of either positive or negative age stereotypes. Those who identify with a negative view of older adults or perceive themselves as "old" and "vulnerable" in a negative sense report poorer health and cognitive abilities as well as a lower self-esteem (Stewart et al., 2012). Furthermore, research shows that older people subjected to infantilization may develop passivity, decreased independence, a withdrawal from responsibility and the acceptance of a marginalized role in society (Grøn, 2016; Hockey & James, 1993; Marson & Powell, 2014; Nilsson et al., 2018; Salari & Rich, 2001). It is plausible that being categorized by state authorities as old and vulnerable could have an impact on the self-image and future health of the individuals within the targeted age group, a potential consequence that was not sufficiently considered in the discussion of how society should deal with the outbreak of the pandemic.

The aim of this study is to investigate how individuals 70 years or older perceived the age-based recommendations in Sweden during the initial phase of the COVID-19 pandemic. It highlights the potential tension between age seen as a productive, equitable and biologically necessary organizing principle and age-based policy seen as irrelevant and illegitimate governmental action.

The purpose is to analyze the effects of governmental considerations of what is best for society in order to shed light on the implicit consequences these considerations may have for individuals. How are age-based recommendations experienced by those targeted by them?

Analytical framework

The state's response to the COVID-19 outbreak is reminiscent of a Foucauldian perspective on power and governance. This is not least due to the fact that for Michel Foucault, the different ways epidemics had been handled historically, more specifically leprosy, the plague, and later smallpox, served as empirical examples to describe three historically different forms of exercising power. Foucault describes a gradual, but partly overlapping, shift from 1) a sovereign force directed at the individual in pre-modern society, to 2) the exercise of power in the form of surveillance and disciplining of the entire population in modern society, what is known today as policy, to 3) the evocation of a new mentality, what Foucault calls "governmentality", among the citizens, through neoliberal individualization and responsibilization in post-modern society, where individuals take increased responsibility for governing themselves (Foucault, 1977, 2007; see Sarasin, 2020).

With the concepts of biopolitics and biopower, Foucault explains the shift in governing strategy in modern society (the second phase) as a process of politicization of the biological, a realization that the biological processes of human beings are crucial for societal development, and thus an issue for political decision making and policy (Foucault, 1977). This shift formed a new relationship between the state and the human, more specifically between the state and the population. The population became the target for a multitude of political techniques: measurement, comparison, categorization and optimization, something that required a parallel process of institutionalization and professionalization (Rose, 1999). The scientific field of epidemiology in general, and the Public Health Agency of Sweden in particular, are institutions that derive from, and still enable, biopolitical governance. In the emergence of the Swedish welfare state from the beginning of the 20th century, the exercise of biopower came to influence all aspects of life into the 1980s, and still does so in many ways up until today.

However, in the contemporary context of neoliberal governmentality (the third phase), power is instead assigned to the population, or more specifically to individual citizens, provided that they are obedient and govern themselves (Rose, 1999). Under the pretext of freedom, it is expected that individuals in this third phase should engage in practices of self-optimization; they should "invest" in themselves and their future health and wellbeing. This, sociologist Nicolas Rose argues, has led to a view of citizens as either active or passive in which the active citizen who takes responsibility for himself or herself sets the example, and the passive citizen living in a dependent relationship is seen as irresponsible and, in some cases, even immoral (Rose, 1999). The "active-aging" and "successful-aging" paradigms are examples of how, in the neoliberal society, health and wellbeing is made the responsibility of the individual (Katz, 2013). In this context, it is plausible that age-based policy will be experienced as a less legitimate governing technique among the population affected.

What, then, has become of biopolitics and biopower? Are they irrelevant concepts, or has the pandemic renewed their relevance (Hannah, 2020)? How would Foucault explain the governmental responses to the COVID-19 pandemic? For the purposes of this paper, the definition of an age-based risk group as established by the Public Health Agency in response to the outbreak of COVID-19 pandemic, the agency's categorization of the vulnerable in terms of age, and the formulation of recommendations specifically targeting this category, are all seen as biopolitical techniques. We investigate individual's experiences when confronted with the sudden exercise of biopolitical governance in a time of neoliberal governmentality, which became a highly visible and pressing issue in the form of explicit age restrictions that trumped the contemporary active aging ideal.

Method

The results derive from a study of how individuals 70 years or older experienced the age-based recommendations that formed a central component of the Swedish response to the COVID-19 pandemic. The study was conducted between April 21–28, 2020. A web-based survey with five closed-ended background questions and three thematic open-ended questions was designed to produce qualitative data using an open-source online survey software. As no personal data nor sensitive data were collected, an ethical review was not required according to Sweden's Act concerning the Ethical Review of Research Involving Humans (SFS 2003). The survey was distributed via snowball sampling in various social media channels and spread more rapidly than expected, which led to the decision to close the survey after one week. At this point, 1,011 anonymous respondents had answered the questionnaire. All quotations reported below derive from the survey.

The respondents consisted of both men and women 70–90 years of age, although most were women (78%) between 70–75 years of age (60%) with a university degree (70%). The fact that a majority of respondents fell on the younger end of the age range is not surprising and may have both methodological and analytical explanations. First, participation required some form of social media presence, which may decline with age (Cowie & Gurney, 2018), and second, it is conceivable that the age-based recommendations aroused a greater deal of thought and emotion in this age group, which may have motivated them to participate in the study. The results of the survey, however, show that, independent of age, gender or health status, the majority of the respondents accepted and adjusted their everyday habits in line with the Public Health Agency's recommendations for people 70 years or older.

The analysis in this paper is based on the responses to one of the three thematic questions, a question specifically addressing the age limit and its impact on self-perception. The respondents were asked to write freely about this theme. Of the total number of responses (n = 1,011), 851 respondents answered this thematic question. These 851 answers were coded manually. Three researchers were involved in the coding process. Initially, the first hundred answers were selected, and the researchers worked individually to search for patterns and categories through Ethnographic Content Analysis. Ethnographic Content Analysis involves a reflexive movement between data selection, coding and interpretation as well as an acceptance of the fact that categories and analytical themes emerge throughout the study (Altheide, 1987). The research group compared proposed categories and discussed how they should be delimited and described for the greatest possible rigor and clarity. This resulted in six different thematically designed categories that were found to be fruitful for answering the purpose of the study. Finally, the total number of responses was coded manually by the researchers based on these six categories. A few answers are coded in more than one category, which becomes clear below, where the number of categorized responses is greater than the number of respondents.

Results

Descriptive results

The following six categories were identified, and the responses coded accordingly:

(1) Accept the age-based recommendation without further elaboration (n = 216)
(2) Accept the age-based recommendation with reference to solidarity (n = 93)
(3) Accept the age-based recommendation but emphasize that it does not apply due to an active and healthy lifestyle (n = 102)
(4) Accept the age-based recommendation with reference to views or experiences of the biological aging body (n = 171)
(5) Accept the age-based recommendation but express ambivalence and a change in self-perception (n = 163)
(6) Reject the legitimacy of age as an organizing principle (n = 127)

Of the 851 responses coded, 31 were included in two categories and two were included in three categories.

Drawing from the responses in both categories 1 and 2, under the subheading "Being proud of the Swedish way", we analyze the notion that Swedes, by definition, are considered to follow governmental recommendations. Under the subheading "At 70, you are not old", we analyze the responses in category 6, which explicitly reject the legitimacy of age as an organizing principle and argue for a perspective of biological age instead of chronological age. In "Active aging as a means to counter infections", drawing from the responses in category 3, we discuss the age restrictions against the backdrop of the active aging ideal. Under the subheading "My lung tissue is 72 years old", we highlight those responses within category 4, which argue for biological age as a natural and necessary organizing principle. In the final section, under the subheading "Aged by restriction", we analyze those responses belonging to category 5 that explicitly describe how the age restriction had an impact on respondents' self-esteem.

Being proud of the Swedish way

One-fourth of the respondents (Category 1, n = 216) found the age-based recommendations reasonable without elaborating further on how the age restriction made them feel as individuals. The risk group had to be defined in one way or another, and age, some wrote, offered a simple way to create clarity: "In Sweden, such an age categorization is practical and easily enforceable, since we are all registered with our personal identity number." For these respondents, the age restriction did not challenge their self-perception. Instead, some wrote that they were "grateful" that they were now viewed by others as belonging to a vulnerable group; this was something they "appreciated." The view that the age restriction was "understandable" indicates that in Sweden, people 70 years or older are accustomed to being subjected to biopolitical interventions; these are seen as "practical and easily enforceable."

One category of respondents (Category 2), represented in eleven percent (n = 93) of the answers, described how they accepted and followed the recommendations out of trust in society and loyalty with the authorities: "I believe you should respect what the authorities say;" "I am loyal to the Public Health Agency and the Government." These answers, too, indicate a strong internalization of the legitimacy of biopower as exercised by the welfare state, an acceptance of being part of the Swedish "population" (see Foucault, 1977; Rose, 1996). The acceptance was strengthened through a reliance on "expertise" in the form of scientific knowledge in general and medical research in particular: "I believe in the researchers;" "I stick to science;" "I think it's a medical question. Experts have said that you become more vulnerable after 70." These arguments are all in line with the Swedish self-image of a people with a firmly rooted trust in scientific knowledge and technological development (Petersén, 2020).

The responses in Category 2 must be viewed in light of the fact that Sweden chose a very different strategy in dealing with the COVID-19 pandemic than the rest of the world. In particular, the Swedish response to the pandemic aroused recurrent criticism in both national and international media for being too soft. For some respondents, mutual trust, the citizens' trust in the authorities and the government's trust in the citizens' willingness to follow recommendations, seemed to be what most distinguished the Swedish response from that of other countries. Trust was something that filled them with pride: "I am proud that in Sweden we have a trust that makes it possible to act wisely without complete lockdown;" "I am pretty proud of the Swedish way of handling this." Even though the respondents themselves were the ones targeted by restrictions in Sweden, "the Swedish way of handling this" was still perceived as being better than the complete lockdown in other countries. In fact, aside from some constitutional restraints, this trust in the authorities, described as being part of the "Swedish culture," was the main reason the government based its strategies on recommendations rather than regulations (Irwin, 2020). As described by state epidemiologist Anders Tegnell, "I think what we're talking about here is the sort of Swedish culture. How they interpret recommendations from authorities … There is a long tradition in Sweden … to follow the advice of the authorities … I think there is a cultural difference" (as cited in Irwin, 2020).

In a paper on the Swedish response to the pandemic, cultural anthropologist Rachel Irwin describes how, in Sweden, following recommendations is not understood to be voluntary, but a duty and a responsibility (Irwin, 2020). Consequently, many of the respondents, though some with a hint of self-irony, described themselves as "cautious,", "obedient" or "well-behaved": "I don't like restrictions, but I am an obedient citizen who realizes that it is not just my health that is protected, but healthcare and society at large." Among these respondents, the term "solidarity" was sometimes used to legitimize compliance with age-based recommendations. The participants felt that "the age restriction is set not only for 'our' sake, but for all members of society." Consideration should be given to those younger than themselves: "The younger generation is the world's future." Limiting social contacts with others was thus a necessary "sacrifice." Failing to follow the recommendations would be "stupid," "selfish" and "irresponsible."

At first glance, the emphasis on solidarity and the argument that older people needed to make sacrifices for both the younger generations and society as a whole appears to be an expression of lower self-determination. However, these arguments could also be seen as a way of turning a passive stance, one of the fragile and dependent elderly, into a more active stance – the position of the adult or even the hero: "We elderly must take responsibility for helping to protect the rest of society;" "It is important that we are up to the task and ride out the storm." Rather than just obediently resigning themselves to isolation and dependency, by adopting a perspective of solidarity, following recommendations became something rather proactive, a way of doing age in a more positive and constructive way (see Laz, 1998).

At 70, you are not old

In only a small percentage of the total number of responses, namely the 15% of responses falling into to Category 6 (n = 127), did respondents view the age limit as problematic to the extent that they explicitly hesitated to follow the recommendations. The answers reported for this group highlight one of the problems with age as an organizing principle, namely the definition of what a certain age should mean. From the perspective of the government and the Public Health Agency, "70 years or older" was intended to mean "vulnerable," "at risk" and "old." This definition of age was opposed by the respondents in this category: "At 70, you are not old. I was a bit offended by this;" "I think age plays too large a role. 70 is the new 50!" Within Category 6, five percent of the respondents (n = 44) would have preferred another age threshold. Ten percent (n = 83) did not accept age at all as a basis for the definition of vulnerability: "In the event of a pandemic outbreak, isn't everyone exposed to the risk of being infected regardless of age?" One argument against age as the organizing principle was that the age-based recommendations risked making other age groups less cautious: "It is wrong to point out a specific age. We should all be observant and careful regardless of age." Another argument stemmed from the large size and heterogeneity of the 70 + age group, which constitute 16% of the Swedish population: "There are about 1.5 million Swedes over 70 years of age. It should have been taken into consideration the variety this means."

Questioning of age as an organizing principle in response to the pandemic highlights the potential conflict between chronological age and biological age (Andersson et al., 2011). Among those who were critical of the age-based recommendation, biological age was considered a more effective tool to define vulnerability than chronological age: "One should distinguish between chronological and biological age. The age demarcation 70+ does not take into account whether you may have a significantly lower biological age." Some respondents used themselves as examples of this reverse biological age and thereby argued for the absurdity of the age–based recommendation: "I used to go to the gym three times a week and felt really well. Now I am not allowed."

Some answers suggest feelings of betrayal after the respondents lived up to the politically advocated active aging ideal: "I go to the gym three times a week and walk a couple of kilometers a day. I have lined up to help children and grandchildren. It feels strange to suddenly be viewed as fragile and in need of help." Some experienced the age limit as contradictory, "not least since the political discourse advocates continued professional activity well into the 70s." The negative reaction could thus be seen as a response to the failure of the age restriction not to provide room for doing age in a way that was in line with the active aging ideal (see Blaakilde, 2007). Instead of the "freedom" to govern themselves in the form of self-improvement and self-optimization (Rose, 1999), they were targeted by a biopolitical state intervention that stood in contradiction to the active lifestyle that was normally promoted.

Consistent with this perspective, some respondents wished that instead of using age as a tool, the decision about who would be subject to specific recommendations would be decided individually: "70-year-olds can be so different. Some, like myself, are energized and active both physically and mentally, while others are less active and feel old. You can't stare blindly at a number; you have to take in the whole picture." The respondents doubted the effectiveness of age as a way of determining who was actually at risk: "The age restriction is too blunt a tool," some argued. Instead, other potential risk factors were highlighted, such as obesity, smoking and underlying illnesses: "Just going by age feels wrong. It is mainly the underlying factors that should be addressed." These arguments reveal the desire to place risk somewhere else, or rather with someone else – in this case with those with underlying illnesses: "Those who are ill and tired may be isolated but not healthy and employable people. Incredible that you can place all the responsibility on a group of people who work in this way."

More specifically, what this study highlights is the inevitable tension between age seen as a productive and necessary organizing principle by some – as "practical and easily enforceable" as it was described in the previous section – and the possibility that age limits are experienced as irrelevant and illegitimate governmental practices by others. Responses in this category include examples of the latter view: "Defining people over 70 a risk group is convenient, but completely arbitrary." For these respondents, the exercise of biopower that was hidden in the recommendations, "under the cover 'It's for your own good,'" as one respondent wrote, was clearly visible.

The equality argument – that an age restriction is "equal" since it will eventually hit all individuals in a certain society – was not applicable since the age limit was temporary. Thus, it is not surprising that some respondents felt discriminated against: "To trap us 70+ within fences feels like discrimination in disguise;" "Healthy people who get imprisoned, that is age discrimination;" "Just one day after turning 70, I was incapacitated." In contrast to the respondents who saw it as their duty to comply with the authorities' recommendations, these respondents refrained from doing so as they perceived the exercise of power to be arbitrary and abusive. The use of words such as "fences," "imprisonment" and "incapacitation" strongly indicate that biopolitical interventions were experienced by some proportion of the target population as illegitimate in contemporary Sweden.

Active aging as a means to counter infections

Twelve percent of the participants (n = 102) supported the age categorization and followed the recommendations but still argued strongly that their vitality was a more important means of avoiding infection (Category 3): "I think the age restriction is reasonable, although ... " was a common way these respondents began description of their particularly healthy and active lifestyle: "The age categorization may be justified, but I am perfectly healthy." Thus, many compared their own health, strength and active lifestyle to that of others, mostly hypothetic others: "I think it is good to have a clear boundary that is easy to follow up on. Even though I could handle the disease better than a normal 60-year-old by virtue of my well-trained body, I can't know for sure."

Instead of feeling incapacitated and discriminated against by being categorized as belonging to an age-based risk group, these respondents utilized their age as a means to distinguish themselves from "a normal person their age." Instead of regarding the age restriction as an exercise of bio-power and feeling forced by the authorities to identify as "old and vulnerable," as was the experience reported in the responses discussed in the previous section, these respondents saw the pandemic as a confirmation that their healthy lifestyle would pay off. Having a well-trained body, they seemed to argue, made them better equipped to resist the virus. It is clear that this group of respondents relate to the age-based recommendation, as well as to the pandemic in general, from a perspective on governmentality and active aging, from the view, or perhaps belief, that it is possible to counter ill health and negative aspects of aging by taking responsibility as an individual (see Katz, 2013; Rose, 1996).

Similar to the last section respondents pointed to the distinction between chronological and biological age to highlight their own ability to counter aging despite acceptance of the age restriction: "The age 70 is not always the same as the biological age. As a healthy 82-year-old, my biological age is maybe 75." The responses in both of these categories (Categories 3 and 6) thus indicate that the age restriction, set "overnight" during the initial phase of the COVID-19 pandemic, seems to have opened the door to reflection on the kind of age definition that should be employed: the chronological age utilized by the state as an organizing principle, or the biological age that could be felt in their own bodies. For some respondents, the choice seemed to come down to the latter: "My biological age does not feel like 70 + . [...] I don't think you should be judged by an age limit." This attitude is not surprising in the prevailing neoliberal context of governmentality emphasizing individual freedom and self-determination.

In the situation created by the pandemic, where, according to some respondents, an overly large and "non-uniform" age group was "bundled together" and defined as a risk group regardless of health status, some responses indicate a need to create a distinction within this group to maintain a self-image as biologically young: "I feel more like I belong to a 'subgroup' within the risk group;" "I understand that most people are in worse condition than I am today, so I accept the 70 limit." By positioning themselves within a "subgroup," they did not experience the same negative consequences for self-esteem due to the age categorization, as compared to the respondents in the previous section (Category 6) They accepted and followed the age-based recommendations, even if they were still convinced that the recommendations did not apply to them. In this way, the biopolitical intervention did not make them feel imprisoned and insulted.

My lung tissue is 72 years old

Twenty percent of respondents (n = 171) accepted and supported the age-based recommendations based on knowledge and/or experiences of the aging body (Category 4). Many described how the cells age, lung capacity is impaired, healing ability slows down, the immune system becomes weaker and susceptibility to disease increases. These were all seen as normal bodily changes resulting from chronological aging, independent of the perceptions of the individual. There was no escape from bodily impairments: "Obviously, cells age and it does not help if you feel healthy and strong. Age will show." Others turned this general knowledge of the aging body into reflections on their own bodies: "My heart has beaten an incredible number of more strokes than the heart of a fifty-year-old person. My lung tissue is 72 years old." For some respondents, the age recommendations set by the Public Health Agency appeared reasonable since bodily aging is not always something conscious: "Even if you are healthy, there are a number of changes in older people that you might not be aware of."

Among these respondents, acceptance seems to be the sentiment that guided their approach to the age-based recommendations. This reveals an opposing view of biology in comparison to the respondents above, who were guided by the active aging ideal (Category 3). While the above respondents understood biology as individual, something they themselves could influence and work with through different lifestyle choices, for the category of responses discussed in this section (Category 4), biological changes were an inevitable process that they simply needed to accept. They described this approach to aging as more realistic. Many expressed feeling surprised and even provoked by those over 70 who did not accept "the facts" of aging, which would inevitably impact their bodies without exception: "I understand that some feel offended by being considered old, but I don't. We are all biological beings."

Some wrote from their own experiences of aging: "My body is not as strong as before, which I noticed when I got the flu last year and got very sick. It was a lesson that the years pass, and life will end one day. It is not sad, but a good reminder." This is the only category of respondents to whom the recommendations did not seem to stand out as a political intervention but an unproblematic objective fact. Thus, it is plausible that the age restriction had no effect on their self-image. Nevertheless, these responses exemplify how governance is hidden behind objectivity and factuality (Rose, 1996, p. 156). In the first section, it was discussed how respondents in Category 2 seemed to base their compliance with the recommendation in part on a trust in science and medical experts. Here (Category 4), however, it does not seem to be faith in the authority of medical facts that guides their views, but their own feelings of what is "objectively true." Consequently, respondents in this category saw those who ignore the bodily signs of aging as absurd: "I think the motto '70 is the new 50' is ridiculous. There is age madness in this country. We must accept that we are getting older and adapt our lives accordingly."

For some, bodily shortcomings and current illnesses made them less prone to relate to the recommendations in terms of age. Having cancer, heart problems, rheumatism, COPD, high blood pressure, diabetes, anemia, asthma, etc., made them feel at risk regardless of age: "Age does not matter for me because I am seriously ill and have poor immune system." For these respondents, age was not relevant for their approach to the COVID-19 pandemic. In fact, what these answers suggest is that underlying illnesses made it easier to accept the age-based recommendations. It seems more justified, and possibly less discriminatory, to be defined as belonging to an age-based risk group if you also feel that you belong to the risk group due to other reasons. In this way, it was not your age that had transformed you from "able" to "disabled" (Kelley-Moore et al., 2006), but illness. How you were defined by society, as vulnerable, was not caused by your status as "old" but by bodily facts that are perhaps not tied to identity in the same way.

Aged by recommendation

The last, but perhaps most relevant, category of responses in answering the aim of this study are the nineteen percent (n = 163) who express ambivalence toward being defined as part of a vulnerable group based on age (Category 5). Above all, the responses showed that regardless of whether the age-based recommendations are acknowledged and accepted, they may still be viewed and experienced as something highly negative by those they target and have severely negative consequences for self-esteem. From a critical perspective on age, where age categories and the meanings that these categories are ascribed form and reproduce a larger power structure, it is evident that categorizations in terms of age affect the self-image of the individual (Krekula & Johansson, 2017). The responses thus reveal that for the individual, biopolitical interventions are never neutral and harmless, regardless of their benefits for the population as a whole. This is clearly reflected in the respondents' answers.

In the vast majority of responses within this category, the age-based recommendations made the respondents think about their age in a new way: "It is a strange feeling to suddenly think of how old you are as if it was the most important thing. We, the eternal teenagers." For some, the age categorization more than anything made it apparent to them that others now viewed them as old: "My experience has probably been, 'Oops, society thinks I am old and a risk to others;'" To be viewed as old felt "strange," "surprising," "breathtaking" and "unpleasant." The respondents were "startled," "perplexed,", "angry and sad," and "humiliated": "I have never before seen myself as old, but now we are bundled together as a package of frail individuals that society must protect." For these respondents, a central aspect of their negative experience with the age-based recommendations was that others defined them as old, that old age was a "stamp" they received.

For others, the age limit formed the basis for a new insight. It made them realize that they were, in fact, old: "The previously vague realization of increased vulnerability was suddenly and brutally concretized." Realizing and accepting one's age is here described as a process instigated by the coronavirus in general and the age-based recommendations in particular. These accounts can be seen as expressions of how age is something that is done in a contextual way (Krekula & Johansson, 2017; Laz, 1998). More specifically, "being old," in the case of these respondents, was a practice resulting from a correspondence between feeling old and being told you are old.

Yet another group, however, described how the age limit had actually turned them old: "I've grown older by this;" "The 70-year limit is reasonable. However, sadly, I feel older than before … The isolation makes me inquire more as to how I feel, which I have not had time for when I was an active retiree." As mentioned in the introduction, research has shown that older people subjected to infantilization may develop passivity, decreased independence, a withdrawal from responsibility and the acceptance of a marginalized role in society (Grøn, 2016; Hockey & James, 1993; Marson & Powell, 2014; Nilsson et al., 2018; Salari & Rich, 2001). The responses that fall into this category support these findings.

Age limits that place the individual in a certain age category inevitably stir up thoughts and feelings that have the potential to change that individual: "To now, as an 80-year-old, be forced to understand that I am the one being referred to when someone speaks of 'our oldest' is revolting." These responses express how the respondents experienced age-based recommendations as being forced to "do age" (Laz, 1998) in a way that had a direct impact on their autonomy and feelings of vulnerability (Nilsson et al., 2018). It is pertinent to reflect on which of these perceived changes in identity will remain after the restrictions are lifted. Will the participants return to their usual lifestyle as active retirees, or has the age limit made a permanent mark on their self-image ?: "It probably affects my view of myself. An example. The other day I gave a super nice summer dress to my granddaughter, who usually want things that I no longer use. This dress had a bare back and I heard myself say, 'Now that I belong to the old group in society, maybe I can't wear dresses with bare back anymore,' though I like that dress very much."

Since many older people were still working at the time of the COVID-19 outbreak, the sudden designation as old, and more specifically the decree to stay home, was seen as something of a paradox: "I work full time, but the age restriction has changed my ability to work;" For some, the opportunity to continue working after reaching retirement age was described as their driving force and joy in life: "I am healthy, and I have been working all these years – up until now! I understand the consideration, but it is DIFFICULT to suddenly be expelled from the work community. I have never felt old until now!" Along with a pervasive promotion of active aging these reactions must be understood in the context of a long-standing policy debate about raising the retirement age in Sweden (Parliament proposition 2019): "The idea has been that before this broke out we were supposed to work until 70 years, and now we are considered 'old.'" In this context, the age limit was perceived as paradoxical.

One aspect some of the respondents specifically addressed in this category was the time frame. Aging is normally understood as a gradual process of increased bodily shortcomings or weaknesses. With the outbreak of COVID-19, the consequences of age were implemented overnight. It was fast and not at all gradual, sudden instead of incremental: "Overnight I turned 'elderly;'" "From one day to the next, I went from being a perfectly normal woman to becoming an 'old old' woman who would need protection." Overnight, the age limit forcefully presumed a change in identity – from "young" to "elderly," from "normal" to "old old." As was discussed previously in relation to Category 6, some experienced this transformation as a form of age discrimination: "Ageism has struck. I am being treated differently, as someone to beware of. Or patronized, as if it was I who put everything into misery."

For some of the respondents, continuous thoughts about age inevitably lead to thoughts about death: "Have not previously considered myself that old, which of course I am. But it feels real now. Have probably been putting my head in the sand. I respect all safeguards and do not defy the restrictions. Still, I am saddened and anxious by this fact, where it is continuously pointed out how old I am. Get death anxiety. Irrational, yes, I know;" These responses show that the age-based recommendations clearly constituted a reminder of the finite nature of life.

Discussion

The objective of this paper has been to describe how age-based policy works in practice. Age restrictions has long been one of the more pervasive biopolitical techniques for shaping the conduct of the population in modern society (Katz, 2013; Rose, 1999). However, political arguments for a particular age restriction always challenge values like individuality, self-determination, and equality. Consequently, ageism and age-discrimination has gained growing scholarly attention in recent decades (Ayalon & Tesch-Römer, 2018; Heikkinen & Krekula, 2008), and in research on the COVID-19 pandemic, this perspective on aging has proved continued relevance (Ehni & Wahl, 2020; Previtali et al., 2020; Reynolds, 2020). Hans-Joerg Ehni and Hans-Werner Wahl stress that negative age stereotyping is currently taking place on a massive scale in light of the COVID-19 pandemic, and that widespread deficit views of old age are dangerous to older citizens and societies at large (Ehni & Wahl, 2020).

The Swedish response to COVID-19 pandemic – the issuance of specific recommendations for the 70 and older age group – unexpectedly challenged values like individuality, self-determination and equality without any discussion or further explanation. The study was called for as the long-term consequences of suddenly being categorized as old and vulnerable by state authorities was perhaps not sufficiently considered at the start of the pandemic. This is particularly relevant since, in a neoliberal society where older people are called upon to take responsibility for their aging through a healthy and active lifestyle, policy based on chronological age may be perceived as a less legitimate organizing principle.

The active aging discourse constructs aging as a dichotomy of either a "success" or "failure." Successful aging means being able to counter the biological aging process with a healthy and active lifestyle, of keeping the biological age low regardless of chronological age (Katz & Calasanti, 2015; Rowe & Kahn, 1997; Stuckelberger, 2008; Timonen, 2016). The background for this distinction is the view on aging as a societal problem, a "threat" that grew to dominate the discourse where the connection between older people and concepts such as ill health, dependence, and inactivity are made almost automatically (Lundgren & Ljuslinder, 2011; Nilsson, 2008; Stewart et al., 2012). In order to counter this negative characterization, an alternative conceptualization was introduced that emphasizes older people's competence and activity (Coupland & Coupland, 1993; Katz, 2000). Since then, activity in old age has become a universal "good" and a political strategy to counter the age threat (FUTURAGE, 2011; Katz, 2000).

In this discursive context, age is relational; more specifically, governmentality opens the door for age to be "done" (Laz, 1998) by distinguishing oneself from the other – the less successful, biologically older other. However, the response to the pandemic meant that the active-aging ideal that is normally politically advocated was abandoned overnight without further explanation. The aim of this study was thus to investigate how age-based recommendations were experienced by those targeted by them and what the consequences were for their self-image.

This study should not be seen as a critique of the Swedish response to the COVID-19 pandemic in general nor the Public Health Agency in particular. In some situations, a population perspective inevitably needs to be prioritized over a perspective focused on the individual, and chronological age is commonly seen as one of the more equal bases for categorization when this is called for. However, from a Foucauldian perspective, it becomes relevant to discuss the legitimacy of "traditional" biopolitical governance, of age-based policymaking, in a time characterized by neoliberal governmentality, as exemplified by the active and successful aging concepts. The state response to the COVID-19 pandemic offered the opportunity to do just that (Hannah, 2020).

The answers to the question of how the age-based recommendations were experienced indicated six different ways of relating to the recommendations. However, the most overwhelming response was the acceptance of and willingness to follow them. Respondents in five of the six categories described how they had made changes in their daily lives in accordance with the recommendations. This acceptance supports the assumption on which the Public Health Agency based its efforts, namely that it is inherent in the "Swedish culture" to willingly follow government recommendations (Irwin, 2020). However, following Foucault's line of reasoning there is no exercise of power without resistance, and we thus set out to investigate how compliance and resistance were expressed.

The responses show that, on the one hand, individuals 70 years or older are familiar with being targeted by biopolitical interventions. Through the 1980s, this had been the common way of governing in Swedish society, and thus something that large segments of the older population were used to and accepting of. As the results show in the responses within Category 2, this tradition was something that filled the respondents with trust and pride. However, the responses in Categories 3 and 6 show that the lives of older people in Sweden today are clearly affected by the neoliberal governmentality that is explicitly apparent in the active aging ideal. For these respondents, the recommendations stood out as more surprising and paradoxical, not to say abusive. This points to an unfamiliarity with being the group targeted by restrictions and governance. On the contrary, this generation has long been viewed as more powerful and dominant in the Swedish society than both previous and following generations (Nilsson, 2011; SVT [Swedish Television], 1984), and as such rather accustomed to targeting others.

The ambivalence and strong feelings of anxiety expressed in the nineteen percent of the responses within Category 5 are the most startling findings in this study. The respondents describe how they had a changed self-image as a result of being categorized as old, how the isolation led to a reduced ability to act, feelings of depression and increased thoughts of death, statements that are consistent with previous research. In a study of how older persons reason about the "finitude of life", Andersson (2020) refers to Jasper's view on borderline situations as a means to analyze the social and embodied experience of the finite nature of life. Examples of borderline situations could be loss of family members or friends or physical deterioration; but being ascribed a particular vulnerability in the context of a pandemic could also be an example of such a borderline situation. Following Andersson's line of reasoning, it is thus not surprising that accounts of increased melancholia emerge when one abruptly identifies oneself as "old."

If these and other negative effects, such as lower self-esteem, passivity, and the acceptance of a marginalized role in society, persist after the restrictions are lifted, it is plausible that individuals within the age group may show poorer health and lower quality of life. There is a clear risk that people will become vulnerable by being labeled vulnerable and to ultimately need help by being forced to receive help (Nilsson et al., 2018). Thus, it is of great importance to continuously track the long-term consequences of the governmental responses to the COVID-19 pandemic.

The rejection of age as an organizing principle shown in the responses in Category 6 can be seen as active and explicit resistance against being positioned as vulnerable and, as such, an understandable defensive reaction to protect self-esteem and ward off depression. However, another interesting finding in this study is that it seems possible to accept the age restriction, and thus follow the recommendations, without being affected or "stricken" by it in terms of a changed identity and self-image. More concretely, it seems possible to actively "protect" oneself from the labels ascribed to the 70 and older age group during the pandemic, such as vulnerability and fragility. Three examples will be highlighted.

First, the analysis of Category 2 shows how solidarity can work as a "counter-concept" with which it became possible for respondents to turn the passive position of the "old" into the active position of the "hero." Second, the analysis of Category 3 demonstrate that the distinction supported in the active-aging paradigm between success (being healthy and active) and failure (being in poor health and passive) could work as a means to place oneself in a "subgroup", an exception, within the age-based risk group, and thus escape being labeled as "vulnerable." Third, the analysis in Category 4 reveals examples whereby having underlying illnesses and experiences of "real" vulnerability make the age-based recommendations feel less applicable as age becomes irrelevant and physical health becomes paramount.

These three examples could be seen as expressions of how compliance and resistance can be parallel practices. Put another way, we argue that compliance in itself could be a form of resistance, and thus we would like to problematize the idea that Swedes, by definition, tend to follow governmental recommendations. In fact, even though the vast majority of respondents wrote that they accepted and followed the recommendations, many described how they did this in a "pragmatic" way which exemplifies resistance. For many, only underlying illnesses seemed to be a legitimate reason for isolation to the extent that they actually felt at risk, even though they were otherwise accepting the age restrictions put into place. This may point to a need to question the effectiveness of age as an organizing principle for policy making.

Limitations

The most obvious limitation is the sampling strategy which involved broadcasting the survey and recruiting respondents via various social media channels. Generalizability of the study results was thus limited because only people who had access and skills to use these media were included in the sample. Furthermore, most respondents were highly educated women in the lower age spectrum, thereby further limiting the potential generalizability of the results. Still, we strove to increase internal validity and transferability of the study findings by providing detailed examples from respondents in each of the six categories identified. By discussing the results in light of relevant concepts and theories we aimed to contribute to dependability and to facilitate the theoretical generalizability of the results. Further, by providing detailed description of study participants we aimed to increase accuracy concerning transferability of the study findings to other contexts.

The interdisciplinary competence among the authors has been a challenge and a strength during the analysis. The researchers in this project have expertise in different disciplines and different research traditions, thus the analysis of the data involved thorough discussions, argumentations and clarifications concerning coherence and differences of the categorizations and interpretations made. We believe that this negotiation contributed to the credibility of the results. The inclusion of quotations and comprehensive examples in the results enhances the ability of readers to assess confirmability and trustworthiness.

Conclusion

The study shows that age is not an unproblematic governing principle, especially not in a time of governmentality, where the exercise of power, to at least some extent, has been transferred from the policy to individual level. By contributing to the field of research on how age limits are experienced, and what consequences they might have for the targeted individual, this study questions the effectiveness of age as a principle for policy making in a neoliberal society. In addition to protecting a vulnerable group, the sudden implementation of an age-based governmental response to the COVID-19 pandemic in Sweden, meant a deprivation of a previously assigned individual responsibility and, consequently, autonomy. The study stresses the importance of tracking the long-term consequences of this policy. If negative effects, such as lower self-esteem, passivity, and the acceptance of a marginalized role in society persist after the restrictions are lifted, it is plausible that individuals within the age group may show poorer health and lower quality of life in subsequent years.

Key points

- Six ways of relating to the age-based recommendations of voluntary quarantine for those 70 years of ageand older were identified.
- The majority of the respondents showed acceptance of, and willingness to follow, therecommendations, however compliance was paired with resistancesIn a time when social responsibility has becomemore individualized, age-based policy may be perceived as less legitimate by those targeted.
- It is important tocontinuously track the long-term consequences of age-based policy to avoid negative self-image and poorer healthamong older adults.

Disclosure statement

No potential conflict of interest was reported by the author(s).

ORCID

Gabriella Nilsson (iD) http://orcid.org/0000-0001-7995-6838
Lisa Ekstam (iD) http://orcid.org/0000-0002-7965-5530
Anna Axmon (iD) http://orcid.org/0000-0002-4539-8337
Janicke Andersson (iD) http://orcid.org/0000-0002-2511-1183

References

Age Cap. (2020). *H70-studien* [the H70 study]. Centre for Ageing and Health, Gothenburg University. https://www.gu.se/agecap/h70-och-vara-andra-befolkningsstudier

Altheide, D. L. (1987). Ethnographic content analysis. *Qualitative Sociology*, *10*(1), 65–77. https://doi.org/10.1007/BF00988269

Andersson, J. (2020) "Att förhålla sig till ändligheten i livet och strategier för 'framgångsrikt döende'", Sociologisk Forskning, 57(3–4), s. 271–287. doi:10.37062/sf.57.20328

Andersson, J., Lukkarinen-Kvist, M., Nilsson, M., & Närvänen, A.-L. (2011). *Att leva med tiden. Samhälls- och kulturanalytiska perspektiv på ålder och åldrande*. [Living with time. Social and cultural analytical perspectives on age and aging]. Studentlitteratur.

Ayalon, L., & Tesch-Römer, C. (2018). *Contemporary perspectives on ageism*. Springer.

Blaakilde, A. L. (2007). Löper Tiden från Kronos? Om Kronologiseringens Betydelse för Föreställningar om Ålder. [Time out for chronos? On the significance of chronology for notions of age]. In *Åldrandets betydelser*. Studentlitteratur; Jönsson, L, -E., Lundin, S., (Eds.), pp 25–51.

Coupland, N., & Coupland, J. (1993). Discourses of ageism and anti-ageism. *Journal of Aging Studies, 7*(3), 279–301. https://doi.org/10.1016/0890-4065(93)90016-D

Cowie, J. M., & Gurney, M. E. (2018). The use of facebook advertising to recruit healthy elderly people for a clinical trial: Baseline metrics. *JMIR Res Protoc, 7*(1), e20. https://doi.org/10. 2196/resprot.7918

Ehni, H.-J., & Wahl, H.-W. (2020). Six propositions against ageism in the COVID-19 pandemic. *Journal of Aging & Social Policy, 32*(4–5), 515–525. https://doi.org/10.1080/ 08959420.2020.1770032

Foucault, M. (1977). *Discipline and punish: The birth of the prison*. Random House.

Foucault, M. (2007). *Security, territory, population. Lectures at the college de france, 1977 – 78*. Palgrave Macmillan.

FUTURAGE. (2011) . *A road map for European ageing research*. The University of Sheffield.

Grøn, L. (2016). Old age and vulnerability between first, second and third person perspectives. Ethnographic explorations of ageing in contemporary Denmark. *Journal of Aging Studies, 39* (39), 21–30. https://doi.org/10.1016/j.jaging.2016.09.002

Hannah, M. (2020). Thinking Corona measures with Foucault.

Heikkinen, S., & Krekula, C. (2008). Ålderism – Ett fruktbart begrepp? [Ageism - a fruitful concept?]. *Sociologisk Forskning, 2008, 45* (2), 18–34. https://sociologiskforskning.se/sf/arti cle/view/19233

Hockey, J., & James, A. (1993). *Infantilization as a social discourse. Growing up and growing old: Ageing and dependency in life course*. Sage Publications.

Irwin, R. E. (2020). Misinformation and de-contextualization: International media reporting on Sweden and COVID-19. *Global Health, 16*(62), 2020. https://doi.org/10.1186/s12992- 020-00588-x

Katz, S. (2000). Busy bodies. activity, aging, and the management of everyday life. *Journal of Aging Studies, 14*(2), 135–152. https://doi.org/10.1016/S0890-4065(00)80008-0

Katz, S. (2013). Active and successful aging. Lifestyle as a gerontological idea. *Recherches sociologiques et anthropologiques, 44*(1), 33–49. https://doi.org/10.4000/rsa.910

Katz, S., & Calasanti, T (2015). Critical Perspectives on Successful Aging: Does It "Appeal More Than It Illuminates"? *The Gerontologist, 55* (1), 26–33.

Kelley-Moore, J. A., Schumacher, J. G., Kahana, E., & Kahana, B. (2006). When do older adults become "disabled"? Social and health antecedents of perceived disability in a panel study of the oldest old. *Journal of Health and Social Behavior, 47*(2), 126–141. https://doi.org/10. 1177/002214650604700203

Krekula, C., & Johansson, B. (2017). *Introduktion till kritisk åldersstudier* [Introducing critical age studies]. Studentlitteratur.

Laz, C. (1998). Act your age. *Sociological Forum, 13*(1), 85–113. https://doi.org/10.1023/ A:1022160015408

Lundgren, A.-S & Ljuslinder, K. (2011). Act your age. The baby-boom is over and the ageing shock awaits' Populist media imagery in news press representations of population ageing. International Journal of Ageing and Later Life, 6, 39–71.

Marson, S. M., & Powell, R. M. (2014). Goffman and the infantilization of elderly persons: A theory in development. *Journal of Sociology and Social Welfare, XLI*(4), 143–158. https:// scholarworks.wmich.edu/jssw/vol41/iss4/8

Meisner, B. A. (2021). Are You OK, Boomer? Intensification of Ageism and Intergenerational Tensions on Social Media Amid COVID-19. *Leisure Sciences*, *43*, 1–2. DOI: 10.1080/01490400.2020.1773983

Nilsson, G. (2011). Age and class in the third age. Talking about life as a mappie. *Etnologia Scandinavica*, *41*(1), 71–88.

Nilsson, G., Ekstam, L., & Andersson, J. (2018). Pushing for miracles, pulling away from risk: An ethnographic analysis of the force dynamics at senior summer camps in Sweden. *Journal of Aging Studies*, *47*(47), 96–103. https://doi.org/10.1016/j.jaging.2018.03.004

Nilsson, M. (2008). Våra Äldre. Om Konstruktioner av Äldre iOffentligheten. Linköping: Linköping University.

Petersén, M. (2020). Den microchippade enhörningsskötaren. Svensk teknikoptimism på 2010-talet [The microchipped unicorn caretaker. Swedish technology optimism in the 2010s]. In V. Höög, S. Kärrholm, & G. Nilsson (Eds.), *Kultur X. 10-talet i kulturvetenskaplig belysning* (pp. 24). Lund studies in arts and cultural sciences.

Press Conference. (2020, March 16). *Folkhälsomyndighetens pressträff* [Public health agency press conferences]. Sweden: the Public Health Agency, .

Previtali, F., Allen, L. D., & Varlamova, M. (2020). Not only virus spread: The diffusion of ageism during the outbreak of COVID-19. *Journal of Aging and Social Policy*, *32*(4–5), 506–514. https://doi.org/10.1080/08959420.2020.1772002

Reynolds, L. (2020). The COVID-19 pandemic exposes limited understanding of ageism. *Journal of Aging and Social Policy*, *32*(4–5), 499–505. https://doi.org/10.1080/08959420.2020.1772003

Rose, N. (1996). *Foucault and political reason: Liberalism, neo-liberalism, and rationalities of government* (A. Barry, T. Osborne, & N. Rose, eds). University of Chicago Press.

Rose, N. (1999). *Powers of freedom: Reframing political thought*. Cambridge University Press.

Rowe, J. W., & Kahn, R. L. (1997). Successful aging. *The Gerontologist*, *37*(4), 433–440. https://doi.org/10.1093/geront/37.4.433

Salari, S. M., & Rich, M. (2001). Social and environmental infantilization of aged persons: Observations in two adult day care centers. *International Journal of Aging and Human Development*, *52*(2), 115–134. https://doi.org/10.2190/1219-B2GW-Y5G1-JFEG

Sarasin, P. (2020, March 31). *Understanding the coronavirus pandemic with foucault?* https://doi.org/10.13095/uzh.fsw.fb.254

SFS. 2003:460. The Ethical Review Act.

Stewart, T. L., Chipperfield, J. G., Perry, R. P., & Weiner, B. (2012). Attributing illness to "old age". *Psychology and Health*, *27*(8), 881–897. https://doi.org/10.1080/08870446.2011.630735

Stuckelberger, A (2008). Anti-ageing medicine: Myths and chances. Zürich: vdf Hochschulverlag AG.

SVT [Swedish Television]. (1984, November 23). Ärligt talat [Honestly speaking]. *Episode*, 8.

the Public Health Agency. (2020). *Information till riskgrupper om covid-19* [Information for risk groups about covid-19]. Sweden: the Public Health Agency, . https://www.folkhalsomyndigheten.se/smittskydd-beredskap/utbrott/aktuella-utbrott/covid-19/skydda-dig-och-andra/rad-och-information-till-riskgrupper/

Living Through the COVID-19 Pandemic: Community-Dwelling Older Adults' Experiences

Bo Xie (ID), Kristina Shiroma, Atami Sagna De Main,
Nathan W Davis, Karen Fingerman, and Valerie Danesh

ABSTRACT

Increasing research is investigating the COVID-19 pandemic's impact on older adults, but relatively little is known about the complexities of community-dwelling older adults' lived experiences during this historical period. This study aimed to address this gap in the literature by taking a bottom-up, theory-generating, inductive approach. Older adults living in Central Texas ($N = 200$; age, 65–92 years, $M = 73.6 \pm 6.33$) responded to a telephone interview during June–August 2020. Data were analyzed using inductive thematic analysis. We identified three key themes: positive, mixed, and negative experiences, with a total of 11 subthemes. A thematic map was developed, illustrating potential connections to mental health. These findings reveal the complexities of older adults' lived experiences during COVID-19 and have implications for developing aging-related policies and community-based interventions during future public health crises. Recognizing the complexities of older adults' lived experiences, tailored policies and interventions can be developed to effectively leverage older adults' effective coping and resilience while at the same time helping overcome negative effects among specific subgroups.

Introduction

Coronavirus disease 2019 (COVID-19) has disproportionally affected older adults, who are at greater risk for developing COVID-19 and experiencing its most severe consequences (Auld et al., 2020; Gupta et al., 2020). To protect older adults and other vulnerable populations, the U.S. Centers for Disease Control and Prevention (2021) has recommended precautions, and senior centers have been closed or have operated on a limited basis (National Council on Aging, 2020). Such changes and modifications to daily life have increased isolation for many older adults, who were already at high risk for social isolation (Cudjoe et al., 2020). Social isolation is a significant risk factor for loneliness (National Academies of Sciences, Engineering and Medicine,

2020), and both social isolation and loneliness are significant risk factors for negative health outcomes (Cacioppo & Cacioppo, 2014; Courtin & Knapp, 2017; Hayashi et al., 2020). During the pandemic, changes in daily activities and community resources may be leading to additional negative health outcomes in older adults.

Since December 2019, COVID-19 has spurred rapid and extensive research (Kang et al., 2020), but this research has focused on specific perspectives with others understudied. Recent studies have used quantitative methods to document older adults' experiences and effective coping during the pandemic (Birditt et al., 2020; Carney et al., 2021; Carstensen et al., 2020; Heid et al., 2021; Whitehead & Torossian, 2021). However, studies have not yet explored the complexities of those experiences. The present study was part of a larger study of community-dwelling older adults' access to information, services, and social interactions during the pandemic. In the larger study, we intentionally did not take a top-down, theory-driven, reductive approach. Instead, we chose to take a bottom-up, theory-generating, inductive approach in this study. These two research paradigms are fundamentally different, but both have value. The COVID-19 pandemic is unprecedented in many ways. As such, we felt that it was necessary to start out the investigation broadly, to understand, from the research participants' perspective, what they are experiencing; and then, grounded in the data, we could then develop a theory (that could be tested in future research – and be used to guide the development of future policy and community interventions). As illustrated in our data and the theoretical framework derived from the data, this inductive approach has led us to discover unique aspects of older adults' lived experiences during the COVID-19 pandemic that otherwise might not have been discovered.

The present paper focuses on older adults' lived experiences. The primary research question that guided the present paper was:

> What are community-dwelling older adults' lived experiences during the COVID-19 pandemic?

Methods

Design

This was a mixed-methods study; data were gathered with both open- and closed-ended questions over the telephone. The study was approved by the Institutional Review Board of the authors' university.

Participants

A convenience sample of community-dwelling older adults in Central Texas (N = 200; age range, 65–92 years; M = 73.6 ± 6.33) participated in this study during June–August 2020. Participants were recruited through local organizations that serve the older population (e.g., senior centers, Meals on Wheels).

Procedure

Interested individuals were contacted by telephone and invited to participate in the study. The interviewer – one of the researchers on the team – asked each potential participant if they would be willing to share their experiences in coping with life during the COVID-19 pandemic. The interviewer then read a brief informed consent paragraph and asked for verbal consent from interested individuals. After obtaining informed consent, a predetermined semi-structured interview script was used to ask open- and closed-ended questions. The interviewer used an online Qualtrics questionnaire to guide the phone interview, entered each participant's responses in Qualtrics during the interview, and cleaned the data after each interview. Each interview lasted 30–45 min but was extended at the participant's request. At the conclusion of the interview, each participant was provided with a $20 Amazon e-gift card for participation in this study.

Materials

We used a predetermined interview guide that contained open- and closed-ended questions, with necessary prompts, to guide the interviews. Each interview began with demographic questions. We then asked an open-ended question "How are you doing?" This question served to elicit participant-driven responses about their general experience during the COVID-19 pandemic. If participants' answers devolved away from their lived experience during COVID-19, the interview protocol allowed for redirection of the question. For example, a follow-up prompt such as "In light of COVID-19, how are you doing?" would redirect a participant who gave a simple "I'm doing fine" answer. The interview protocol also allowed for interviewers to probe deeper into shorter, less descriptive answers as necessary. Other questions included in the interview guide focused on experiences with technology such as video chat, telehealth, and online grocery shopping during the pandemic; experiences with obtaining COVID-19 related information; and experiences with keeping in touch with family and friends. We asked participants about how their life experience helped them cope with the current health situation, what they felt was the most challenging about life during a pandemic, and what they felt would be the best way to help them get through the situation. Participants were eager and enthusiastic to engage in this research. They carefully considered our interview questions and offered deep insights. Participants offered such rich data across all of the interview questions that we were forced to report our findings in multiple manuscripts. The data presented in this manuscript focused on participants' responses to our questions about their general experience in the first 3–5 months of the pandemic, which offered rich comprehensive insights into the lived experience of older adults during those first few months of COVID-19.

Data analysis

Demographic data were exported from Qualtrics to SPSS and analyzed with descriptive statistics. The qualitative data were analyzed using inductive thematic analysis (Braun & Clarke, 2006). Data analysis was first performed by one of the researchers on our team, who was experienced with qualitative data analysis techniques including inductive thematic analysis. A second team member, also experienced with qualitative data analysis, independently reviewed the same data and verified the first researcher's data analysis results. Differences between these two researchers were resolved through discussions and modifications were made to the framework to reflect these discussions. The rest of the team then reviewed the themes and suggested further revisions, which were incorporated into the final framework.

Specifically, following the guidelines of inductive thematic analysis, the first step was to read and reread the text to familiarize ourselves with the data. Second, we generated initial codes and assigned them to the appropriate text; the initial codes we generated at this step included: doing great/excellent; okay with reservation; hard at first, okay now; negative/bitter complains; and fine at first/hard now. Third, we collated similar codes into themes; specifically, we collated 3 of the initial codes (okay with reservation; hard at first, okay now; and fine at first/hard now) into the theme of mixed experiences, while developing the other initial codes, doing great/excellent and negative/bitter complains, into the themes of positive and negative experiences, respectively.

Fourth, we reviewed the themes and related codes to develop a "thematic map" that illustrated the specifics of each theme, including each theme's definition, the subthemes under it, and their relationships. Specifically, during this step we refined the definitions of positive, mixed, and negative experience as experience showing the overall tone being clearly positive with no major concern; doing well in some respects but with major concerns or complaints in other respects; and contained entirely or mostly strong, negative feelings and concerns, respectively. These definitions were intended to be mutually exclusive. Under each theme, we identified specific subthemes with each subtheme representing a unique phenomenon or variable related to its theme. As we lined up the themes and subthemes, it became clear to us that these themes might align with mental health. Specifically, positive experiences were more likely to align with mental wellness; negative experiences were more likely to align with poor mental wellness; and mixed experiences were more likely to align with a position in between mental wellness and illness. As such, the thematic map also illustrated the themes' relationships to each other, as laid out in their relative positions on the projected mental health spectrum.

Fifth, we iteratively refined the thematic map by further defining and naming the themes, subthemes, and their relative positions on the potential alignment with mental health. As one example, initially we had used solid lines in the thematic map to illustrate the mental health spectrum; upon further examination of the data and deliberation among our team members, we decided to change the solid lines to dotted lines to indicate that it was a "possible" spectrum and that a more definite relationship would require further investigation in future research. Finally, we wrote this report, with vivid, compelling quotes selected from the data, organized by the thematic map, and followed by our interpretation of their meanings and implications, as we situate our findings within the literature.

Results

Participants' responses varied greatly, ranging from a few words, e.g., "I'm doing fine," to lengthy responses. However, we found that life during a pandemic was at the focal point of our participants' thoughts and the majority of responses were rich with extensive details. Participants' experiences fell into 3 types or themes: positive, mixed, and negative. Approximately half of the participants ($n = 98$; 49.5%) had positive experiences; 70 (35%) had mixed experiences; and 30 (15%), negative experiences. Participants' characteristics are summarized in Table 1.

Theme 1: positive experiences

We coded a response as a "positive experience" if its overall tone was clearly positive with no major concern. Positive experiences comprised four subthemes: (1) perception that the pandemic had not changed one's lifestyle; (2) adjusting well – particularly with the aid of technology; (3) being positive in perspective; and (4) the "loner advantage" – having been a "loner" before the pandemic was advantageous during the pandemic.

Perception that the pandemic had not changed one's lifestyle
Some older adults reported that the pandemic had not changed their lifestyles. Exemplary quote:

Table 1. Participant demographics.

Characteristics	Participant n (%)
Gender	
Female	138(69)
Male	62(31)
Ethnicity	
Hispanic	23(11.5)
Non-Hispanic	177(88.5)
Race	
American Indian/Alaska Native	4(2.0)
African American	16(8.0)
Asian	10(5.0)
White Caucasian	146(73.0)
Other	24(12.0)
Education	
Less than high school graduate	2(1)
High school graduate/GED/Vocational training	24(12)
Some college/Associate degree	50(25)
Bachelor's degree	60(30)
Graduate degree	64(32)
Annual household income	
Less than $20,000	22(11)
$20,000 – $29,999	17(8.5)
$30,000 – $39,999	9(4.5)
$40,000 – $49,999	12(6)
$50,000 – $59,999	11(5.5)
$60,000 – $69,999	12(6)
$70,000 – $99,999	24(12.0)
$100,000 or more	19(9.5)
Do not know for certain	9(4.5)
Do not wish to answer	65(32.5)

*Some data are missing; percentages shown are valid percentages.

We are doing fantastic. We are very blessed here. We live in a small town population-wise and it really hasn't affected us at all. Psychologically we are doing great. Physically we are doing great. It really hasn't changed our lifestyle all that much.

Adjusting well – particularly with the aid of technology

Adjustments were necessary during the pandemic, given that most activities had to be confined to the home setting. Developing new hobbies – or, rather, continuing old hobbies in new ways – was an important adjustment. Some older adults explicitly mentioned technology in their adjustment to the "new normal":

I think fine. Um, one adjusts ... I'm getting very, very good at the computer. It is one benefit. I find that between the iPad and the iPhone I can amuse myself for a long time.

I'm doing fine. Actually, there's been quite a bit of things going on here. Zoom trivia, Zoom bingo ... I had a Zoom book club. I love Zoom. I'm doing a family Zoom tomorrow. I'm hosting that one.

Being positive in perspective

Some older adults felt positive when they compared their own situations with (their perceptions of) those of their peers – everything was in perspective.

Uh, I think well, compared to what I think everybody else is.

I think we're doing well if not better than most folks. It's, yeah, yeah, we are doing better than most folks, although I don't know most folks.

The "loner advantage"

Some older adults reported that they were used to be loners pre-pandemic, which was seen as advantage in a pandemic that necessitated quarantine, sheltering in place, and social isolation, and being alone did not make them feel lonely.

I feel pretty well because I am used to being by myself. I live alone so it's a little bit easier because I'm already accustomed to being home alone.

I'm doing fine. I'm kind of a loner so being alone isn't hard for me. It's just a part of who I am, and I think that helps—if you can be alone, it really is an asset when you have to be alone.

Theme 2: mixed experiences

We coded responses as "mixed experiences" if participants reported doing okay in some respects but with major concerns or complaints in other respects; four subthemes were identified: (1) doing well but unhappy about having to change lifestyle routines (e.g., travel); (2) doing well but unhappy about not having in-person interactions with family and friends; (3) doing well but frustrated by witnessing absence of social distancing or facemask use by others; and (4) maintaining physical health with fluctuating symptoms of depression or anxiety.

Doing well but unhappy about having to change lifestyle routines

Some older adults reported doing fine, but they also expressed dissatisfaction about having to change their routines, particularly travel.

Hanging in there. Not much choice. Doing fine. Wish the isolation or the self-quarantine was lifted and biggest disappointment is not being able to travel.

Generally pretty well. It's been a hassle because I can't go and do things that I used to do. We go and do what we need to do. I hate suiting up to go into the store, but it is what it is."

Doing well but unhappy about not having in-person interactions

Some participants reported doing okay but explicitly stated how much they missed in-person interactions with family (especially grandchildren) and friends.

I would say I'm doing pretty well ... The hardest part for me is not getting hugs and kisses from my family members. Because I live on my own and human touch is just so important but we do what we have to do.

We are doing fine ... We wish that we get together with friends but unfortunately, we cannot do it anymore. We missed it very much. We missed very much our friends. It's kind of tough when we cannot see our friends.

Doing well but frustrated by others' behaviors

Some participants were adamant about witnessing others who did not follow proper prevention guidelines, risking everyone's health and safety.

Health is fine. You know, I get a little frustrated sometime over the ways some people are taking it—just the number of people who are not social distancing and wearing masks ... We live in a neighborhood where we get together every now and then; we have one person who hasn't been taking this seriously. We usually keep our groups to five or six people and she invited about 12. No one was wearing a mask; people were hugging. A lot of people were in their 30s or 40s ... .That's frustrating to me that they are not observing ...

They are putting themselves at risk and others and the infection rate is spiking.

Maintaining physical health with fluctuations of isolation and symptoms of depression or anxiety

Some participants reported being healthy physically but felt bored, frustrated, lonely, and depressed. As one person stated: "I'm doing ok, physically. I get bored and depressed." These self-reports of isolation and depression fluctuated, with some days good and other days bad: "Some days better than others. Some days are very hard. I just sit all day. I don't care if I eat, I don't care if I read, don't care if I watch TV. On the good days, there's a couple of news shows I try to catch just to keep up a little bit ... "

Theme 3: negative experiences

We coded a response as a "negative experience" if it contained entirely or mostly strong, negative feelings and concerns; three subthemes were identified: (1) bitter about others (including society and government) not caring for older adults; (2) feeling isolated, bored, and powerless; and (3) worsening as time goes by.

Bitter about others (including society and government) not caring for older adults

Some older adults expressed bitterness and disappointment in how other individuals, society, and the government handled the pandemic, and in how little concern had been shown for high-risk groups like older adults by not following proper protocols. As one person stated: "there are few people that have respect for older adults. If it is ok for us to die in assisted living and long-term care and the administration does not seem to care." Another person explained: "It's horrible, for us seniors; they've cut us off at the knees ... I don't feel government is doing anything to protect us … .It's the worst thing I've been through."

Feeling isolated, bored, and powerless

This subtheme recalled the subtheme of maintaining physical health with fluctuations of isolation and symptoms of depression or anxiety, but it *featured* isolation, depression, and anxiety. Without reference to physical health, this subtheme showed no mention of anything positive; negativity under this subtheme was strong. Exemplary quotes from three different participants: "The isolation is daunting"; "I am kind of getting a little bit bored. I don't go anywhere and staying in"; and "the feeling of so much powerlessness to control my environment."

Worsening as time goes by

Some older adults mentioned that their lived experiences had changed, increasingly worsening as the pandemic dragged along. Mental health was of most concern as depression developed, along with cognition. As one participant stated: "Was doing okay, but starting to get really depressed as of last week. Had trouble sleeping. It's been challenging."

Thematic mapping

Based on the preceding findings, we developed the thematic map (Figure 1) to illustrate themes, subthemes, and their relationships (i.e., the degree to which these themes might be associated with differing degrees of mental health).

Discussion

In this paper, we have explored the complexities of community-dwelling older adults' lived experiences during the pandemic. Our data-driven, inductive thematic analysis generated three key themes – positive, mixed, and negative experiences – with 11 subthemes. These findings may inform interventions to support older adults' access to digital information, services, and social interaction during future societal crises and to build their strengths in coping with crises.

Recent quantitative studies (Birditt et al., 2020; Carstensen et al., 2020; Heid et al., 2021; Whitehead & Torossian, 2021) have revealed effective coping among older adults during the pandemic. Theme 1 in our study, *positive experiences*, presents novel insights into the strategies older adults use to cope. One key to these positive experiences consisted of older adults' positive attitudes toward adaptions and adjustments based on COVID-19 prevention guidelines. Indoor hobbies helped them keep busy while staying home. Some mentioned technology as an important means that enabled routines in a new

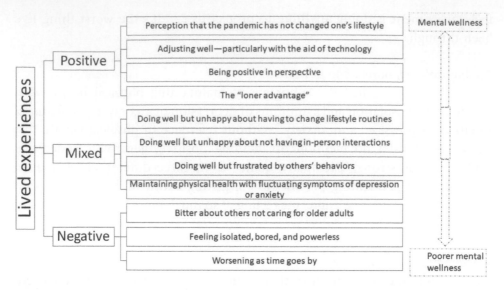

Figure 1. Thematic map: older adults' lived experiences during the COVID-19 pandemic.

form. These findings are in line with a recent online survey that found family/ friends, digital interaction, and hobbies to be the top three sources of joy among older adults (Whitehead & Torossian, 2021). They also echo another study in which staying busy (e.g., with hobbies), communication with family and friends (e.g., using technology to stay in touch), and having a positive mind-set were effective coping strategies for older adults during COVID-19 (Fuller & Huseth-Zosel, 2021).

During the COVID-19 pandemic, obtaining information, services, and social interaction via digital means has become necessary more than ever (Xie et al., 2020). Several types of apps for older adults during the pandemic have been reviewed, most of them utility oriented (Banskota et al., 2020; McGarrigle et al., 2020; McGarrigle & Todd, 2020). Such apps will be essential for future societal upheavals, but our findings suggest a need for hobby-oriented apps that might incorporate pandemic-related adaptations to help older adults continue current hobbies as well as develop new ones.

Nearly half of participants in the present study reported positive experiences with no major concerns or challenges during the pandemic. This percentage differs with one study in which only 6% of participants reported that "nothing" was stressful (Whitehead & Torossian, 2021) and another study in which 87% of participants reported their coping as positive (Fuller & Huseth-Zosel, 2021). Measurement differences between these studies make direct comparison impossible. Longitudinal research is already emerging (Daly et al., 2020; O'Connor et al., 2020; Pierce et al., 2020), but we need research with standardized measures to better understand older adults' effective coping strategies and resilience.

Evidence shows that, compared with younger adults, older adults exhibited lower degrees of stress, change in lifestyles, social isolation, and negative emotions during the pandemic's first few months (Birditt et al., 2020; Carney et al., 2021; Carstensen et al., 2020). We do not yet know whether these patterns continue to hold. Nonetheless, increased age is associated with increased strengths related to positive appraisal of stressful events and successful coping (Scott et al., 2013). Because older adults have experienced significant life stressors over the years (e.g., economic crises, wars), they have likely accumulated personal resources to deal with such stressors and developed ways to cope with them.

Theme 2, *mixed experiences*, included responses of doing well but with some major concerns or complaints. Challenges identified under this theme echo those in another study in which social relationships, activity restrictions, and psychological challenges were found to be the most difficult for older adults during the pandemic (Heid et al., 2021). Rich evidence shows that factors such as leisure, social activity engagement, and interaction with family and friends support health in older adulthood (Hornby-Turner et al., 2017). Although mobile apps for social networking connect older adults with their family and friends (Banskota et al., 2020), such "virtual" interactions may not suffice to meet older adults' needs for "physical" touch. Future research should examine whether more advanced technology (e.g., virtual reality) might provide a more "real," more acceptable form of social interaction among older adults.

This "mixed experience" theme also suggests that, while coping is feasible during a pandemic, older adults' ambivalence about their experiences suggests that there are compounding effects of sustained stressors and psychosocial challenges. Older adults could demonstrate resilience and positive emotional regulation early on, yet their overall well-being may face longstanding effects of the pandemic's stressors and difficulties, leading to greater psychological distress, depression, and anxiety (Carney et al., 2021). It will be important to investigate if, to what extent, and in what ways the mixed experience might evolve over time.

Theme 3, *negative experiences*, included responses entirely or mostly negative. Older adults in this group provided lengthy, detailed narratives of strong, negative experiences – primarily in the form of symptoms of depression or anxiety – with little or no positivity in their responses. Participants who contributed to Theme 2 described fluctuation from day to day, but those who contributed to Theme 3 suggested a more steady "trend" toward symptoms of depression or anxiety. Low mood, a sense of isolation, and worsening mental emotions over time, which can translate into clinical diagnoses of depression, anxiety, or suicidal thoughts, have been characterized as the pandemic's fourth wave, with an increasing number of older adults expected to be impacted over time (Hamm et al., 2020).

Our thematic map suggests that the spectrum of lived experiences may align with the spectrum of mental wellness, in which people who report positive experiences show no symptoms of depression or anxiety, whereas those who report negative experiences seem to show intensifying symptoms. The literature shows that COVID-19 has profound, likely long-lasting, effects on the behavioral, psychological, and social well-being of various populations including healthcare workers (Kleinpell et al., 2020; Luo et al., 2020; Pappa et al., 2020), younger adults (Liu et al., 2020; Shi et al., 2020), and older adults (Abdelbasset, 2020; Alves et al., 2020; Banskota et al., 2020; D'cruz & Banerjee, 2020; Edwards et al., 2020; Hajek & König, 2020; McGarrigle et al., 2020; McGarrigle & Todd, 2020; Sher, 2020; Tegeler et al., 2020). The pandemic has affected several factors, including social isolation, financial stress, insomnia, and gun sales, all of which are risk factors for suicide (Edwards et al., 2020). It is critical to have strategies at the community level (e.g., wellness calls, low-tech remote programming for activities, remote home monitoring for older adults with comorbid conditions) to maintain mental health and social connections while respecting public health guidelines.

Ageism was common before the pandemic, and it appears to have increased with the pandemic and will likely last (Ayalon et al., 2021; D'cruz & Banerjee, 2020). The exclusion of older adults from clinical trials of SARS-CoV-2 vaccines (Sacco et al., 2020) and age-based care when hospitals reach capacity illustrates challenges that older adults face (Farrell et al., 2020). Participants described frustration related to ageism, suggesting that this had contributed to their negative feelings during the pandemic. Older adults' social and health needs must be prioritized; they are one of most vulnerable populations, and we need educational campaigns to lessen ageism and stigma, risk factors for social isolation, and barriers to care. Innovative ways to ensure older adults' social integration during and after the pandemic are needed to overcome marginalization.

The sample for this study was larger than the typical sample for a qualitative study. We recruited participants from the same local organizations that we had been working with for years on other research projects (Davis et al., 2021), and many participants of the present study had participated in our prior studies and engaged in extensive in-person interactions with the same researchers before the pandemic. This facilitated trust and rapport, which likely contributed to the participants' open, candid responses.

The key themes reported in this paper serve as a foundation for follow-up investigations where we explore, in particular, characteristics of older adults who had varying experiences. Factors such as age, gender, communication with family and friends, education, income may be predicative of older adults' positive, mixed, and negative experiences during the pandemic. Understanding these predictive factors – and their relative predicting power – will help develop effective policy and community interventions designed for specific subgroups of older adults.

Limitations and future research directions

This study has limitations. We used a convenience sample of older adults; our findings may not generalize to the U.S. older adult population (e.g., we had a high percentage of highly educated older adults in our sample; also, 37% of our participants did not report their income, making it difficult to compare with other samples on income). Future research will benefit from using nationally representative samples. The study design was cross-sectional, specific to the time of data collection (June–August 2020). Such a snapshot view is invaluable in not only documenting a historical period but also helping understand the development of long-term impacts of the pandemic. Building on the insights gained from this snapshot view investigation, we plan to conduct follow-up research to understand, from a longitudinal point of view, potential changes over time in older adults' lived experiences during and after the COVID-19 pandemic.

Also, in our interview questions we did not include specific questions related to mental health. This was in line with our research design: we intentionally designed the study to be inductive, bottom-up, that is, to expect the themes to be grounded in the data. The strength of this approach is that our findings were more convincing when mental health spontaneously emerged from the data (versus being elicited by researchers). The tradeoff, however, is that we were unable to measure mental health or link the themes to varying levels of mental health. However, our findings can inform future research taking a reductive approach to examining potential relationships between the themes and mental health (and the strength of each relationship) quantitatively.

Conclusion

We found that community-dwelling older adults might have positive, mixed, or negative experiences during a pandemic. The present study echoes other studies' findings (those of Heid et al., 2021; Whitehead & Torossian, 2021), but it reveals novel phenomena that, to our best knowledge, have not been reported elsewhere. First, we identified the "loner advantage," whereby older adults who were used to being alone did not feel affected by the pandemic. Second, a useful coping mechanism some older adults used was to explicitly compare their own situations with (their perceptions of) those of their peers and felt positive as a result. Third, some older adults felt frustrated with others who did not observe prevention protocols or with a lack of support from society and government. These findings are worth further investigation for insights (e.g., regarding effective coping strategies) to inform the development of policy and community-based interventions to improve older adults' well-being. In particular, aging-related policies and community-based interventions should be tailored to leverage older adults' effective coping and resilience during the pandemic while at the same time overcoming negative effects among specific subgroups. The COVID-19 pandemic has likely long-lasting impacts on older adults' mental health that require attention from policy-makers, practitioners, and researchers.

Key points

- Community-dwelling older adults' experiences during the COVID-19 pandemic are complicated, ranging from positive, mixed, to negative experiences.
- Aging-related policies and community-based interventions should leverage older adults' effective coping and resilience during the pandemic while overcoming negative effects.
- Community-dwelling older adults' experiences during the COVID-19 pandemic are complicated, ranging from positive, mixed, to negative experiences.
- Aging-related policies and community-based interventions should leverage older adults' effective coping and resilience during the pandemic while overcoming negative effects.
- The COVID-19 pandemic has likely long-lasting impacts on older adults' mental health that require attention from policymakers, practitioners, and researchers.

Acknowledgments

The authors wish to thank our research participants for sharing their lived experiences with us and the local organizations for assisting our participant recruitment. Editorial service for this manuscript was provided by the Cain Center in the School of Nursing.

Disclosure statement

No potential conflict of interest was reported by the author(s).

Funding

This work was supported by The University of Texas at Austin (UT Austin) Office of the Vice President for Research, with matching funds from UT Austin School of Nursing and School of Information to Bo Xie.

ORCID

Bo Xie ⓘ http://orcid.org/0000-0002-6016-6008

References

Abdelbasset, W. K. (2020). Stay home: Role of physical exercise training in elderly individuals' ability to face the COVID-19 infection. *Journal of Immunology Research, 2020,* Article 8375096. https://doi.org/10.1155/2020/8375096

Alves, G. S., Casali, M. E., Veras, A. B., Carrilho, C. G., Costa, E. B., Rodrigues, V. M., & Dourado, M. C. N. (2020). A systematic review of home-setting psychoeducation interventions for behavioral changes in dementia: Some lessons for the COVID-19 pandemic and post-pandemic assistance. *Frontiers in Psychiatry, 11,* Article 577871. https://doi.org/10.3389/fpsyt.2020.577871

Auld, S. C., Caridi-Scheible, M., Blum, J. M., Robichaux, C., Kraft, C., Jacob, J. T., Jabaley, C. S., Carpenter, D., Kaplow, R., Hernandez-Romieu, A. C., Adelman, M. W., Martin, G. S., Coopersmith, C. M., & Murphy, D. J.; Emory COVID-19 Quality and Clinical Research Collaborative. (2020). ICU and ventilator mortality among critically ill adults with coronavirus disease 2019. *Critical Care Medicine, 48*(9), e799–e84. https://doi.org/10.1097/CCM.0000000000004457

Ayalon, L., Chasteen, A., Diehl, M., Levy, B. R., Neupert, S. D., Rothermund, K., Tesch-Römer, C., & Wahl, H.-W. (2021). Aging in times of the COVID-19 pandemic: Avoiding ageism and fostering intergenerational solidarity. *The Journals of Gerontology Series B: Psychological Sciences and Social Sciences, 76*(2), e49–e52. https://doi.org/10.1093/geronb/gbaa051

Banskota, S., Healy, M., & Goldberg, E. M. (2020). 15 smartphone apps for older adults to use while in isolation during the COVID-19 pandemic. *The Western Journal of Emergency Medicine, 21*(3), 514–525. https://doi.org/10.5811/westjem.2020.4.47372

Birditt, K. S., Turkelson, A., Fingerman, K. L., Polenick, C. A., & Oya, A. (2020). Age differences in stress, life changes, and social ties during the COVID-19 pandemic: Implications for psychological well-being. *The Gerontologist, 61*(2), 205–216. https://doi.org/10.1093/geront/gnaa204

Braun, V., & Clarke, V. (2006). Using thematic analysis in psychology. *Qualitative Research in Psychology, 3*(2), 77–101. https://doi.org/10.1191/1478088706qp063oa

Cacioppo, J. T., & Cacioppo, S. (2014). Older adults reporting social isolation or loneliness show poorer cognitive function 4 years later. *Evidence-Based Nursing, 17*(2), 59–60. https://doi.org/10.1136/eb-2013-101379

Carney, A. K., Graf, A. S., Hudson, G., & Wilson, E. (2021). Age moderates perceived COVID-19 disruption on well-being. *The Gerontologist, 61*(1), 30–35. https://doi.org/10.1093/geront/gnaa106

Carstensen, L. L., Shavit, Y. Z., & Barnes, J. T. (2020). Age advantages in emotional experience persist even under threat from the COVID-19 pandemic. *Psychological Science, 31*(11), 1374–1385. https://doi.org/10.1177/0956797620967261

Centers for Disease Control and Prevention. (2021). *People at increased risk, and other people who need to take extra precautions.* COVID-19 website. https://www.cdc.gov/coronavirus/2019-ncov/specific-groups/high-risk-complications.html

Courtin, E., & Knapp, M. (2017). Social isolation, loneliness and health in old age: A scoping review. *Health and Social Care in the Community, 25*(3), 799–812. https://doi.org/10.1111/hsc.12311

Cudjoe, T. K. M., Roth, D. L., Szanton, S. L., Wolff, J. L., Boyd, C. M., & Thorpe, R. J. (2020). The epidemiology of social isolation: National health and aging trends study. *The Journals of Gerontology Series B: Psychological Sciences and Social Sciences, 75*(1), 107–113. https://doi.org/10.1093/geronb/gby037

D'cruz, M., & Banerjee, D. (2020). "An invisible human rights crisis": The marginalization of older adults during the COVID-19 pandemic—An advocacy review. *Psychiatry Research*, *292*, Article 113369. https://doi.org/10.1016/j.psychres.2020.113369

Daly, M., Sutin, A. R., & Robinson, E. (2020). Longitudinal changes in mental health and the COVID-19 pandemic: Evidence from the UK household longitudinal study. *Psychological Medicine*, 1–10. https://doi.org/10.1017/S0033291720004432

Davis, N. W., Shiroma, K., Xie, B., Yeh, T., Han, X., & De Main, A. 2021. Designing eHealth tutorials with and for older adults. In *Proceedings of the 84th annual meeting of the Association for Information Science and Technology* (p. 13). October 30-November 2, 2021, Salt Lake City, Utah.

Edwards, E., Janney, C. A., Mancuso, A., Rollings, J. H., VanDenToorn, A., DeYoung, M., Halstead, S., & Eastburg, M. (2020). Preparing for the behavioral health impact of COVID-19 in Michigan. *Current Psychiatry Reports*, *22*(12), Article 88. https://doi.org/10.1007/s11920-020-01210-y

Farrell, T. W., Francis, L., Brown, T., Ferrante, L. E., Widera, E., Rhodes, R., Rosen, T., Hwang, U., Witt, L. J., Thothala, N., Liu, S. W., Vitale, C. A., Braun, U. K., Stephens, C., & Saliba, D. (2020). Rationing limited healthcare resources in the COVID-19 era and beyond: Ethical considerations regarding older adults. *Journal of the American Geriatrics Society*, *68*(6), 1143–1149. https://doi.org/10.1111/jgs.16539

Fuller, H. R., & Huseth-Zosel, A. (2021). Lessons in resilience: Initial coping among older adults during the COVID-19 pandemic. *The Gerontologist*, *61*(1), 114–125. https://doi.org/10.1093/geront/gnaa170

Gupta, S., Hayek, S. S., Wang, W., Chan, L., Mathews, K. S., Melamed, M. L., Brenner, S. K., Leonberg-Yoo, A., Schenck, E. J., Radbel, J., Reiser, J., Bansal, A., Srivastava, A., Zhou, Y., Sutherland, A., Green, A., Shehata, A. M., Goyal, N., Vijayan, A., & David, E. L., & for the STOP-COVID Investigators. (2020). Factors associated wiith death in critically ill patients with coronavirus disease 2019 in the US. *JAMA Internal Medicine*, *180*(11), 1436–1446. https://doi.org/10.1001/jamainternmed.2020.3596

Hajek, A., & König, -H.-H. (2020). Social isolation and loneliness of older adults in times of the COVID-19 pandemic: Can use of online social media sites and video chats assist in mitigating social isolation and loneliness? *Gerontology*, *67*(1), 121–124. https://doi.org/10.1159/000512793

Hamm, M. E., Brown, P. J., Karp, J. F., Lenard, E., Cameron, F., Dawdani, A., Lavretsky, H., Miller, J. P., Mulsant, B. H., Pham, V. T., Reynolds, C. F., Roose, S. P., & Lenze, E. J. (2020). Experiences of American older adults with pre-existing depression during the beginnings of the COVID-19 pandemic: A multicity, mixed-methods study. *The American Journal of Geriatric Psychiatry*, *28*(9), 924–932. https://doi.org/10.1016/j.jagp.2020.06.013

Hayashi, T., Umegaki, H., Makino, T., Huang, C. H., Inoue, A., Shimada, H., & Kuzuya, M. (2020). Combined impact of physical frailty and social isolation on rate of falls in older adults. *The Journal of Nutrition, Health & Aging*, *24*(3), 312–318. https://doi.org/10.1007/s12603-020-1316-5

Heid, A. R., Cartwright, F., Wilson-Genderson, M., & Pruchno, R. (2021). Challenges experienced by older people during the initial months of the COVID-19 pandemic. *The Gerontologist*, *61*(1), 48–58. https://doi.org/10.1093/geront/gnaa138

Hornby-Turner, Y. C., Peel, N. M., & Hubbard, R. E. (2017). Health assets in older age: A systematic review. *BMJ Open*, *7*(5), Article e013226. https://doi.org/10.1136/bmjopen-2016-013226

Kang, M., Gurbani, S. S., & Kempker, J. A. (2020). The published scientific literature on COVID-19: An analysis of PubMed abstracts. *Journal of Medical Systems, 45*(1), Article 3. https://doi.org/10.1007/s10916-020-01678-4

Kleinpell, R., Ferraro, D. M., Maves, R. C., Kane Gill, S. L., Branson, R., Greenberg, S., Doersam, J. K., Raman, R., & Kaplan, L. J. (2020). Coronavirus disease 2019 pandemic measures: Reports from a national survey of 9,120 ICU clinicians. *Critical Care Medicine, 48* (10), e846–e855. https://doi.org/10.1097/CCM.0000000000004521

Liu, C. H., Zhang, E., Wong, G. T. F., Hyun, S., & Hahm, H. C. (2020). Factors associated with depression, anxiety, and PTSD symptomatology during the COVID-19 pandemic: Clinical implications for U.S. young adult mental health. *Psychiatry Research, 290*, Article 113172. https://doi.org/10.1016/j.psychres.2020.113172

Luo, M., Guo, L., Yu, M., Jiang, W., & Wang, H. (2020). The psychological and mental impact of coronavirus disease 2019 (COVID-19) on medical staff and general public—A systematic review and meta-analysis. *Psychiatry Research, 291*, Article 113190. https://doi.org/10.1016/j.psychres.2020.113190

McGarrigle, L., Boulton, E., & Todd, C. (2020). Map the apps: A rapid review of digital approaches to support the engagement of older adults in strength and balance exercises. *BMC Geriatrics, 20*, Article 483. https://doi.org/10.1186/s12877-020-01880-6

McGarrigle, L., & Todd, C. (2020). Promotion of physical activity in older people using mHealth and eHealth technologies: Rapid review of reviews. *Journal of Medical Internet Research, 22*(12), Article e22201. https://doi.org/10.2196/22201

National Academies of Sciences, Engineering, and Medicine. (2020). *Social isolation and loneliness in older adults: Opportunities for the health care system.* The National Academies Press. https://doi.org/10.17226/25663

National Council on Aging. (2020, March 10). *COVID-19 resources for senior centers.* https://www.ncoa.org/news/ncoa-news/national-institute-of-senior-centers-news/covid-19-resources-for-senior-centers

O'Connor, R. C., Wetherall, K., Cleare, S., McClelland, H., Melson, A. J., Niedzwiedz, C. L., O'Carroll, R. E., O'Connor, D. B., Platt, S., Scowcroft, E., Watson, B., Zortea, T., Ferguson, E., & Robb, K. A. (2020). Mental health and well-being during the COVID-19 pandemic: Longitudinal analyses of adults in the UK COVID-19 mental health & wellbeing study. *The British Journal of Psychiatry.* https://doi.org/10.1192/bjp.2020.212

Pappa, S., Ntella, V., Giannakas, T., Giannakoulis, V. G., Papoutsi, E., & Katsaounou, P. (2020). Prevalence of depression, anxiety, and insomnia among healthcare workers during the COVID-19 pandemic: A systematic review and meta-analysis. *Brain, Behavior, and Immunity, 88*, 901–907. https://doi.org/10.1016/j.bbi.2020.05.026

Pierce, M., Hope, H., Ford, T., Hatch, S., Hotopf, M., John, A., Kontopantelis, E., Webb, R., Wessely, S., McManus, S., & Abel, K. M. (2020). Mental health before and during the COVID-19 pandemic: A longitudinal probability sample survey of the UK population. *The Lancet Psychiatry, 7*(10), 883–892. https://doi.org/10.1016/S2215-0366(20)30308-4

Sacco, G., Célarier, T., Gavazzi, G., & Annweiler, C. (2020). Older adults should not be omitted from inclusion in clinical trials of SARS-CoV-2 vaccines. *Maturitas, 146*, 63-64. https://doi.org/10.1016/j.maturitas.2020.10.002

Scott, S. B., Sliwinski, M. J., & Blanchard-Fields, F. (2013). Age differences in emotional responses to daily stress: The role of timing, severity, and global perceived stress. *Psychology and Aging, 28*(4), 1076–1087. https://doi.org/10.1037/a0034000

Sher, L. (2020). The impact of the COVID-19 pandemic on suicide rates. *QJM: An International Journal of Medicine, 113*(10), 707–712. https://doi.org/10.1093/qjmed/hcaa202

Shi, L., Lu, Z.-A., Que, J.-Y., Huang, X.-L., Liu, L., Ran, M.-S., Gong, Y.-M., Yuan, K., Yan, W., Sun, Y.-K., Shi, J., Bao, Y.-P., & Lu, L. (2020). Prevalence of and risk factors associated with mental health systems among the general population in China during the coronavirus disease 2019 pandemic. *JAMA Network Open*, *3*(7), e2014053. https://doi.org/10.1001/jama networkopen.2020.14053

Tegeler, C., Beyer, A.-K., Hoppmann, F., Ludwig, V., & Kessler, E.-M. (2020). Current state of research on psychotherapy for home-living vulnerable older adults with depression. *Zeitschrift für Gerontologie und Geriatrie*, *53*(8), 721–727. https://doi.org/10.1007/s00391-020-01805-3

Whitehead, B. R., & Torossian, E. (2021). Older adults' experience of the COVID-19 pandemic: A mixed-methods analysis of stresses and joys. *The Gerontologist*, *61*(1), 36–47. https://doi.org/10.1093/geront/gnaa126

Xie, B., Charness, N., Fingerman, K., Kaye, J., Kim, M. T., & Khurshid, A. (2020). When going digital becomes a necessity: Ensuring older adults' needs for health information, services, and social inclusion during COVID-19. *Journal of Aging & Social Policy*, *32*(4–5), 460–470. https://doi.org/10.1080/08959420.2020.1771237

"We Are Saving Their Bodies and Destroying Their Souls.": Family Caregivers' Experiences of Formal Care Setting Visitation Restrictions during the COVID-19 Pandemic

Whitney A. Nash (ID), Lesley M. Harris,
Kimberly E. Heller, and Brandon D. Mitchell

ABSTRACT

This study aims to explore the experiences of family caregivers during the COVID-19 pandemic-imposed visitation restrictions at formal care settings (FCS) such as assisted living centers and traditional nursing homes. Participants (N = 512) were recruited from an international caregiving social media site that was developed at the beginning of the COVID-19 pandemic. Descriptive data was collected on the family caregivers, the care recipient and facility. Respondents also provided a single feeling word describing their experience and an open-ended question allowed for further exploration. Caregivers were predominantly daughters (n = 375). The most common reported feeling words were sadness (n = 200), trauma (n = 108), anger (n = 65), frustration (n = 56), helplessness (n = 50), and anxiety (n = 36). Thematic analysis revealed four overarching themes: 1) isolation 2) rapid decline 3) inhumane care and 4) lack of oversight. This study highlights the importance of addressing the mental, emotional and physical needs of *both* care recipient *and family* caregiver during this challenging time. Caregiver visitation policy reform that includes the care recipient and family caregiver is also discussed.

Introduction

Formal care setting (FCS) residents (care recipients) have been one of the most negatively impacted populations by the COVID-19 pandemic. For the purposes of this study FCS care recipients are defined as those individuals residing in any level of long-term care setting where they are receiving some type of nursing care. Their advanced age and the high prevalence of preexisting conditions placed them at an increased risk for severe illness and mortality from the coronavirus. Furthermore, the congregate setting allowed for the rapid spread of the disease. One measure taken to mitigate the virus's spread was visitation restrictions mandated by federal, state, and local officials (Soergel, 2020); this led to many unintended consequences. One of which was the increase in social isolation within FCS facilities. Beyond the established impact of isolation on the FCS care recipient, family caregivers suffered in part due to their lack of access to their care recipient. The focus of this paper explores the experiences of these caregivers during the COVID-19 pandemic-imposed FCS visitation restrictions.

At the beginning of the pandemic, restrictions related to attempts to mitigate the spread of COVID-19 were much harsher and strictly prohibited any visitors or non-essential healthcare personnel from entering facilities. Some exceptions were made for compassionate care, such as end-of-life situations. As of May 2020, FCSs accounted for 42% of COVID-19 deaths despite limiting visitation (Abrams et al., 2020). Beginning in March and updated periodically, the Centers for Medicare and Medicaid Services (CMS) released guidance for visitation restrictions and reopening through a multiphase approach (Quality, Safety and Oversight Group, 2020). Many facilities could not meet the benchmark guidelines outlined by CMS and therefore continued significant restrictions. In September 2020, federal officials revised guidance and encouraged facilities to allow visitation with a preference for outdoor visits (Soergel, 2020). To date, all but two states have lifted their mandates though many FCSs continued to prohibit or excessively restrict visitation. These mandates and their associated isolation continued to add stress to the caregiver role and contribute to negative outcomes for individuals. Anecdotal physicians' experiences within FCSs suggest that individuals may have died prematurely due to the lack of socialization and stimulation (Abbasi, 2020). Indeed, loneliness, which can occur from social isolation, has been shown to increase the likelihood of mortality by 26% (Holt-Lunstad et al., 2015). Loneliness has also been associated with a 29% increase in coronary heart disease incidence and a 32% increase in risk for stroke (National Academies of Sciences, Engineering and Medicine, 2020). In individuals with dementia, loneliness can lead to further cognitive decline (Chu et al., 2020). Family and friends with care recipients experiencing cognitive decline fear that these restrictions will lead to their care recipients no longer recognizing them once restrictions are removed (Simard & Volicer, 2020). This finding is one of very few that acknowledges the family caregiver perspective in this crisis.

Though emerging data continues to focus on the physical and social well-being of those residing in FCSs, there has been limited investigation exploring the impact that restrictions have had on caregivers. A reported one in five adults in the U.S. is involved in the caregiving of a friend or family member with a health problem or disability (National Association of Chronic Disease Directors, 2018). These individuals play a crucial role in their care recipient's well-being; as an advocate, sharing, if not directing, decision-making, and often providing basic care (e.g., feeding, hygiene, and socialization) during their visits. Despite much of the literature focusing on caregiving stress, research also suggests that caregivers may derive mental health benefits from their role (Beach et al., 2000; Picot, 1994; Wolff et al., 2007). When the caregiving role changes, either by the death of the patient or changes in the ability of the caregiver, there may be alterations in sleep quality (Arber & Venn, 2011; Carter, 2005; Corey & McCurry, 2018) along with further changes in the physical and mental well-being of the caregiver (Aneshensel et al., 2004; Bodnar & Kiecolt-Glaser, 1994; Corey & McCurry, 2018; Tweedy & Guarnaccia, 2008).

What is left unknown is how the COVID-19 visitation restrictions in FCSs have impacted the family caregivers during this interruption in their role. The purpose of this study was to explore the emotions and experiences of family caregivers affected by the visitation restrictions at FCSs during the 2020 COVID-19 pandemic.

Methods

Study sample

This study included 518 adults, who self-identified as a caregiver for a person living in residential care during the time of the COVID-19 pandemic. The study link and description were posted on the Facebook group "Caregivers for Compromise ... Because Isolation Kills Too." This group was launched on July 6, 2020 and was created as a space to allow members to share information, garner support and rally for improved access to their care recipient in FCSs during the COVID-19 pandemic. There are currently over 14,000 members of this group.

Sampling strategy and recruitment

Following approval from the Facebook group's administrators, a description of the study, survey link, and principal investigator's contact information was shared with the group members. The survey was live for two weeks (September 25 to October 9, 2020). Respondents did not have to be members of the group to participate, and members were encouraged to share the study link. Individuals who were unpaid, usually family caregivers for a care recipient in a FCS during the COVID-19 pandemic were eligible to complete the survey. The care recipient did not have to currently be living for the caregiver to participate. Individuals were eligible to participate even if their care recipient had transitioned to home or other living arrangement. Questions were focused on their experience while their care recipient was in a FCS during the COVID-19 pandemic. No incentives for completing the survey were provided.

All study procedures were approved by the Institutional Review Board at the University of Louisville.

Data collection

Respondents completed a survey that included questions regarding personal demographic characteristics and health status, demographics, and the health status of the care recipients, as well as information about their care recipients' facility. This included questions about whether they had reported concerns to facility leadership or government officials. Also included was a specific question regarding their concern about retaliation should they report a concern. Additionally, respondents provided a one-word response to, *"Please list any feelings that you have had in regard to the reduced visitation of your loved one (care recipient), and please use one word to describe each feeling."* Following this question, family caregivers were asked to write a response to the prompt, *"Please use this space to communicate anything else about your experience with your loved one (care recipient) who resided in a formal care setting during the COVID-19 pandemic."* The data from the survey, and the responses to the prompts were exported from Qualtrics into Excel for data analysis.

Data analysis

The open-ended responses were coded for inductive themes using an applied thematic approach (Guest et al., 2012) informed by the constant comparative method of qualitative analysis (Boeije, 2002). First, the research team read all of the feeling words from the open-ended responses in their entirety. Then half of the responses were coded line by line. After the first half was coded, initial codes were clustered together by topic to develop thematic codes.

For the feeling word responses, the research team organized them into seven thematic categories, which represented each emotion. For the responses to the prompt asking about caregiver experiences, the most frequent and significant focused codes were used to construct a codebook of nine codes with definitions.

Next, two research team members used Dedoose software to inductively code one hundred percent of the responses. Themes in the data were discussed and finalized in consensus building discussions with the full study team, including topic and method experts. The number of times the themes were mentioned in the transcripts was tabulated.

Three additional steps were taken to ensure credibility and confirmability of our research findings (Lincoln & Guba, 1985). For triangulation of data, we used two sources of data, both the emotion word and the written narratives of caregivers to understand the phenomenon of separation at a deeper level. Additionally, the research team performed a negative case analysis to search for data that did not support our main findings. This came in the form of five caregivers who reported full trust and satisfaction with the FCS in which the care recipient was living. Upon closer examination of these data, we learned that the caregivers were not living within the same location as their family member, and therefore had to rely more on a long distance, trusting relationship with the FCS. They were also more likely to already communicate with their family member using phone or technology, so therefore the long-distance caregivers did not experience as drastic of a change in communication. Lastly, as a research team, we used peer debriefing with the two authors who were not involved in the data analysis (WN and KH) as a way to engage analytical probing. This process also led to conversations on taken for granted assumptions and perceptions on behalf of the two members of the analytic team (LH and BM). This support helped refine the analysis in terms of clarifying our emerging findings.

Results

Care recipient

The majority of caregivers' care recipients were still living at the time of survey completion (90.4%). The most frequently cited reason for admission was a diagnosis of Alzheimer's disease or related dementia (ADRD) (33%). This was followed by experiencing a fall (13.4%). When asked if their care recipient was able to make their needs known verbally, 61.2% felt they could, while 28.4% reported their care recipient was unable or needed an assistive device. Of those who were able to communicate their needs, 55% expressed concern regarding their care at their facility. Greater than 92% of caregivers reported that their care recipient had experienced an injury or a decline in their health during the COVID-19 pandemic with 11.4% diagnosed with COVID-19.

Caregivers

The majority of caregivers were female (96.5%) with 77.6% being the daughter of the care recipient (Table 1). Questions regarding the caregivers' health status revealed that although 40.3% of individuals reported "feeling fine" when asked if they had experienced a change in their health status during the COVID-19 pandemic, additional data presented a different picture. Over 38% of caregivers reported a current diagnosis of a mental health diagnosis (anxiety/depression) with 24% reporting a new or worsening mental health condition. Anxiety and depression were the top two health conditions reported (38%) followed by "other" (9.1%) and weight gain of more than 10% (6.4%). Nearly 11% had a significant medical event such as a surgery or

Table 1. Demographic characteristics of caregivers and their loved ones.

Characteristic	Resident (n = 522)	Caregiver (n = 518)
Age (M, SD)	84.3 (10.3)	59.7 (8.9)
Gender (%)		
Male	29.5	2.9
Female	70.3	96.5
Race/Ethnicity (%)		
Caucasian	97.3	96.3
African American	1.2	1.2
Other	1.2	1.2
Facility Type (%)		
Nursing Home	78.4	–
Assisted Living	17.2	–
Other	4.3	–
Relationship to Loved One (%)		
Child	–	77.8
Spouse	–	10.2
Sibling	–	3.1
Other	–	8.6
Employment (%)		
Full-time	–	31.4
Part-time	–	9.5
Self-employed	–	6.9
Retired	–	36.1
Laid off since March 2020	–	2.4
Other	–	13.8

a new serious medical diagnosis, although these were not clearly defined. Fifteen caregivers (2.90%) had been diagnosed with COVID-19.

Experiences with FCSs during the COVID-19 pandemic

Prior to the COVID-19 imposed visitation restrictions, 87% of caregivers visited their care recipient at least once a week with 29.9% of those going daily. As part of those visits 58.1% provided some type of personal care including feeding and hygiene. This all changed in March 2020. Visitation restrictions have evolved repeatedly during the pandemic. Table 2 demonstrates the wide range of strategies that were being implemented at the time of this survey. According to an AARP report (Markowitz, 2020), Indiana was the

Table 2. Visitation strategies implemented for family caregivers.

Visitation Strategy	n	%
No visitation allowed	82	8.0
Telephone/video chat	232	22.7
Window visits only	210	20.6
Patio visits only	154	15.1
Scheduled visits in facility with PPE and social distancing	73	7.1
In-person visits with ability to care for loved one with precautions [a]	53	5.2
In-person visits with negative COVID-19 test result	32	3.1
Allowed out for medical appointments	89	8.7
Other	81	7.9

N = 518. Responses reflect family-caregiver reported visitation policies at time of survey completion. Respondents were able to select multiple responses. PPE = Personal Protective Equipment.
[a]Precautions include PPE and hygiene practices.

first state (June 2020) that authorized an essential caregiver program that allowed individuals that had previously provided some level of care to a care recipient in a FCS to continue in an abbreviated capacity. By the time this survey was conducted four more states had joined this effort.

Most participants (87%) were unaware of any State Board of Nursing, State Board of Health or CMS infractions or citations against the FCS where their care recipient resides/resided. Participants were not asked if they knew how to access that information. Although 58.1% of caregivers reported that they were fearful that if they raised a concern their care recipient may be retaliated upon, 77.6% still brought their concern to the facility's administrator. Beyond the FCS, 33.4% of caregivers brought concerns to the state ombudsman and 54.6% felt compelled enough to reach out to their state representative for assistance.

Feelings regarding reduced visitation

Responses to the question, *"Please list any feelings that you have had in regard to the reduced visitation of your loved one (care recipient), and please use one word to describe each feeling",* were categorized by type of emotion (Table 3). The most common reported emotion was sadness ($n = 200$), which included feeling words such as heartbroken, sorrow and devastation. This was followed by trauma ($n = 108$) which included words such as horrified, panic, and desperate. Other categories of emotion included anger ($n = 65$) (i.e., mad and rage), frustration ($n = 56$) (i.e., unfair and annoyed), helplessness ($n = 50$) (i.e., debilitating and inadequate), and anxiety ($n = 36$) (i.e., stressed and worried).

Thematic analysis of the opened question revealed four overarching themes including: 1) isolation 2) rapid decline 3) inhumane care and 4) lack of oversight.

Table 3. Participants one-word response to describe their feelings with the Covid-19 visitation restrictions.

	N	%
Anger	60	11.83
Sad	58	11.44
Frustration	53	10.45
Helplessness/Hopeless	50	9.86
Devastated	47	9.27
Heartbroken	38	7.50
Despair/Desperation	20	3.94
Abuse/Criminal/Cruel/Neglect	17	3.35
Worried/Stressed	16	3.16
Depressed	14	2.76
Fear/Frightened/Terrified	12	2.37
Anxious	11	2.17
Concerned	7	1.38
Other	104	20.53

Responses accounting for less than 1% of the total were categorized as "Other."

Theme 1 isolation

Isolation was the most commonly applied code ($n = 246$) and the highest rate of code co-occurrence. Participants defined isolation as seeing their care recipient confined to their room, with no activities, visitors, or communal dining for months at a time. Isolation was also conceptualized as mutual, being that many caregivers experienced the detrimental effects of isolation, because they had previously been engaged in socializing and receiving emotional support from their care recipient. Caregivers described isolation as being *"inhumane"* due to the length of time (over 6 months when these data were collected). Another respondent gave an example of what isolation looks like within her mother's facility, *"Although her facility has done most everything they can to ensure safety for residents from COVID and almost no effort has been made to ensure their mental health due to the isolation. Staff rarely stay and visit with Mom, no special in-room activities or stimulation has been attempted."* From the negative effects of isolation came suggestions for policy changes related to the status of family caregivers. One participant stated, *"We should be recognized as essential caregiver and be allowed into our loved one's facility using the same safety precautions as staff to provide physical, emotional support . . . because isolation kills too."*

Theme 2 rapid decline

Many participants ($n = 203$) reported a rapid decline in their care recipient's mental and physical state as soon as lock down began. One caregiver reported, *"The decline due to isolation was dramatic, alarming and devastating."* Caregivers equated the deterioration to a lack of mental, physical, emotional and social stimulation. Participants stated that they were often the key person who their care recipient turned to provide stimulation, despite being in assisted living or other FCS.

One participant reflected, *"To think in her final year(s) when she is most vulnerable and most in need of love and support from her children & was denied this for 6 months is in my opinion is devastating. I would rather my Mom died of COVID with me by her side than deteriorating and suffering emotionally with no family advocate holding her hand."*

In situations where family members were able to visit via online platforms, they noticed decline in their care recipient's physical and mental condition. One caregiver reflected, *"We watched her decline before our eyes at the video visits. She didn't understand what was happening. She thought she did something wrong. The anxiety and worry cause horrible depression."*

Theme 3 inhumane care

The third most frequently applied code was the inhumane environment their care recipient was being subjected to during the COVID-19 pandemic ($n =150$). One participant stated, *"We are saving their bodies and destroying their souls."* Another participant said, *"They are being treated like caged animals."* Caregivers expressed heartbreak over seeing relatives, who often had diagnosis of Alzheimer's or dementia, experience isolation without being able to comprehend why their family members could not enter the facility or their room. Caregivers were sometimes allowed visits through an online platform or a glass window, which for many triggered feelings of being in prison, and often led to an increase in agitation behaviors and emotional outbursts. One caregiver explained that her mother, *"doesn't understand why we can't come in. She has lost over 41 lbs since COVID and now has stopped eating and drinking. Starting Monday, she will be in Hospice. Why do we have to wait until they are almost dying before we can see them! It is inhumane! Everyone needs love!"*

Theme 4 lack of oversight

Participants (*n* = 126) reported a lack of oversight in terms of the facility in which their care recipient was residing. The lack of oversight created an environment of neglect due to short staffing as one caregiver explained, *"Facility never has sufficient staffing leaving the residents laying in their own waste all night. Numerous large bruises neglect. Mom has lost 11lbs in 3 months. She has mentally and physically declined making her dementia worse."* Family members would witness the neglect through their window visits. A daughter visiting her mother from outside of the facility described the scene, *"Dementia patients need consistent routines in order to stay stimulated. This is the most heartbreaking thing that has been agonizing to see in the 90-degree temperatures outside a window."*

The impact of the COVID-19 pandemic caused many CNAs to quit their job due to the high rates of the illness within their facilities. The short staffing and lack of oversight from management led to emotional distress and infections. One daughter describes the panic experienced by her father's phone call, *"He called crying he has been calling nurse and CNA and they would not come to take him to bathroom. He was discharged (dc) with urinary tract infections (UTIs) 6x in 7 months. I cannot even imagine what he went through."*

As a final resort, 30 participants reported that they decided to provide care outside of the FCS and bring their care recipient home. One caregiver reported on how these events unfolded, *"It became very clear that I was providing at least 20% of my mother's care in the facility prior to quarantine. She did not get that personal care during quarantine. She failed to thrive, so I brought her to my home."* At times, family members were too late to nurse their care recipient back to health, as demonstrated by the following caregiver, *"We could tell she was failing to thrive. We watched helplessly through her window. Finally, we took her home and she died 5 hours later with no mention she was at end of life."* One concerning aspect about caregivers providing care in this manner is geography. One husband spoke about taking his wife out of her facility, *"I filed a lawsuit after I was evicted from our assisted living for being a nonessential spouse. It went nowhere. After 10 weeks of separation, I brought my wife to our mountain cabin to live with me, with no caregiving help."*

Some families were equipped to administer care to their care recipient, but experienced training delays due to short staffing, which delayed their ability to bring their family member home. However, not all home caregiving situations have proven to be successful. One caregiver reported how she struggled to care for her father within her home, *"I removed my dad from his memory care facility mid-March, cared for him in my home alone, until August. It has ONLY been a month back at the facility, but he has ended up in the hospital once, he lost weight and his clothes are covered in fecal matter regularly. He is fading from a lack of my care and advocacy."* Situations such as this could create more stress for care recipients and family due to the inability to successfully provide care at home, while re-exposing the care recipient to a failing system of care.

Discussion

Based on this study's findings, the interruption of the family caregiving role due to the COVID-19 FCS visitation restrictions has significantly impacted both the care recipient and the caregiver. This study further validates Holt-Lunstad et al. (2015) work demonstrating the impact that social isolation has on an individual's well-being. In the current study, this includes both the caregiver and care recipient. Each group has members that have experienced a decline in mental and physical health. This decline was self-reported in the caregiver's case, but in many cases, the decline of the care recipient was directly observed by the caregiver or reported to them by facility staff.

Prior to the imposed visitation restrictions, 87% of caregivers visited their care recipient weekly, with nearly 30% going daily. Caregiver responses indicate that part of this time was spent giving personal care, advocating for their care recipient, and monitoring care delivery. Due to the visitor restrictions during the COVID-19 pandemic, informal caregiving support disappeared, which exacerbated the existing challenges related to staff shortages in nursing homes (McGilton et al., 2020).

The wide range of revised visitation procedures changed how the caregiving role was implemented. Caregivers expressed high levels of frustration with their limited access to their care recipient. Many expanded the advocate domain of the caregiving role by reaching out beyond the facility to state authorities. Crossing the Quality Chasm (Institute of Medicine (IOM), 2001) emphasizes patient-centered care as a critical element in quality health care delivery. This approach includes the family as well as the patient. It is apparent from the personal accounts of caregivers in this study that planning for limiting COVID-19 facility spread did not fully take into account the physical and mental health needs of the care recipient. Other sources, including the

Institute for Patient- and Family-Centered Care and The National Quality Forum's National Priorities Partnership support the need for including family and patients in key decision-making. This should extend to how care can be continued even during a pandemic.

Implications

Policy/practice

Much has been learned regarding the crucial role family caregivers play in helping ensure the needs of their care recipients are met during a time of crisis. These results support the previously established impact that can occur when family caregivers are excluded from the process. Older adults are at risk when patient- (or person-) centered care is not continued in FCSs even during challenging times. It is important to note that FCSs were under federal mandate to impose restrictions to visitation early on in the pandemic and many struggled to obtain clear guidance in interpreting and implementing these restrictions.

The results revealed that caregivers deemed that isolation was just as deadly as the pandemic for their care recipients. They reported that the severed ties with their care recipient led to a rapid decline in health. They viewed the social and physical health provided through their caregiving as critical, even when faced with risk factors associated with spreading the virus. As caregivers diminish in presence, this may have led to cascading and deteriorating health status of individuals residing in the facility. Research has already established the link between the psychological impacts of isolation and neglect and the rapid deterioration of health, including mortality (Dong et al., 2009; Pantell et al., 2013), which has been compounded by COVID-19 risk factors.

Our results indicate many caregivers perceived that many deaths were not COVID-related from a medical standpoint but were related to care changes in light of COVID-19. In order to rebuild trust, their concerns should be recognized as a failure of the formal care system to respond and quickly implement policies that enabled safer visitation. This crisis has given way to recommendations grounded in our participants' experiences and by reviewing literature from the Centers for Medicare and Medicaid Services (2020) and the Centers for Disease Control and Prevention (2020). We recommend that a) FCS administrators onboard their residents and staff to technology that facilitates frequent communication between caregivers and care-recipients (e.g., video calls, text messages, e-mail, and phone calls), b) protocols established during compassionate care visits be evaluated and potentially expanded to include ways to include essential caregivers, and c) frequent and scheduled visits which include parades of cars, high-quality visits through glass windows, and outdoor visits which make accommodations for the weather (e.g., umbrellas, heat lamps, etc.) be implemented to ensure greater comfort for all parties.

Research has established that addressing complex grief will be needed among healthcare workers during the COVID-19 pandemic (Greenberg et al., 2020). Recent studies have suggested that nursing home workers will face additional guilt and distress related to their role in transmitting the virus under enormously stressful working conditions, including understaffing (McGilton et al., 2020). Less is known about how grief is experienced by family caregivers who lost their ability to deliver care. Although a care recipient's death in FCSs is typically a normative expectation, the COVID-19 pandemic has altered the meaning-making experiences surrounding death. Grief may be further complicated with trauma and feelings of betrayal. In their article addressing bereavement during the COVID-19 pandemic, Carr et al. (2020) suggest that COVID-19 related deaths exemplify "bad deaths" and support expanded, active advanced care planning that includes respect for the older adults' wishes. We recommend that efforts be made to rebuild trust between family members and nursing homes and that hospice services join the efforts to deliver tailored bereavement services that address families who have lost a care recipient under these circumstances.

Unfortunately, this will most likely not be the last public health crisis that will impact the care recipients' in FCSs. The COVID-19 pandemic, not unlike the aftermath of Hurricane Katrina in 2005, has brought to light the lack of preparedness to deal with the safety and health of our elderly during a crisis (Adams et al., 2011). The authors propose a significant post-pandemic assessment of the physical and emotional health of the individuals in FCSs as well as their informal caregivers. Evidence-based decision-making regarding how best to adapt must be evaluated prior to the next crisis.

Future direction

Although person-centered care has been well established as a critical framework for positive care outcomes, further research is needed to evaluate the balance between providing person-centered care and the need to provide for the safety of all residents, staff, visitors, and the general public when a crisis such as the COVID-19 pandemic occurs. This future research should include input from care recipients, family caregivers as well as formal/paid caregivers and administrators of FCSs. Although some families in this study were able to pivot to administer home health in times of crisis quickly, they experienced delays in being trained on how to administer home health care by staff. Families who transitioned to caring for their care recipient at home successfully during the COVID-19 pandemic may provide valuable insight for disaster preparedness planning. Lastly, much focus has been placed on the role of residential staff in spreading COVID-19. Less attention has been given to how family members have contributed to the spread of COVID-19 during the pandemic. Future studies can look at how visitation policies have been implemented across various regions to determine how family members may have contributed to the virus's spread. This research might serve as a mechanism for repairing relationships between families and residential care through delivering evidence as to why some "lockdown" procedures were necessary.

Limitations

The current study is limited in part due to the potential for selection bias. Although participants did not have to be a member of the caregiver advocacy group to participate in the survey and respond to the prompts, we recognize that many of the participants were previously engaged in caregiver activism around issues of isolation. It is certainly possible that individuals who were not members of the Facebook page used for recruitment may have had different experiences than those who participated in the study. Additionally, the prompt of asking for a one-word feeling about the reduced visitation experience may have limited the participants' sharing of how and why they expressed the identified sentiment. Finally, 9.6% of the respondents' care recipients had died prior to the completion of the survey. Potential negative feelings toward the FCS regarding the circumstances of the death may have influenced the responses. Future research will explore the connection between experiences and emotional responses of caregivers during the COVID-19 pandemic.

Conclusion

In these unprecedented times, there is a need to ensure that trust remains between FCSs and families. Leadership in the field must acknowledge the harm created by implementing policies that severed family ties while communicating that restrictions were designed to minimize the virus's impact on all parties (i.e., residents, staff, and families). This pandemic has amplified existing problems within FCSs and offered opportunities to rethink the future of long-term care, such as enhanced disaster preparedness, integration of technology for communication, and inclusive planning.

Key points

- Older adults residing in FCSs are at increased risk for decline in health status related to isolation.
- COVID-19 related visitation restrictions increase social isolation for both the care recipient and family caregiver.

- Family caregivers have role disruption and experience stress due to imposed restrictions
- Policy development regarding the needs of *both* the care recipient and family caregiver is critical

Acknowledgments

The authors of this paper would like to thank the members and administrators of the Caregiver for Compromise . . . .Because Isolation Kills Too FB group for their willingness to share their stories with the authors and facilitate recruitment of others.

Disclosure statement

No potential conflict of interest was reported by the author(s).

Funding

The authors received no financial support for the research, authorship, and/or publication of this article.

ORCID

Whitney A. Nash ⓘ http://orcid.org/0000-0002-0372-0594

References

Abbasi, J. (2020). Social isolation-the other COVID-19 threat in nursing homes. *Journal of the American Medical Association*, 324(7), 619–620. https://doi.org/10.1001/jama.2020.13484

Abrams, H. R., Loomer, L., Gandhi, A., & Grabowski, D. C. (2020). Characteristics of U.S. nursing homes with COVID-19 cases. *Journal of American Geriatric Society*, 68(8), 1653–1656. https://doi.org/10.1111/jgs.16661

Adams, V., Kaufman, S. R., Van Hattum, T., & Moody, S. (2011). Aging disaster: Mortality, vulnerability, and long-term recovery among Katrina survivors. *Medical Anthropology*, 30 (3), 247–270. https://doi.org/10.1080/01459740.2011.560777

Aneshensel, C. S., Botticello, A. L., & Yamamoto-Mitani, N. (2004). When caregiving ends: The course of depressive symptoms after bereavement. *Journal of Health and Social Behavior*, 45 (4), 422–440. https://doi.org/10.1177/002214650404500405

Arber, S., & Venn, S. (2011). Caregiving at night: Understanding the impact on carers. *Journal of Aging Studies*, 25(2), 155–165. https://doi.org/10.1016/j.jaging.2010.08.020

Beach, S. R., Schulz, R., Yee, J. L., & Jackson, S. (2000). Negative and positive health effects of caring for a disabled spouse: Longitudinal findings from the caregiver health effects study. *Psychology and Aging*, 15(2), 259–271. https://doi.org/10.1037/0882-7974.15.2.259

Bodnar, J. C., & Kiecolt-Glaser, J. K. (1994). Caregiver depression after bereavement: Chronic stress isn't over when it's over. *Psychology and Aging*, 9(3), 372–380. https://doi.org/10.1037/0882-7974.9.3.372

Boeije, H. R. (2002). A purposeful approach to the constant comparative method in the analysis of qualitative interviews. *Quality and Quantity, 36*, 391–409. https://doi.org/10.1023/A:1020909529486

Carr, D., Boerner, K., & Moorman, S. N. (2020). Bereavement in the time of coronavirus: Unprecedented challenges demand novel interventions. *Journal of Aging & Social Policy, 32* (4–5), 425–431. https://doi.org/10.1080/08959420.2020.1764320

Carter, P. A. (2005). Bereaved caregivers' descriptions of sleep: Impact on daily life and the bereavement process. *Oncology Nursing Forum, 32*(4), E70–75. https://doi.org/10.1188/05.ONF.E70-E75

Centers for Disease Control and Prevention. (2020). *Coronavirus disease 2019 (COVID-19): Supporting your care recipient in a long-term care facility.* https://www.cdc.gov/coronavirus/2019-ncov/downloads/supporting-loved-one-in-long-term-care-facility.pdf

Centers for Medicare and Medicaid Services. (2020, December). *Toolkit on state actions to mitigate COVID-19 prevalence in nursing homes (version 16).* U.S. Department of Health and Human Services. https://www.cms.gov/files/document/covid-toolkit-states-mitigate-covid-19-nursing-homes.pdf

Chu, C. H., Donato-Woodger, S., & Dainton, C. J. (2020). Competing crises: COVID-19 countermeasures and social isolation among older adults in long-term care. *Journal of Advanced Nursing, 76*(10), 2456–2459. https://doi.org/10.1111/jan.14467

Corey, K. L., & McCurry, M. K. (2018). When caregiving ends: The experiences of former family caregivers of people with dementia. *The Gerontologist, 58*(2), e87–e96. https://doi.org/10.1093/geront/gnw205

Dong, X., Simon, M., Mendes de Leon, C., Fulmer, T., Beck, T., Hebert, L., Dyer, C., Paveza, G., & Evans, D. (2009). Elder self-neglect and abuse and mortality risk in a community-dwelling population. *Journal of American Medical Association, 302*(5), 517–526. https://doi.org/10.1001/jama.2009.1109

Greenberg, N., Docherty, M., Gnanapragasam, S., & Wessely, S. (2020). Managing mental health challenges faced by healthcare workers during COVID-19 pandemic. *BMJ, 368*, 1–4. https://doi.org/10.1136/bmj.m1211

Guest, G., MacQueen, K. M., & Namey, E. E. (2012). *Applied thematic analysis.* Sage Publications.

Holt-Lunstad, J., Smith, T. B., Baker, M., Harris, T., & Stephenson, D. (2015). Loneliness and social isolation as risk factors for mortality: A meta-analytic review. *Perspectives on Psychological Science, 10*(2), 227–237. https://doi.org/10.1177/1745691614568352

Institute of Medicine. (2001). *Crossing the quality chasm: A new health system for the 21st century.* The National Academies Press. https://doi.org/10.17226/10027

Lincoln, Y. S., & Guba, E. G. (1985). *Naturalistic inquiry.* Sage Publications.

Markowitz, A. (2020, October 30). *When can visitors return to nursing homes?* AARP. https://www.aarp.org/caregiving/health/info-2020/nursing-home-visits-after-coronavirus.html)/

McGilton, K. S., Escrig-Pinol, A., Gordon, A., Chu, C. H., Zuniga, F., Sanchez, M. G., Boscart, V., Meyer, J., Corazzini, K. N., Jacinto, A. F., Spilsbury, K., Backman, A., Scales, K., Fagertun, A., Wu, B., Edvardsson, D., Lepore, M. J., Leung, A. Y. M., Siegel, E. O., Noguchi-Watanabe, M., ... Bowers, B. (2020). Uncovering the devaluation of nursing home staff during COVID-19: Are we fuelling the next health care crisis? *Journal of the American Medical Directors Association, 21*(7), 962–965. https://doi.org/10.1016/j.jamda.2020.06.010

National Academies of Sciences, Engineering, and Medicine. (2020). *Social isolation and loneliness in older adults: Opportunities for the health care system.* The National Academies Press. https://doi.org/10.17226/25663

National Association of Chronic Disease Directors. (2018). *Caregiving for family and friends – A public health issue.* Centers for Disease Control and Prevention. https://www.cdc.gov/aging/agingdata/docs/caregiver-brief-508.pdf

Pantell, M., Rehkopf, D., Jutte, D., Syme, S. L., Balmes, J., & Adler, N. (2013). Social isolation: A predictor of mortality comparable to traditional clinical risk factors. *American Journal of Public Health, 103*(11), 2056–2062. https://doi.org/10.2105/AJPH.2013.301261

Picot, S. J. (1994). Choice and social exchange theory and the rewards of African American caregivers. *Journal of National Black Nurses' Association, 7*(2), 29–40. PMID: 9128531.

Quality, Safety and Oversight Group. (2020, September 28). *Guidance for infection control and prevention of coronavirus disease 2019 (COVID-19) in nursing homes (Ref: QSO-20-14-NH).* U.S. Department of Health and Human Services, Centers for Medicare and Medicaid Services. https://www.cms.gov/files/document/qso-20-14-nh-revised.pdf

Simard, J., & Volicer, L. (2020). Loneliness and isolation in long-term care and the COVID-19 pandemic. *Journal of the American Medical Directors Association, 21*(7), 966–967. https://doi.org/10.1016/j.jamda.2020.05.006

Soergel, A. (2020, December 16). *Track the status of nursing home visits in your state.* AARP (American Association of Retired Persons). https://www.aarp.org/caregiving/health/info-2020/nursing-home-visits-by-state.html

Tweedy, M. P., & Guarnaccia, C. A. (2008). Change in depression of spousal caregivers of dementia patients following patient's death. *OMEGA, 56*(3), 217–228. https://doi.org/10.2190/OM.56.3.a

Wolff, J. L., Dy, S. M., Frick, K. D., & Kasper, J. D. (2007). End-of-life care: Findings from a national survey of informal caregivers. *Archives of Internal Medicine, 167*(1), 40–46. https://doi.org/10.1001/archinte.167.1.40

Long-Term Care System Impacts

Prevalence of COVID-19 in Ohio Nursing Homes: What's Quality Got to Do with It?

John Bowblis and Robert Applebaum

ABSTRACT

With nursing homes being hit hard by the COVID-19 pandemic, it is important to know whether facilities that have any cases, or those with particularly high caseloads, are different from nursing homes that do not have any reported cases. Our analysis found that through mid-June, just under one-third of nursing homes in Ohio had at least one resident with COVID-19, with over 82% of all cases in the state coming from 37% of nursing homes. Overall findings on the association between facility quality and the prevalence of COVID-19 showed that having any resident case of the virus or even having a high caseload of residents with the virus is not more likely in nursing homes with lower quality ratings.

Introduction

Almost every day across the nation, news stories describe the high rates of COVID-19 being reported in our nation's nursing homes (New York Times, Washington Post, Huffington Post). In Ohio, almost one-half (46%) of all deaths in the state from COVID-19 occurred in nursing homes (Ohio Department of Health, COVID-19 Dashboard, May 20, 2020). For many experts the higher prevalence rates and associated deaths in nursing homes are not necessarily a surprise. Nursing home residents are among the frailest members of U.S. society. Nursing homes are primarily staffed with a direct care workforce who do not have the luxury of being able to social distance either in their commute to work, or once on the job as nursing home care is a high touch intervention. Combining these factors with an initial shortage of personal protection equipment in nursing homes highlights the vulnerability of nursing home residents and staff.

The media coverage about the impact of COVID-19 on nursing home residents has included differing perspectives. Some media stories have concluded that the high nursing home prevalence and the subsequent death rate are not a surprise and is driven by who nursing homes care for rather than individual provider quality (Associated press with Yu & Felman, 2020 and Dayton daily news with Schroeder, 2020). Others have raised questions about whether facilities with lower quality have higher COVID-19 prevalence (Nonprofit quarterly (Kahn, 2020); NPR (Jaffe, 2020); New York Times (Goldstein et al., 2020) & Los Angeles Times (Dolan & Mejia, 2020)). Although there is no shortage of media stories about the impacts of COVID-19 on nursing home residents, there have been only a limited number of peer-reviewed papers about this topic and very little work linking prevalence and quality (Applegate & Ouslander, 2020; Grabowski & Joynt Maddox, 2020; Li et al., 2020; Tan & Seetharaman, 2020).

Examining just released COVID-19 prevalence data in Ohio nursing homes, this work asks whether the presence of COVID-19 cases in nursing homes is associated with facility quality after controlling for other factors that may be associated with exposure to the virus, such as being located in an urban environment. To examine this question, we combined data on COVID-19 nursing home residents reported by the Ohio Department of Health (ODH) with the latest data on facility quality. We examine reports from multiple months in order to examine how the experience of COVID-19 in nursing homes changed throughout the pandemic.

Method

Data

Multiple sources of data were used to construct the analytic sample. The cumulative number of residents infected by COVID-19 in each nursing home came from the Ohio Department of Health. Each nursing home is mandated by the State of Ohio to report the number of coronavirus cases in long-term care facilities to the county's health department. This information is then forwarded to the ODH, which aggregates and publishes this information weekly. The cumulative number of resident cases in each weekly report represents the number of resident cases recorded from April 15, 2020. We utilized the weekly reports released on April 28, May 14, and June 17 for this analysis.

The ODH resident data were merged with two publicly available sources from the Centers for Medicare and Medicaid Services [CMS]. The first of these datasets is the February 2020 monthly Nursing Home Compare archive database. The archive contains summary information about each nursing home, including select measures of facility structure (e.g., ownership, number of beds), nursing staff levels, substantiated complaints, health deficiencies, and Nursing Home Compare star ratings. This information is updated regularly by CMS and it contains the most recent publicly available information regarding facilities. The second of these datasets is the Payroll-Based Journaling (PBJ) data from the third quarter of 2019. The PBJ data contains daily information regarding nursing home staff and we utilized this data to calculate the proportion of agency nursing staff utilized by the facility in the third quarter of 2019. To capture rurality, we merged the CMS public datasets with rural-urban commuting area (RUCA) based on zip code (WWAMI Rural Health Research Center, 2020).

A limitation of the public CMS datasets is the lack of information about the residents in the facility during or just prior to the pandemic. To capture a snapshot of each facility's payer-mix and resident case-mix prior to the pandemic, data were included from the Certification and Survey Provider Enhanced Reporting (CASPER) system. CASPER includes data collected as part of initial and annual recertification inspections of all Medicare and Medicaid certified nursing homes, with these inspections occurring every 9 to 15 months. Because CASPER is available with a lag, we utilized the most recent inspection for each facility that occurred from August 2018 through October 2019 (with a median date of March 28th, 2019). We also incorporated information on racial/ethnic composition of the nursing home from the Minimum Data Set from calendar year 2017.

After merging all of these datasets, our analytic sample included all 942 nursing homes in Ohio that were certified for Medicare and/or Medicaid that were operating as of February 2020. This sample excluded hospital-based units. Because some nursing homes did not report staffing data in the publicly available CMS datasets, our regression analyses were restricted to a sample of 921 that did not have missing information for staffing covariates. These 21 excluded facilities were not statistically different from facilities included in the regression analyses.

Dependent variables

The Ohio Department of Health data reported the number of cumulative resident cases of COVID-19 that have occurred since April 15. From this information, we constructed two dependent variables. The first dependent variable was a binary indicator for whether the nursing home had at least one resident case of COVID-19. This dependent variable measures how many nursing homes had the virus confirmed in their resident population.

The second dependent variable measured the spread of the virus within a nursing home. Among nursing homes with at least one case, we constructed a binary measure for whether the nursing home had a high number of COVID-19 cases. The definition of a high number of cases is having a cumulative number of resident cases that are equal to or greater than 20% of the number of licensed beds in the facility (i.e., having at least 2 cases per every 10 beds). We utilized a case per bed metric because utilizing number of cases does not account for larger facilities having more residents that could be exposed to the virus. Furthermore, we utilized the licensed beds as the denominator because we do not know the number of residents in the facility at the start of the pandemic or how many residents were admitted to the nursing home during the pandemic. Finally, because there is likely measurement error as testing is imprecise and we do not really know the number of unique residents that could have been exposed to the virus, our measure of high vs. low caseload is less likely to suffer from measurement error.

Nursing staff and quality measures

In one set of regression analyses, the key explanatory variables of interest are measures of nursing staff and quality. Nursing staffing levels are measured in hours per resident day (HPRD) of registered nurses, licensed practical nurses, and certified nurse aides. HPRD reflects the number of hours per resident staff that is available to care for residents and perform administrative duties. Because this information is obtained from the monthly Nursing Home Compare archives, registered nurses include those with administrative duties and certified nurse aides include medication assistants (Centers for Medicare and Medicaid Services [CMS], 2019). One theory for COVID-19 spread is that staff may be treating residents at multiple facilities. This pattern is most likely to occur if a facility is utilizing temporary staff that provides services to multiple nursing homes. Measures of temporary staff, also called agency or contracted staff, were included in two ways in our model: the percentage of agency staff (Specification 1) and the use of any agency staff (Specification 2). We utilized both measures because less than half of nursing homes use agency staff, but for the nursing homes that use agency staff, the proportion can be skewed.

To measure quality, we include two variables that reflect nursing home quality via the regulatory process. The first of these was the number of substantiated complaints. The second was the deficiency score the facility received in their most recent recertification inspection. These measures were obtained from the Nursing Home Compare archives.

In a second set of regression analyses, we examined quality as measured by the overall 5-star rating of the facility because the overall 5-star rating is a metric of quality commonly cited in recent news reports. The overall 5-star rating is a composite measure of quality computed by CMS that ranges from 1 (lowest quality) to 5 (highest quality). This composite measure combines quality information from deficiencies issues during state recertification and complaint inspections, nursing staff levels, and quality indicators calculated from other administrative datasets (CMS, 2019). For this reason, when the overall 5-star rating is included in the model, the nursing staff and quality measures described in this section are not included as covariates. The overall

5-star rating is utilized is each facility's rating reported on the Nursing Home Compare website as of February 2020.

Additional covariates

In all regression analyses, we include four sets of additional covariates. The first of these is facility structure. Facility structure includes the number of beds (measured in increments of 10), ownership, chain affiliation, being part of a continuing care retirement community (CCRC), and having a dementia or other special care unit. It is our expectation that larger facilities may have greater risk of having any case and having a high number of cases as they require more staff and cross-contamination across units may be easier. Research also suggests that for-profit nursing homes have lower quality (Grabowski et al., 2013), and we may find this to be associated with COVID-19 cases. Chain affiliated nursing homes may have more COVID-19 cases because the facility is sharing staff across locations or they have greater resources to obtain testing.

The second and third sets of covariates were primarily obtained from CASPER and included measures of financial resources (e.g., occupancy and payer-mix) and resident case-mix prior to the pandemic. Facilities with higher occupancy rates may have greater risk of COVID-19 spread, but at the same time have more financial resources for testing and identifying residents with COVID-19. Similarly, Medicare reimbursement rates and charges to private pay residents are significantly higher than Medicaid, affecting financial resources to identify and prevent the virus. Resident population and case-mix may also have an effect on outcomes if certain residents are more susceptible to the virus. Nursing homes that have a greater share of residents who are Black, Indigenous, or other Persons of Color (BIPOC) may be at greater risk for COVID-19 (Shippee et al., 2020). Therefore, we included the proportion of BIPOC residents constructed from newly admitted residents in the 2017 Minimum data set. For the few facilities that this could not be calculated, these nursing homes were coded as 0 for the racial/ethnic composition variable and identified with an indicator variable for missing race/ethnicity information. Measures of resident case-mix include an Activities of Daily Living Score, as well as the percentage of residents with dementia, serious mental illness, depression, and developmental disabilities.

Finally, because COVID-19 is more common in urban areas, we included a measure of rurality. In particular, we utilized Categorization B from the WWAMI Rural Health Research Center (2020) which defines a zip code as being an urban metropolitan area, micropolitan (i.e., rural city), and a small or isolated small rural town (i.e., rural).

Analytic approach

Separate analyses were conducted using the number of cumulative cases in the April 28, May 14, and June 17 reports. The purpose of examining multiple reports is the April 28 report reflects the status in an earlier phase of the pandemic, when concerns regarding the virus in nursing homes were attracting additional national attention. The May 14 report reflects the more intermediate term as these concerns turned into policies and action. The June 17 report reflects the state of pandemic during a period when nursing home visitation was still restricted, but our knowledge regarding the risk to nursing home residents was better known. For each report, our analytic approach started with utilizing information from the 942 freestanding nursing homes in Ohio to describe the distribution of residents with COVID-19 in the state.

To understand which factors predict having at least one resident with COVID 19, and among nursing homes with at least one resident case, whether the facility had a high number of residents with COVID-19, defined as 20% or higher of licensed beds, we estimated logit regressions. The analytic sample includes the 921 nursing homes that have information for all covariates. In our initial set of regression analyses, each logit model included nursing staff, the two quality measures of number of substantiated complaints and deficiency score, as well as other covariates described earlier. We estimated two specifications based on how agency staff are included in the model. In our second set of regression analyses, we examined whether there was an association between COVID-19 and the composite indicator of facility quality as measured by the overall 5-star rating. This regression analysis included all the covariates as the initial specification, except the nursing staff variables and the two individual quality measures. Nursing staff and the two deficiency quality measures were excluded because they are used in calculating the overall 5-star rating.

To make the interpretation of the logit models easier, all coefficient estimates were converted to marginal effects. Also, standard errors were adjusted to account for the clustering of nursing homes within counties. The county is the appropriate unit of clustering because COVID-19 information is first handled by the county health department before being forward to the state-level.

Results

Results presented in Table 1 show the cumulative number of residents with COVID-19 as reported by the Ohio Department of Health on April 28, May 14, and June 17. In the April 28 report, there were 1,873 nursing home residents in 138 (14.6%) facilities that tested positive for COVID-19 out of 942 facilities. The May 14 report had 3,607 nursing home residents testing positive in 187 (19.9%) facilities. Consistent with an expansion of the virus into more

Table 1. COVID-19 prevalence in Ohio: Number of nursing homes and residents.

Number of Cases	Number of Nursing Homes	% of Nursing Homes in State	% of Nursing Homes With Cases	% of Resident Cases
Panel A: Cumulative Cases in the April 28th Report				
1	24	2.5%	17.4%	1.3%
2 to 3	25	2.7%	18.1%	3.4%
4 to 5	12	1.3%	8.7%	2.9%
6 to 10	19	2.0%	13.8%	7.5%
11 to 19	24	2.5%	17.4%	19.6%
20+	34	3.6%	24.6%	65.3%
Any Case	138	14.6%	100.0%	100.0%
Panel B: Cumulative Cases in the May 14th Report				
1	26	2.8%	13.9%	0.7%
2 to 3	26	2.8%	13.9%	1.8%
4 to 5	14	1.5%	7.5%	1.7%
6 to 10	22	2.3%	11.8%	4.4%
11 to 19	32	3.4%	17.1%	13.0%
20+	67	7.1%	35.8%	78.3%
Any Case	187	19.9%	100.0%	100.0%
Panel C: Cumulative Cases in the June 17th Report				
1	64	6.8%	21.9%	1.1%
2 to 3	37	3.9%	12.7%	1.6%
4 to 5	18	1.9%	6.2%	1.4%
6 to 10	28	3.0%	9.6%	3.8%
11 to 19	38	4.0%	13.0%	10.3%
20+	107	11.4%	36.6%	81.9%
Any Case	292	31.0%	100.0%	100.0%

Information is based on data reported to Ohio Department of Health and released to the public on April 28, May 14, and June 17, 2020. The Ohio Department of Health notes that the number of cumulative cases are preliminary and reflect the cumulative cases since April 15, 2020. Data is restricted to all free-standing nursing homes in the state that where resident cases at "nursing homes" that could be identified and merged with archived Nursing Home Compare data for February 2020, Payroll-based Journaling Data, and their most recent CASPER survey.

facilities as the pandemic progressed, the June 17 report had 5,714 resident testing positive in 292 (31.0%) facilities. There was also expansion in intensity among nursing homes that had at least one resident case of the virus. In the April 28 report, facilities with 1 to 5 residents with COVID-19 made up 44% of nursing homes with at least one case, accounting for 7.6% of cases. By the June 17 reports, this decreased to 31% of nursing homes and 4.1% of cases. The growth in the intensity of virus is most evident among nursing homes with 20 or more residents with COVID-19. In the April 28 report, these facilities comprised 25% of all nursing homes with at least one case but 65.3% of resident cases. In contrast, by the May 14 and June 17 reports, nursing homes with 20 or more cases made up 35.8% and 36.6% of facilities and 78.3% and 81.9% of residents with COVID-19, respectively.

To gain a better understanding of the impact of COVID-19 in Ohio nursing homes we examined prevalence in the context of various facility and pre-pandemic resident characteristics. Table 2 reports the summary statistics and the marginal effects for our initial regression analyses associated with having at

Table 2. Summary statistics and factors associated with having at least one resident with COVID-19.

	Summary Statistics	April 28th Report		May 14th Report		June 17th Report	
		Spec. 1	Spec. 2	Spec. 1	Spec. 2	Spec. 1	Spec. 2
Summary Statistics of Dependent Variable		0.147 (0.354)		0.200 (0.400)		0.311 (0.463)	
Facility Structure							
Number of Beds (10s)	9.236 (4.025)	-0.004 (0.003)	-0.004 (0.003)	-0.002 (0.003)	-0.002 (0.003)	0.004 (0.004)	0.004 (0.004)
Government Ownership (Ref = For-profit)	0.016 (0.127)	-0.028 (0.133)	-0.029 (0.136)	0.104 (0.102)	0.100 (0.106)	0.311** (0.136)	0.307** (0.139)
Not-for-profit Ownership (Ref = For-profit)	0.190 (0.393)	-0.027 (0.039)	-0.018 (0.042)	-0.078** (0.039)	-0.067 (0.041)	-0.051 (0.040)	-0.053 (0.042)
Chain Affiliated	0.701 (0.458)	0.061** (0.026)	0.061** (0.027)	0.111*** (0.026)	0.110*** (0.027)	0.094*** (0.031)	0.095*** (0.032)
Continuing Care Retirement Community	0.157 (0.364)	-0.005 (0.035)	-0.008 (0.034)	0.024 (0.036)	0.021 (0.037)	0.020 (0.037)	0.019 (0.038)
Dementia Special Care Unit	0.269 (0.444)	0.036* (0.022)	0.037* (0.021)	0.052** (0.026)	0.052** (0.026)	0.040 (0.031)	0.037 (0.031)
Other Special Care Unit	0.117 (0.322)	0.011 (0.030)	0.004 (0.030)	-0.015 (0.036)	-0.022 (0.036)	0.028 (0.038)	0.026 (0.037)
Prior Occupancy and Payer-mix							
Occupancy Rate	82.377 (12.737)	-0.000 (0.001)	-0.000 (0.001)	-0.000 (0.001)	-0.000 (0.001)	0.002 (0.001)	0.002 (0.001)
% Medicaid (Ref = % Private Pay/Other)	59.924 (20.063)	0.000 (0.001)	0.000 (0.001)	0.001 (0.001)	0.001 (0.001)	0.000 (0.001)	0.000 (0.001)
% Medicare (Ref = % Private Pay/Other)	10.075 (10.373)	-0.002 (0.002)	-0.002 (0.002)	-0.002 (0.002)	-0.003 (0.002)	-0.000 (0.002)	-0.000 (0.002)
Prior Resident Population and Case-Mix							
% of BIPOC Residents	12.691 (19.068)	0.001 (0.001)	0.001 (0.001)	0.002* (0.001)	0.001* (0.001)	0.003*** (0.001)	0.003*** (0.001)
Activities of Daily Living Score	10.121 (0.999)	-0.008 (0.011)	-0.009 (0.011)	0.001 (0.016)	0.000 (0.016)	-0.003 (0.018)	-0.005 (0.018)
% Dementia	43.580 (15.143)	0.000 (0.001)	0.000 (0.001)	0.000 (0.001)	0.000 (0.001)	-0.000 (0.001)	-0.000 (0.001)
% Serious Mental Illness	41.607 (18.005)	-0.000 (0.001)	-0.000 (0.001)	-0.001 (0.001)	-0.001 (0.001)	-0.000 (0.001)	-0.000 (0.001)
% Depression	52.695 (21.629)	-0.001* (0.001)	-0.001* (0.001)	-0.001 (0.001)	-0.001 (0.001)	-0.002** (0.001)	-0.002** (0.001)
% Intellectual Disability	1.974 (3.614)	0.002 (0.003)	0.001 (0.002)	0.001 (0.003)	0.001 (0.003)	-0.002 (0.004)	-0.002 (0.004)

(Continued)

Table 2. (Continued).

	Summary Statistics	April 28th Report		May 14th Report		June 17th Report	
		Spec. 1	Spec. 2	Spec. 1	Spec. 2	Spec. 1	Spec. 2
Nursing Staff							
Registered Nurse HPRD	0.601	0.091	0.103*	0.195***	0.208***	0.153**	0.161**
	(0.281)	(0.059)	(0.056)	(0.050)	(0.050)	(0.070)	(0.070)
Licensed Nurse HPRD	0.930	0.104**	0.103**	0.089**	0.090**	0.091*	0.091*
	(0.273)	(0.052)	(0.051)	(0.040)	(0.041)	(0.050)	(0.050)
Certified Nurse Aides HPRD	2.076	-0.016	-0.024	0.004	-0.003	0.008	0.004
	(0.460)	(0.030)	(0.028)	(0.033)	(0.032)	(0.044)	(0.042)
Agency Registered Nurses (%)	1.920	-0.009**		-0.006***		-0.003	
	(6.145)	(0.004)		(0.002)		(0.002)	
Agency Registered Nurses (Any)	0.322		-0.023		-0.031		-0.040
	(0.468)		(0.026)		(0.025)		(0.026)
Agency Licensed Practical Nurses (%)	3.031	0.005***		0.003*		0.001	
	(7.585)	(0.002)		(0.002)		(0.002)	
Agency Licensed Practical Nurses (Any)	0.319		0.057		0.056		0.072
	(0.466)		(0.040)		(0.035)		(0.059)
Agency Certified Nurse Aides (%)	3.225	-0.001		0.001		0.001	
	(7.532)	(0.002)		(0.002)		(0.002)	
Agency Certified Nurse Aides (Any)	0.308		-0.055*		-0.054*		-0.018
	(0.462)		(0.030)		(0.028)		(0.041)
Indicators of Quality							
Number of Substantiated Complaints	3.976	0.002	0.002	0.001	0.001	0.001	0.001
	(5.744)	(0.002)	(0.002)	(0.002)	(0.002)	(0.003)	(0.003)
Deficiency Score	59.667	-0.000	-0.000	0.000	0.000	-0.000	-0.000
	(69.025)	(0.000)	(0.000)	(0.000)	(0.000)	(0.000)	(0.000)
Rurality							
Micropolitan	0.186	-0.144***	-0.141***	-0.180***	-0.178***	-0.164***	-0.160***
	(0.389)	(0.043)	(0.043)	(0.053)	(0.054)	(0.059)	(0.060)
Rural	0.100	-0.127**	-0.132**	-0.129**	-0.134**	-0.117**	-0.118**
	(0.300)	(0.058)	(0.058)	(0.058)	(0.058)	(0.057)	(0.057)
Sample size	921	921	921	921	921	921	921

The first column reports summary statistics as the mean and standard deviation in parentheses. All other columns report marginal effects for a logit regression with a dependent variable of having at least one resident case reported by the public release of data reported in each column. This logit model includes all covariates in the table plus an indicator variable for observation in which the the % of BIPOC residents could not be calculated. There are two model specifications. Specification 1 includes the % of agency nursing staff. Specification 2 includes an indicator for any agency nursing staff. Marginal effects are evaluated at the mean and all standard errors are reported in parentheses and are adjusted for clustering of nursing homes within counties.

HPRD = Hours Per Resident Day; BIPOC = Black, Indigenous, and Persons of Color.

*** $p < 0.01$; ** $p < 0.05$; * $p < 0.10$

least one resident test positive for COVID-19 in the three reports. Among facility structure covariates, the only effect that is statistically significant in all specifications is chain affiliation. Compared to independent facilities, chains are associated with an increased likelihood of having at least one resident with the virus (6.1–11.1% points depending on the report). A facility having a dementia special care unit increased the probability of having a resident with the virus in the first two reports, but the effect was no longer statistically significant in the June 17 report. Occupancy, payer-mix, and most resident case-mix covariates prior to the pandemic have no statistically significant association on having a resident with the virus. Facilities with a greater proportion of BIPOC residents initially did not have a higher probability of having a resident with the virus, but this changed as the pandemic progressed. By the June 17 report, a 10% increase in the proportion of BIPOC residents was associated with a 3% point increase in having at least one resident with the virus.

Generally, higher staffing levels are associated with a higher probability of having at least one resident test positive for the virus, while we find mixed associations with the use of agency staff. For example, a greater proportion of agency-registered nurses decreases the likelihood of having a resident with the virus whereas a greater proportion of licensed practical nurses increases the likelihood in the first two reports. Moreover, the marginal effects for using any agency registered and licensed practical nurses are not statistically significant, but the use of any agency certified nurse aides is associated with a reduced likelihood of having a resident with COVID-19 in the first two reports. None of the agency staff variables were found to be statistically significant in the June 17 report. Overall, we find no consistent effects for these covariates. As expected, nursing homes in rural areas, including rural cities, were less likely to have a resident with COVID-19. Finally, indicators of quality are not associated with having a resident in the facility with COVID-19.

The marginal effects of the initial regression analyses on facilities reporting a high number of residents with COVID-19 (defined as having a cumulative number of cases that exceeds 20% of total beds) among nursing homes with at least one case are reported in Table 3. While there are a number of covariates that are statistically significant, the covariates that are statistically significant in the April 28 report are generally not significant in the May 14 or June 17 report and vice versa. The only exception is facilities with more beds are less likely to report a high number of cases in the May 14 and June 17 reports. There is no statistically significant association between rurality and having a high number of cases.

Finally, to further link COVID-19 cases and quality we examined the association between resident infections and the overall Nursing Home Compare Five-Star Rating (Table 4) after controlling for facility structural, occupancy and payer-mix, resident and case-mix characteristics, and rurality.

Table 3. Factors associated with having a high number of residents with COVID-19 in facilities with a case.

	April 28th Report		May 14th Report		June 17th Report	
	Spec. 1	Spec. 2	Spec. 1	Spec. 2	Spec. 1	Spec. 2
Summary Statistics of Dependent Variable	0.263		0.432		0.409	
	(0.442)		(0.497)		(0.493)	
Facility Structure						
Number of Beds (10s)	−0.012	−0.013	−0.025**	−0.028**	−0.032***	−0.033***
	(0.010)	(0.009)	(0.012)	(0.014)	(0.007)	(0.008)
Government Ownership (Ref = For-profit)			0.446*	0.463*	0.307	0.303
			(0.247)	(0.246)	(0.212)	(0.199)
Not-for-profit Ownership (Ref = For-profit)	0.064	0.006	0.106	0.071	−0.075	−0.081
	(0.107)	(0.119)	(0.099)	(0.106)	(0.067)	(0.080)
Chain Affiliated	−0.139	−0.105	0.037	0.050	0.100*	0.101*
	(0.098)	(0.102)	(0.086)	(0.088)	(0.051)	(0.056)
Continuing Care Retirement Community	0.058	0.020	−0.062	−0.070	0.113	0.102
	(0.090)	(0.095)	(0.162)	(0.155)	(0.084)	(0.076)
Dementia Special Care Unit	−0.254***	−0.225***	0.017	0.020	0.056	0.067
	(0.074)	(0.082)	(0.083)	(0.087)	(0.079)	(0.077)
Other Special Care Unit	−0.313*	−0.317*	−0.051	−0.041	−0.111	−0.116
	(0.171)	(0.172)	(0.151)	(0.142)	(0.090)	(0.090)
Prior Occupancy and Payer-mix						
Occupancy Rate	0.004	0.003	0.002	0.002	−0.000	−0.000
	(0.003)	(0.003)	(0.003)	(0.003)	(0.002)	(0.002)
% Medicaid (Ref = % Private Pay/Other)	−0.002	−0.002	−0.001	−0.001	−0.001	−0.001
	(0.003)	(0.003)	(0.003)	(0.003)	(0.003)	(0.003)
% Medicare (Ref = % Private Pay/Other)	0.006	0.006	0.008	0.007	0.001	−0.000
	(0.006)	(0.005)	(0.005)	(0.005)	(0.004)	(0.004)
Prior Resident Population and Case-Mix						
% of BIPOC Residents	−0.001	−0.001	−0.000	−0.000	0.000	−0.000
	(0.002)	(0.002)	(0.002)	(0.001)	(0.001)	(0.001)
Activities of Daily Living Score	0.030	0.024	0.041	0.034	0.051**	0.047**
	(0.040)	(0.038)	(0.041)	(0.040)	(0.024)	(0.024)
% Dementia	−0.000	−0.001	0.002	0.002	−0.002	−0.002
	(0.003)	(0.003)	(0.002)	(0.002)	(0.002)	(0.002)
% Serious Mental Illness	0.005*	0.004	0.004	0.004	0.004	0.004
	(0.003)	(0.003)	(0.003)	(0.003)	(0.003)	(0.003)
% Depression	0.003*	0.002	−0.001	−0.001	−0.001	−0.000
	(0.002)	(0.002)	(0.002)	(0.002)	(0.002)	(0.002)
% Intellectual Disability	−0.029	−0.034	−0.004	−0.007	−0.005	−0.007
	(0.021)	(0.022)	(0.019)	(0.020)	(0.014)	(0.014)
Nursing Staff						
Registered Nurse HPRD	−0.121	−0.084	−0.305	−0.292	−0.082	−0.055
	(0.201)	(0.188)	(0.211)	(0.211)	(0.115)	(0.115)
Licensed Nurse HPRD	0.162	0.145	0.119	0.109	−0.011	−0.016
	(0.105)	(0.101)	(0.119)	(0.116)	(0.104)	(0.104)
Certified Nurse Aides HPRD	−0.161*	−0.161	−0.058	−0.063	−0.029	−0.029
	(0.096)	(0.103)	(0.080)	(0.083)	(0.054)	(0.054)
Agency Registered Nurses (%)	−0.011		−0.007		−0.006	
	(0.025)		(0.008)		(0.005)	
Agency Registered Nurses (Any)		−0.018		−0.052		−0.038
		(0.084)		(0.102)		(0.073)
Agency Licensed Practical Nurses (%)	0.006		0.005		0.005	
	(0.005)		(0.004)		(0.005)	
Agency Licensed Practical Nurses (Any)		−0.048		0.024		−0.024
		(0.127)		(0.115)		(0.107)

(Continued)

Table 3. (Continued).

	April 28th Report		May 14th Report		June 17th Report	
	Spec. 1	Spec. 2	Spec. 1	Spec. 2	Spec. 1	Spec. 2
Agency Certified Nurse Aides (%)	−0.011		−0.003		−0.004	
	(0.008)		(0.005)		(0.005)	
Agency Certified Nurse Aides (Any)		0.000		0.061		0.016
		(0.095)		(0.110)		(0.066)
Indicators of Quality						
Number of Substantiated Complaints	0.004	0.003	0.012*	0.012*	0.001	0.001
	(0.004)	(0.005)	(0.007)	(0.007)	(0.006)	(0.006)
Deficiency Score	−0.001	−0.001	−0.000	−0.000	0.001	0.001
	(0.001)	(0.001)	(0.001)	(0.001)	(0.001)	(0.001)
Rurality						
Micropolitan	−0.019	−0.018	0.223	0.215	−0.041	−0.046
	(0.128)	(0.120)	(0.161)	(0.168)	(0.104)	(0.107)
Rural	0.026	0.027	−0.027	−0.023	−0.120	−0.129
	(0.196)	(0.202)	(0.190)	(0.191)	(0.129)	(0.131)
Sample size	133	133	183	183	286	286

The table reports marginal effects of a logit regression with a dependent variable of having a high number of cases (defined as number of cases equal to at least 20% of beds) among facilities with at least one case. This logit model includes all covariates in the table plus an indicator variable for observation in which the % of BIPOC residents could not be calculated. There are two model specifications. Specification 1 includes the % of agency nursing staff. Specification 2 includes an indicator for any agency nursing staff. Marginal effects are evaluated at the mean and all standard errors are reported in parentheses and are adjusted for clustering of nursing homes within counties. HPRD = Hours Per Resident Day; BIPOC = Black, Indigenous, and Persons of Color.
*** $p < 0.01$; ** $p < 0.05$; * $p < 0.10$

Table 4. Overall 5-star ratings and nursing homes with COVID-19 residents.

	% Point Difference Relative to 1-Star Facilities			
	2-star	3-star	4-star	5-star
Panel A: Nursing Homes Having at Least One Resident COVID-19 Case				
April 28th Report	0.025	0.045*	0.031	0.071**
May 14th Report	0.008	0.046	0.047	0.050
June 17th Report	0.029	0.070	0.106**	0.089*
Panel B: Nursing Homes with High Number of Cases Among Nursing Homes with at Least One Case				
April 28th Report	−0.072	−0.133	0.124	−0.178*
May 14th Report	0.031	−0.038	0.084	−0.137
June 17th Report	−0.002	−0.028	0.082	−0.006

Relative to 1-star nursing homes, the table reports the % point difference in the probability of the facility having at least 1 resident COVID-19 case and among facilities with at least one case, the probability of having a high number of cases (defined as number of cases equal to at least 20% of beds) based on the facility's overall 5-star rating. These differences in probabilities were calculated based on the number of cumulative cases reported on April 28, May 14, and June 17, 2020. All statistics reports were estimated from logit models that controlled for ownership, chain affiliation, being part of a continuing care retirement community, presence of special care units, prior occupancy rate, payer-mix, race/ethnic composition of the facility, case-mix, and rurality. All statistical tests are adjusted for clustering of nursing homes within counties.
*** $p < 0.01$; ** $p < 0.05$; * $p < 0.10$

Compared to 1-star facilities, Panel A reports the difference in the probability in percentage points (measured 0–1) of having at least one resident with COVID 19. In the regressions for having at least one case, all of the coefficient estimates are positive, though only some are statistically significant. These results show that nursing homes with higher overall star ratings have a higher probability or are not statistically different from 1-star facilities in the probability of having at least one resident with the virus. In fact, by the June 17 report, facilities with 4 and 5-star are between 8.9% and 10.6% points more likely to report having a resident with the virus than a 1-star nursing home. Panel B of Table 4 reports the difference in the probability of having a high proportion of cases relative to 1-star facilities. Among the facilities with at least one case, 5-star rated nursing homes were less likely to report a high caseload, but this was only significant at the 10% level. All other coefficient estimates reported are not statistically significant. In summary, there is not a statistically significant association between having a higher overall 5-star rating and better COVID-19 outcomes (i.e., less likely to have a case and if a case is present, having a lower caseload).

Discussion

There is no question that residential long-term service settings face considerable challenges in efforts to control COVID-19. Currently, about one in three Ohio nursing homes have at least one resident with coronavirus. While the number of nursing homes with a resident with COVID-19 has increased, most of the increase in COVID-19 in Ohio nursing homes has been in nursing homes that already have the virus. Of the nursing homes with at least one resident with COVID-19, one-quarter were classified as having a high caseload (defined as COVID 19 residents accounting for 20% or more of licensed beds) on April 28, 43% on May 14, and 40.9% on June 17. The most recent data suggest the infection is spreading to more nursing homes, with 105 new facilities reporting at least one case from May 14 to June 17.

Our comparison of facilities with no reported residents with COVID-19 to those with residents with the infection, showed higher quality facilities were not less likely to report having a resident with the virus. Even those facilities classified in the high caseload group did not have worse quality for any of the quality measures examined. The media and the public in general want to be able to blame someone for the tragedies that are now occurring across the nation's nursing homes. Yet, a recent editorial in the Washington Post (Grabowski et al., 2020) describing results from three independent studies, suggests results in-line with our study – that both poor and high-quality nursing homes are equally effected by coronavirus after accounting for factors that increase the risk of coronavirus infection, such as community prevalence. To be sure, there are likely poorly managed nursing homes who are not providing adequate care in this time of crisis. The isolation of residents combined with potential staff shortages means that residents and families in some facilities are suffering. But, there are also facilities that are well-run, that are attempting to protect their residents and staff, and despite all of their effects, have still been hit hard by the virus due to no fault of their own.

Therefore, the simple notion that any nursing home that has had a resident with coronavirus or high number of cases of the virus is not adequately protecting their residents and staff is not justified by our study results. The story is more complex and requires an understanding of the unique circumstances of each facility, including availability of testing and personal protection equipment, which many facilities reported not being able to get in the early days of the pandemic even though they request it. Publicly available quality data in Ohio indicate that the virus is not associated with quality ratings.

To this point, the data suggest that the nature and structure of nursing home care in general are the primary drivers in the spread of the coronavirus in Ohio nursing homes. This means throughout the rest of 2020, the nursing home industry is going to be faced with many challenges. As states allow visitation to nursing homes for the first time in months, it is going to be impossible without low cost and rapid testing to assure a visitor does not have the virus or is in a contagious state. Moreover, the re-opening of the economy and recent increases in coronavirus cases in states like Florida and Texas have only increased the risk for nursing home residents in those states, and provide a warning for other states re-opening their economies. Without regulations that require rapid testing of nursing home managers, front-line workers, suppliers, and potentially even their family members, there is no way to guarantee a staff member or visitor will not bring the virus into a nursing home. Policies that would require nursing home personnel and members of their household to remain in isolation are expensive and would likely induce a shortage of nursing home workers. Therefore, it is imperative to continue aggressive social distancing strategies, because it appears that as long as the pandemic is present, nursing home residents and the individuals who care for them will remain the most vulnerable members of society.

In the longer term, nursing homes are constrained by the policies and reimbursement system in which they operate, limiting their resources to combat the coronavirus. Increasing expenditures over the last decade, along with the deficits many states now face because of stay-at-home orders, will exacerbate the financial pressure faced by states. In the past, the typical response by states has been to either lower Medicaid reimbursement rates or to turn to managed care plans in an attempt to control costs. In this environment, efforts to curtail expenditures place extreme pressure on facilities in their efforts to deliver quality care. As states attempt to balance budgets by reducing reimbursement rates to nursing homes, not only will staffing levels potentially be cut, but nursing homes will not have the resources to invest in personal protective equipment and other measures to prevent the spread of this and future viruses. Therefore, policymakers need to be fully aware of the balancing act that is going to play out between adequately assuring high quality in nursing homes while addressing competing budgetary needs.

Limitations

We must acknowledge that there are reporting challenges with these data as they rely on a chain of communications between facility, county, and state that is imperfect. Virus case information is updated weekly and the response of facilities is fluid. To minimize potential measurement error in our statistical models, we defined facilities as having low or high caseloads using a cumulative number of cases equal to 20% licensed beds as a threshold for low and high caseloads. While this addresses potential measurement error, the 20% threshold, while based on input from industry experts, is subject to debate. For sensitivity analyses, we utilized 10% and 25% as a threshold and found qualitatively similar results (results not shown). We also estimated the model with number of residents per 10 beds and drew similar conclusions (results not shown).

Another limitation that needs to be emphasized is serving an individual with the coronavirus should not be viewed as a negative outcome for some nursing homes, as some facilities are welcoming transfers from hospitals and other settings. There is also variation in the availability and intensity of testing and availability of personal protective equipment across facilities that may affect the reported number of cases, including some nursing homes that may have created dedicated wings to care for individuals with COVID-19 from the community. We lack information on access to testing, personal protective equipment, and which facilities that may focus on admitting COVID-19 positive individuals from hospitals. While information about the number of staff that tested positive for the virus is available, the relationship between staff and resident infections is complex and is beyond the scope of this paper.

Finally, we have attempted to measure covariates as close to the start of the pandemic as possible, with most of our covariates reflecting information that is generally within one year before the start of the pandemic. However, some variables, such as racial/ethnic composition, are based on data from 2017. Therefore, our results provide a first look at this data, but these comparisons will need to be examined again once contemporaneous data are available to better understand prevalence rates and their link to quality and other facility factors.

Conclusion

A high number of COVID-19 cases in the pandemic have occurred among individuals living in nursing homes. Even so, our results show that two-thirds of Ohio nursing homes do not report having a resident with the virus, yet trends suggest that the virus is spreading. Nursing homes that had any case and a high number of cases do not have lower quality during the three time periods examined, indicating that facilities that are of poor quality are not more or less susceptible to the virus than high quality-rated nursing homes. While nursing homes could improve their infection-control procedures, coronavirus is far from being contained and requires system-wide efforts to stop the spread to nursing homes. As states consider restarting family visitation to nursing homes and continue re-opening their economies, policymakers should be aware that the risk to residents in these nursing homes and other congregate living settings will only increase.

Key points

- Nursing homes face considerable challenges in efforts to control COVID-19.
- The effect COVID-19 is having on nursing homes is not a surprise.
- Having any COVID-19 cases and a high caseload is not associated with quality ratings.
- The nature of nursing home care is the primary driver of coronavirus spread.

Acknowledgments

John R. Bowblis provides litigation-consulting services to the health care industry, which sometimes include long-term care providers.

Disclosure statement

All other authors report no known conflicts of interest.

References

Applegate, W. B., & Ouslander, J. G. (2020). COVID-19 presents high risk to older persons. *Journal of the American Geriatrics Society, 68*(4), 681. https://doi.org/10.1111/JGS.16426

Centers for Medicare and Medicaid Services [CMS]. (2019, April). *Design for nursing home compare five-star quality rating system: Technical users' guide.*

Dolan, J., & Mejia, B. (2020, April 14). Coronavirus is attacking nursing homes with poor infection track records in L.A. County. *Los Angeles Times.* https://www.latimes.com/california/story/2020-04-14/coronavirus-nursing-homes-infections-past-violations-citation

Goldstein, M., Silver-Greenberg, J., & Gebeloff, R. (2020, May 7). The New York Times. *Push for profits left nursing homes struggling to provide care.* Retrieved May 7, 2020, from https://www.nytimes.com/2020/05/07/business/coronavirus-nursing-homes.html

Grabowski, D. C., Feng, Z., Hirth, R., Rahman, M., & Mor, V. (2013). Effect of nursing home ownership on the quality of post-acute care: An instrumental variables approach. *Journal of Health Economics, 32*(1), 12–21. https://doi.org/10.1016/j.jhealeco.2012.08.007

Grabowski, D. C., & Joynt Maddox, K. E. (2020, March 25). Postacute care preparedness for COVID-19: Thinking ahead. *JAMA, 323*(20), 2007. https://doi.org/10.1001/jama.2020.4686

Grabowski, D. C., Kontezka, R. T., & Mor, V. (2020, June 25). Washington Post.*We can't protect nursing home from COVID-19 without protecting everyone.* Retrieved June 28, 2020, from https://www.washingtonpost.com/opinions/2020/06/25/we-cant-protect-nursing-homes-covid-19-without-protecting-everyone/

Jaffe, I. (2020, May 12). *Coronavirus pandemic exposes cracks in nursing home system*. NPR. https://www.npr.org/2020/05/12/854363905/coronavirus-pandemic-exposes-cracks-in-the-nursing-home-system

Kahn, K. (2020, May 12). Nonprofit Quarterly. *Nursing home system failure: 25,000 COVID-19 deaths and counting*. https://nonprofitquarterly.org/nursing-home-system-fail-25k-covid-19-deaths-and-counting/

Li, Y., Temkin-Greener, H., Gao, S., & Cai, X. (2020). COVID-19 infections and deaths among Connecticut nursing home residents: Facility correlates. *Journal of the American Geriatrics Society, 68*(9), 1899–1906. https://doi.org/10.1111/jgs.16689

Schroeder, K. (2020, May 1). Dayton Daily News. *Access to COVID-19 testing in Ohio nursing homes 'still spotty'*. Retrieved May 11, 2020, from https://www.daytondailynews.com/news/local/access-covid-testing-ohio-nursing-homes-still-spotty/0V3ywyhojR8sI1IZb1X27N/

Shippee, T. P., Akosionu, O., Ng, W., Woodhouse, M., Duan, Y., Thao, M. S., & Bowblis, J. R. (2020). COVID-19 pandemic: Exacerbating racial/ethnic disparities in long-term services and supports. *Journal of Aging & Social Policy, 32*(4–5), 323–333. in press. https://doi.org/10.1080/08959420.2020.1772004

Tan, L. F., & Seetharaman, S. (2020). Preventing the spread of COVI-19 to nursing homes: Experience from a Singapore geriatric centre. *Journal of the American Geriatrics Society, 68*(5), 942. https://doi.org/10.1111/jgs.16447

WWAMI Rural Health Research Center. (2020). https://depts.washington.edu/uwruca/ruca-data.php

Yu, A., & Feldman, N. (2020, May 6). *'It's a profession that does not love you back': Nursing home staffs bear witness to staggering death tolls*. WHYY PBS. Retrieved May 6, 2020, from https://whyy.org/articles/its-a-profession-that-does-not-love-you-back-nursing-home-staffs-bear-witness-to-staggering-death-tolls/

The Impact of COVID-19 on Nursing Homes in Italy: The Case of Lombardy

Marco Arlotti ⓘ and Costanzo Ranci ⓘ

ABSTRACT

Italy was the first western country strongly hit by the COVID-19 outbreak. This Perspective focuses on the large number of deaths that occurred in nursing homes during the first wave of the pandemic, and the weak capacity of public policy to provide them with adequate protection. The analysis focuses on the case of the Lombardy Region, where the mortality rate due to COVID-19 in nursing homes was the highest in Europe. In the search for possible causes, we investigate the situation of such facilities before the pandemic. Two aspects are analyzed: their institutional embeddedness and recent trends in their management. We conclude by arguing that the negative impact of COVID-19 stems from the poor development of long-term care policy and from the marginality of residential institutions within the healthcare system.

Introduction

Italy was the first western country to be strongly hit by the COVID-19 outbreak. The first two relevant clusters of infection were officially registered in two northern Italian regions (Codogno, in Lombardy and Vò Euganeo in Veneto) on February 21. At that time, the scientific information about COVID-19 and its potential dangers was still very scarce. The WHO did not proclaim COVID-19 as a "high global risk" until February 28: on that same day, Italy already had 888 officially infected persons, 345 hospitalized COVID-19 patients, 105 patients in intensive therapy, and 21 deaths. In the first wave of the outbreak (March-June 2020), most of the deaths occurred in the Northern part of the country, especially in Lombardy (around 50% of total cases; Ministero della Salute, 2020), the richest (highest GDP) and most populated region (10 million inhabitants, the same size as Sweden or the Czech Republic) in the country. Not only was Lombardy the first western region to face this tremendous health risk with no adequate information or indications from other countries or international organizations, it was also the most hit by the pandemic in terms of deaths, with 135.97 deaths caused by COVID-19 per 100,000 inhabitants in the first wave against an average COVID-19 EU regional mortality rate of 21.6 (Kapitsinis, 2020).

In this context, the nursing homes located in Lombardy were probably the first residential institutions in the western world to be hit by the pandemic. The same situation happened in many other countries (Comas-Herrera et al., 2020; Daly, 2020) at a later time. The diffusion of the infection in such institutions became visible and alerted public opinion (and policy makers) only *one month after* the outbreak began: this strong delay in the capacity of the system to acknowledge the problem had a tremendous impact in terms of number of deaths, especially among older people.

In this Perspective, we look for possible causes of such negative outcomes. We consider the case of Lombardy useful to highlight to what extent the harsh impact of COVID-19 on nursing homes has been the result of inadequate policy, both at regional and national levels, addressing the long-term care needs of frail older people, and the financial and management difficulties already faced by these institutions *before* the pandemic came. After providing some empirical evidence of COVID-19 impacts on nursing homes in Lombardy and Italy, we explore the institutional context in which nursing homes are embedded in Italy and Lombardy, and the recent trends affecting the governance and management of these institutions. In the conclusion, we highlight how policy legacy might be considered as a crucial explanatory factor of the tremendous impact that COVID-19 had on nursing homes.

The outcome: a huge number of deaths

The spread of infection in nursing homes has been documented by a national survey conducted in 1,356 nursing homes (41% of the total number of nursing homes in the country), carried out in April-May 2020 by Istituto Superiore di Sanità (ISS, 2020), a national scientific institution responsible for providing data and consultancy on public health. The mortality rate due to COVID-19 was calculated to be 3.8% at the national level, but rose to 7.5% in Lombardy. Southern regions were only partially affected by the pandemic, with mortality rates lower than the national average (ISS, 2020). According to an ILPN (International Long-term care Policy Network, based at the London School of Economics) study (Comas-Herrera et al., 2020), the only source for comparative data on the impact of COVID-19 on LTC systems (https://ltccovid.org/), mortality rates due to COVID-19 in nursing homes ranged between 0.5% in Germany and 6.2% in Spain (France: 2.5%, Sweden: 3.3%, UK: 5.1%). The mortality rate in Lombardy was higher than in any other European country (Figure 1). Moreover, it has been estimated that deaths in nursing homes represent 34% of the total number of COVID-19 deaths in the country

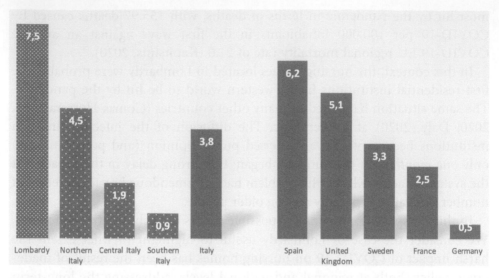

Figure 1. Mortality rates due to COVID-19 in residential structures by country and region (Italy) March-April 2020 (data per 100 hospitalized patients). Source: Istituto Superiore Sanità, National Survey Report, May 14 2020 (ISS, 2020); ILPN study (Comas-Herrera et al., 2020).

(Pesaresi, 2020). Even though these figures are only partially reliable, they show that mortality in nursing homes has been very high and significantly contributed to the total number of COVID-19 deaths in Lombardy.

The policy strategy both at the national and regional levels has been characterized by strong delays in coping with the emergency (Berloto et al., 2020). A national lockdown of nursing homes regarding the access of relatives and external visitors – a crucial measure in order to prevent possible transmission of infection – was established only on March 4 by the Central government, about two weeks after the infection had begun spreading and a national ban for visitors to hospitals was introduced. Though other Northern Italian regions hit by the pandemic (like Veneto and Emilia-Romagna) rapidly introduced the lockdown of nursing homes before the end of February, in the case of Lombardy this decision was postponed and taken only when the national lockdown was declared. Furthermore, for many weeks little attention was paid to testing and monitoring the virus among healthcare staff and patients, a priority for the implementation of such preventive activities in nursing homes was established only at the beginning of April.

While the pandemic therefore invaded nursing homes, these institutions were unable not only to prevent or limit the entry of the virus into their structures but also to provide personal protective equipment for their workers and adequate medical care to their COVID-19 patients. Indeed, according to the ISS survey more than 70% of nursing homes struggled with a lack of personal protective equipment during the pandemic (ISS, 2020).

Nursing homes patients were actually on lockdown in institutions that were clearly unable to take care of them. There is no surprise, therefore, that in April, when the number of deaths became significant and protests arose from workers and patients' relatives, several legal prosecutions started to investigate these situations with the aim of clarifying causes and responsibilities (Corriere della Sera, 2020; La Repubblica, 2020). At this time (January 2021), legal prosecutions are open against the management of nursing homes or regional policy makers.

Exploring

The strong spread of the pandemic in nursing homes has been undoubtedly favored by the high concentration of frail older people in these structures (Gardner et al., 2020). On the other hand, services specializing in providing health care to such frail people should have offered particular protection aimed at limiting infection and related mortality.

A specific investigation of the risk management policy process is necessary to understand the main reasons behind such a tragic impact. In the search for possible causes, below we investigate what the structural situation in such institutions was before the beginning of the epidemic. The underlying hypothesis is that policy legacy factors, coupled with a weak and problematic policy strategy during the pandemic, have played an important role in the way nursing homes have (poorly) dealt with the pandemic. The lack of public knowledge about the spread of the virus in these structures, and the weak response they could give to the pandemic, are to be seen as the result of the poor development of long-term care policy in Italy and of the marginality of these institutions within the healthcare system.

The institutional context

In 2016 (last available data), there were 1,724 residential structures in Lombardy (of 12,500 in Italy) with 66,000 patients over age 64 (285,000 in Italy; see I.Stat online database, http://dati.istat.it/): a highly fragmented sector with huge differences in size and level of specialization among structures (Fosti & Notarnicola, 2018; NNA – Network non autosufficienza, 2011). Nursing homes are classified according to the level of intensity of their health care services, ranging from low (structures that only provide social care services) to high health intensity (structures able to provide highly specialized and intensive health services such as mechanical ventilation or parenteral nutrition). The overall figure is that beds in residential structures covered 3.0% of the entire population of Lombardy in 2016. At the national level, the coverage was 2.2% (see I.Stat online database, http://dati.istat.it/). These figures are much lower than those of other European countries. If we consider the OECD

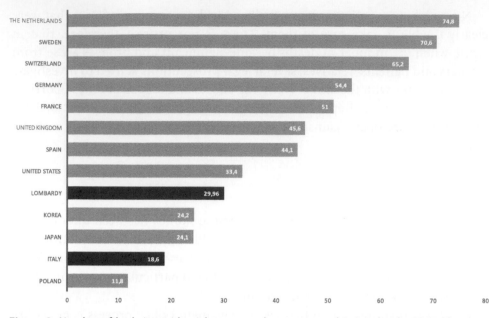

Figure 2. Number of beds in residential structures by country and in Lombardy, 2017 (data per 1,000 over 64-year-old residents). Source: OECD Health Statistics online database; I.Stat online database

Health Statistics data (Figure 2), the coverage in Lombardy (and even more in Italy) is much lower than in Spain or in Germany and less than half that in Sweden or the Netherlands. Japan, Korea, and even the United States surpass Italy.

The poor development of elderly residential care structures in Lombardy and Italy is linked to the centrality of strong family networks and the important role recently played by migrant care workers in providing in-house care. Both these factors have greatly favored aging in place (Bettio et al., 2006; Saraceno, 2016). However, this interpretation is only partially adequate. The OECD data shows that in other countries characterized by strong family ties (such as Spain and Germany), the coverage rate of residential beds is considerably higher than in Lombardy. A complementary explanation is that in Italy long-term care policies have been characterized by strong dominance of monetary transfers to families, under-development of care services (both home care and residential care services), and administrative tolerance for the growth of a huge informal care market based on the supply of undocumented migrant domestic care workers (Ranci et al., 2021; Da Roit & Sabatinelli, 2013). All these facts together explain why Italy's coverage rate of residential services is the lowest of western European countries. The situation in Lombardy basically reproduces this national pattern, with some peculiarities (Table 1). While other regions of Northern Italy (in particular Veneto and Emilia Romagna) have significantly invested in domiciliary care services aimed to

Table 1. Residential and home care services. Coverage rates (over 100 over-64 residents) of the most important regions of Northern Italy, 2016.

	Residential care	Health home care services	Social home care services	Care services (total)	Share of residential services over total coverage
Piedmont	3.7	4.1	0.7	8.6	43.8
Lombardy	3.0	6.1	1.5	10.6	27.9
Veneto	3.0	8.9	1.1	13.0	23.4
Emilia-Romagna	2.5	10.8	1.2	14.5	17.4
Italy	2.1	5.8	1.0	8.9	23.8

Source: I.Stat online database, Ministero della Salute (2019).

support aging in place, Lombardy is affected by a weak development of such type of interventions, which has paved the way for a huge growth of a private in-house (mainly irregular) care market.

In this context, nursing homes are not only residually provided but they also face enormous organizational difficulties. The regulation of this sector is strongly decentralized in the hands of regional governments, with a limited and rather vague coordination provided by the central state that concerns only the funding mechanism for nursing homes providing medium-to-high intensity health services (see below) (Arlotti, 2015). Hence at the sub-national level nursing homes tend to be highly differentiated as far as the coverage and the intensity of care standard (NNA – Network non autosufficienza, 2011).

Over the years, in the wake of population aging, the need for residential structures providing highly specialized long-term treatments to severely impaired people has hugely grown. Given the general low and steady trend in coverage rate, in Lombardy the existing nursing homes have been overwhelmingly occupied by very old people (in 2016, 79% were over 80) with little or no autonomy in daily life and requiring permanent, intensive care (see I.Stat online database, http://dati.istat.it/). In Lombardy, in 2016 97% of patients were cared for in nursing homes with medium-to-high health intensity, while 42% were placed in high-intensity healthcare facilities (see I.Stat online database, http://dati.istat.it/). In this region, nursing homes are supposed to provide long-term health care services to people with a strong loss in their autonomy and physical integrity (Gori, 2018). These structures are mainly considered a long-term health service rather than a housing solution for elderly people (as it happens in other European countries).

It is true that nursing homes providing medium-to-high intensity health services are recognized to be part of the National Health System (NHS).

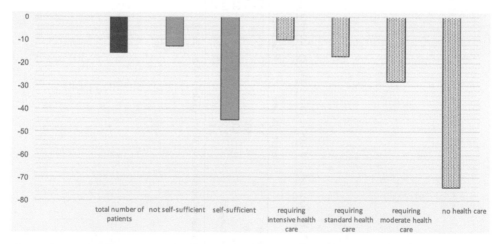

Figure 3. Lombardy: percentage changes 2009-16 in the number of hospitalized patients in nursing homes by category. Source: I.Stat online database

However, according to a national law, the funding mechanism does not cover all their health care expenditures (Arlotti, 2015). While health care provided in hospitals is fully covered by the NHS, funding in nursing homes is split into two parts, with 50% of total costs per capita paid by the NHS and 50% paid through private fees. Local municipalities pay fees only for patients in extreme poverty and there is a family obligation for relatives to support their elders who cannot pay the fee. In spite of their affiliation with the NHS, therefore, these structures permanently lack adequate public funding, with obvious consequences for the quality of their services, especially when their services are targeted to lower and middle-class patients (Arlotti & Aguilar-Hendrickons, 2018; Gori, 2018). Even though nursing homes are integrated into the healthcare sector, they still play a marginal role in this system.

Finally, most of the nursing homes in Lombardy as well as in Italy are very small (the national average number of patients for each structure is only 22) and highly dispersed in the national territory. Moreover, a large number of them are run by private bodies: in 2016, 89% of the total beds in residential institutions provided in Lombardy were owned by private entities (I.Stat online database, http://dati.istat.it/). Such entities include traditional – mostly church-related, nonprofit institutions – and new for-profit enterprises that have recently entered this market. One of the main implications is that funding and control mechanisms are highly complex and expensive, leaving large room not only for differentiation in size and quality, but also for illegality and abuses (Il Fatto Quotidiano, 2020; Senato della Repubblica, 2013). If regulation and

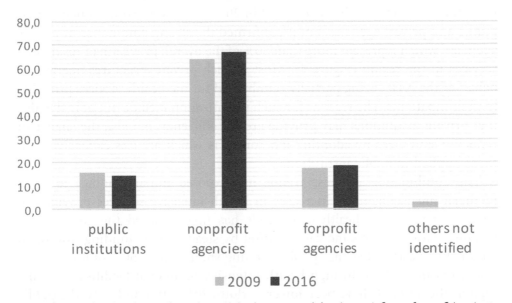

Figure 4. Lombardy: share of residentual beds managed by (nonpriofit or forprofit) private agencies, public institutions, or others not identified, 2009 and 2016. Source: I.Stat online database

control are highly difficult, policy making has to be developed in a context of a high plurality of actors.

Recent trends

Recent trends in Lombardy, documented by data provided by ISTAT (the National Institute for Statistics), highlight the critical nature of this situation. In the face of population aging and the related increase in the need for long-term care, the number of hospitalized patients in nursing homes decreased by 15.8% in the period 2009–2016 (last year available), equal to −12,400 people (Figure 3). The decrease was much higher for self-sufficient patients (−45%) and for older people only requiring moderate (−28%) or no health care (−74%), and more moderate for severely impaired people requiring intensive care (−10%). Such changes in the number and profile of inpatients had been accompanied by an organizational change of the residential structures, which increasingly were transformed into "high health-intensive residential facilities", i.e. nursing homes providing intensive treatments that are essential for the support of the vital functions of their patients. However, no changes have been introduced in the funding system, which is still based on the split mechanism described above.

The form of management of nursing homes had also undergone a profound change. First, in 2009–2016 there was *a huge reduction in the staff of residential institutions*: −20,500 people, equal to −19.9% of the total personnel, a loss not compensated by an increase of 4,000 volunteers. Second, in Lombardy the reduction in residential beds occurred in 2009–2016 was proportionate across public and private agencies, but it confirmed the strong dominance of private agencies, which represent more than 80% of the overall provision of residential services in the region (Figure 4). Most of such private structures operate on behalf of the NHS, being partially reimbursed for the health services provided to their inpatients. The reasons for such privatization include not only the idea that private institutions may provide greater efficiency, but also the chance of reducing staff costs by adopting job contracts which are less expensive than those applied in public institutions.

The combination of these trends has exposed nursing homes to great financial unsustainability. Increases in health-intensive services provided to patients with strong health care needs has hugely raised the costs of the facilities. However, this increase is offset by steady public funding. Although national law establishes that public funding should cover 50% of hospitalization costs in medium to high health-intensive residential facilities, in many regions the amounts have been lower (Arlotti, 2015). In Lombardy, the public funding per user paid to the facilities is on average 41.3 euros per day, while the fee paid by users is between 60 and 69 euros per day (Tidoli & Melzi, 2019). Tight in the grip between rising costs and insufficient public funding, many structures have rationed the expenses through increases in fees (at the expense of the poorest users), cuts in medical personnel, or non-renewal of equipment.

Conclusion

Italy was peculiarly characterized by a very high incidence of deaths in nursing homes in the first crucial months of the pandemic. Lombardy, the Italian region with the highest per capita income and the most efficient health system in the country, showed the highest mortality rate due to COVID-19 in Europe in such institutions.

In this paper, we have advanced the hypothesis that this result might be related to policy legacy factors. The high diffusion of COVID-19 in nursing homes and its extreme mortality have been strongly favored by the low financial public investments in long-term care, and especially in residential structures. As comparative research has clearly shown, while in the last decades most of the European countries have introduced important innovations in this policy field (Leon, 2014; Ranci & Pavolini, 2013), Italy has been peculiarly characterized by a prolonged institutional inertia (Costa, 2013; Naldini & Saraceno, 2008). Care to frail older people is still mainly provided by family members and/or migrant care workers, with a very limited support of public care services (Saraceno, 2016). Finally, Lombardy has never invested in public (either residential or home) care services, letting frail older people rely on informal or irregular care arrangements.

Given this situation, nursing homes had to face both internal and external problems during the pandemic. On the internal side, they had to face the entry of the virus into their structures with inadequate medical staff and insufficient resources and capacity to implement preventive actions. They were also unable to provide adequate health care to their COVID-19 patients, and very often unable to send them to hospitals. On the external side, their situation was ignored for a long time by policy makers, who were mainly focused on handling the emergency in hospitals (Declercq et al., 2020).

We have shown that most of such criticalities came from lack of political investment in long-term care and the preexistent difficult condition of these institutions. The more nursing homes have specialized in the intensive treatment of seriously non-self-sufficient elderly patients, the lower the quality of their services have become due to very precarious financial and organizational conditions, co-determined by the lack of adequate public funding. The COVID-19 emergency has not only determined the death of thousands of nursing homes patients. We argue that such a "focusing event" (Beland & Marier, 2020) has clearly shown the structural weakness of this sector and the main critical problems affecting it, as well as the need for better recognition of the strategic importance of nursing homes within the NHS, which has long been too much neglected by public health policy.

Key points

- Italy was the first western country strongly hit by the COVID-19 outbreak
- In Lombardy, the richest region of the country, mortality in nursing homes was the highest in Europe during the first wave of the pandemic
- Policies showed a very weak capacity to protect people in these facilities
- This reflects the poor development of long-term care policy and the structural marginality of nursing homes in the National Health System.

Disclosure statement

No potential conflict of interest was reported by the author(s).

ORCID

Marco Arlotti (iD) http://orcid.org/0000-0002-5720-5651
Costanzo Ranci (iD) http://orcid.org/0000-0002-1068-4683

References

Arlotti, M. (2015). Missed recalibration or retrenchment? The development of long term care policies for dependent elderly people in Italy. In S. Romano & G. Punziano (Eds.), *The European social model adrift. Europe, social cohesion and economic crisis* (pp. 73–87). Ashgate.

Arlotti, M., & Aguilar-Hendrickons, M. (2018). The vicious layering of multilevel governance in Southern Europe: The case of elderly care in Italy and Spain. *Social Policy & Administration, 52*(3), 646–661. https://doi.org/10.1111/spol.12351

Beland, D., & Marier, P. (2020). COVID-19 and Long-Term CarePolicy for Older People in Canada. *Journal of Aging & Social Policy, 32*(4-5), 358–364. https://doi.org/10.1080/08959420.2020.1764319

Berloto, S., Notarnicola, E., Perobelli, E., & Rotolo, A. (2020). *Italy and the COVID-19 long-term care situation.* Country report in LTC covid.org, International Long Term Care Policy Network, CPEC-LSE, 31st July 2020.

Bettio, F., Simonazzi, A., & Villa, P. (2006). Change in care regimes and female migration: The "Care Drain" in the Mediterranean. *Journal of European Social Policy, 16*(3), 271–285. https://doi.org/10.1177/0958928706065598

Comas-Herrera, A., Zalakain, J., Litwin, C., Hsu, A. T., Lane, N., & Fernandez, J.-L. (2020). *Mortality associated with COVID-19 outbreaks in care homes: Early international evidence.* LTCcovid.org, International LongTerm Care Policy Network, CPEC-LSE, https://ltccovid.org/wp-content/uploads/2020/10/Mortality-associated-with-COVID-among-people-living-in-care-homes-14-October-2020-3.pdf

Corriere della Sera. (2020). *Case di riposo, offensiva dei pm,* 14th April. https://www.politicanews.it/quotidiani/corriere-della-sera-case-di-riposo-offensiva-dei-pm-3556

Costa, G. (2013). Long-term care Italian policies: A case of inertial institutional change. In C. Ranci & E. Pavolini (Eds.), *Reforms in long-term care policies in Europe. Investigating institutional change and social impacts* (pp. 221–241). Springer.

Da Roit, B., & Sabatinelli, S. (2013). Nothing on the move or just going private? Understanding the freeze on care policies in Italy. *Social Politics, 20*(3), 430–453. https://doi.org/10.1093/sp/jxs023

Daly, M. (2020). COVID-19 and care homes in England: What happened and why? *Social Policy & Administration.* https://onlinelibrary.wiley.com/doi/full/10.1111/spol.12645

Declercq, A., De Stampa, M., Geffen, L., Heckman, G., Hirdes, J., Finne-Soveri, H., Lum, T., Millar, N., Morris, J. N., Onder, G., Szczerbińska, K., Topinkova, E., & Van Hout, H. (2020). *Why, in almost all countries, was residential care for older people so badly affected by COVID-19?*, OSE Working Paper Series, Opinion Paper No. 23. Brussels, European Social Observatory. Belgium.

Fosti, G., & Notarnicola, E. (Eds). (2018). *L'innovazione e il cambiamento nel settore della Long Term Care. 1° Rapporto Osservatorio Long Term Care.* Egea.

Gardner, W., States, D., & Bagley, N. (2020). The coronavirus and the risks to the elderly. *Journal of Aging & Social Policy, 32(4-5)*, 310–315. https://doi.org/10.1080/08959420.2020.1750543

Gori, C. (Ed.). (2018). *Il welfare delle riforme? Le politiche lombarde tra norme ed attuazione.* Maggioli.

Il Fatto Quotidiano. (2020). *Rsa, da marzo 700 ispezioni: Gravi irregolarità in una su 4*, 30th April. Editoriale Il Fatto S.p.A. https://www.ilfattoquotidiano.it/in-edicola/articoli/2020/04/30/rsa-da-marzo-700-ispezioni-gravi-irregolarita-in-una-su-4/5786831/

ISS. (2020). *Survey nazionale sul contagio COVID-19 nelle strutture residenziali e sociosanitarie*, Istituto Superiore di Sanità (National Institute of Health). https://www.epicentro.iss.it/en/coronavirus/sars-cov-2-survey-rsa

Kapitsinis, N. (2020). The underlying factors of the COVID-19 spatially uneven spread. Initial evidence from regions in nine EU countries. *Regional Science Policy & Practice, 12*(6), 1027–1045. https://doi.org/10.1111/rsp3.12340

la Repubblica. (2020). *Coronavirus, l'epidemia insabbiata: Al Trivulzio di Milano si indaga su settanta morti*, 4th April. https://rep.repubblica.it/pwa/generale/2020/04/04/news/coronavirus_l_epidemia_insabbiata_al_trivulzio_di_milano_si_indaga_su_settanta_morti-253156789/

Leon, M. (Ed.). (2014). *The transformation of care in European societies.* Palgrave Macmillan.

Ministero della Salute. (2019). Annuario Statistico del Servizio Sanitario Nazionale - Assetto organizzativo, attività e fattori produttivi del SSN - Anno 2016, http://www.salute.gov.it/portale/documentazione/p6_2_2_1.jsp?lingua=italiano&id=2859

Ministero della Salute (2020). *COVID-19. La situazione in Italia*, aggiornamento 24 settembre, https://raw.githubusercontent.com/pcm-dpc/COVID-19/master/schede-riepilogative/regioni/dpc-covid19-ita-scheda-regioni-latest.pdf

Naldini, M., & Saraceno, C. (2008). Social and family policies in Italy: Not totally frozen but far from structural reforms. *Social Policy & Administration, 42*(7), 733–748. https://doi.org/10.1111/j.1467-9515.2008.00635.x

NNA –Network non autosufficienza. (2011). *L'assistenza agli anziani non autosufficienti in Italia. 3° Rapporto. Il monitoraggio degli interventi e il punto sulla residenzialità.* Maggioli.

Pesaresi, F. (2020). *Il Covid-19 nelle strutture residenziali per anziani*, I luoghi dell cura. https://www.luoghicura.it/dati-e-tendenze/2020/05/il-covid-19-nelle-strutture-residenziali-per-anziani/

Ranci, C., Arlotti, M., Cerea, S., & Cordini, M. (2021). Migrant and/or care workers? Debating the ethnicization of the elderly care market in Italy and the United Kingdom. *Social Politics: International Studies in Gender, State & Society, 28*(1), Spring 2021, 47–70. https://doi.org/10.1093/sp/jxz002

Ranci, C., & Pavolini, E. (Eds.). (2013). *Reforms in long-term care policies in Europe. Investigating institutional change and social impacts.* Springer.

Saraceno, C. (2016). Varieties of familialism: Comparing four southern European and East Asian welfare regimes. *Journal of European Social Policy, 26*(4), 314–326. https://doi.org/10.1177/0958928716657275

Senato della Repubblica. (2013). *Commissione parlamentare di inchiesta sull'efficacia e l'efficienza del Servizio sanitario nazionale. Relazione finale sull'attività della Commissione.* Tipografia del Senato. https://www.senato.it/service/PDF/PDFServer/BGT/698049.pdf

Tidoli, R., & Melzi, A. (2019). Rette RSA: Cosa si "nasconde" dietro ai numeri? *Lombardia Sociale,* http://www.lombardiasociale.it/2019/06/20/rette-rsa-cosa-si-nasconde-dietro-ai-numeri/

COVID-19 and Long-Term Care Policy for Older People in Japan

Margarita Estévez-Abe (ID) and Hiroo Ide

ABSTRACT

Japan's initial response to COVID-19 was similar to that of the US. However, the number of deaths in Japan has remained very low. Japan also stands out for the relatively low incidence of viral transmission in Long-Term Care Facilities (LTCFs) compared to both European countries and the United States. We argue that Japan's institutional decision to lockdown Long-Term Care facilities as early as mid-February – weeks earlier than most European countries and the US – contributed to lowering the number of deaths in LTCFs. We highlight a few lessons from the Japanese experience: (i) the presence of hierarchically organized government agencies whose sole missions are elderly care; (ii) the presence of effective communication channels between LTCFs and the regulatory authorities; and (iii) the well-established routine protocols of prevention and control in LTCFs.

Introduction

Experts and journalists have asked why the COVID-19 death tolls in East Asia are so much lower than in Europe and the United States (Sachs, 2020). Japan in particular poses a big puzzle. Japan's initial political reaction to the COVID-19 resembled that of the United States. Unlike other East Asian countries whose governments moved swiftly and decisively to contain the spread of the new virus. Japan was a global laggard in testing and in its lack of national political leadership. Even after the United States began scaling up its testing capacity, Japan still did very little testing. Japan has conducted by far the smallest number of tests of all wealthy democracies. Furthermore, Japan never adopted a strict nation-wide lockdown like seen in many Western countries. According to the Japan National Tourism Office, roughly one million Chinese tourists visited Japan in January and February. Travel from Europe remained unrestricted until March 21. Combined with Japan's high population density, the potential for the spread of the new virus was very high. Japan's COVID-19 mortality rate, however, remains closer to the low figures found in countries like South Korea and Taiwan than those found in Europe and the United States.

How could a country that was so hesitant to act nonetheless avert a disaster? Professor Omi, the Vice Chairman of the Expert Panel that advises the Japanese government on COVID-19, attributes Japan's small death toll to the society-wide use of facial masks (Reynolds, 2020). While we do not deny the importance of wearing face masks, we highlight another factor: Japan's early lockdown of Long-Term Care facilities (LTCFs).

We claim that an early lockdown of LTCFs in Japan during the initial uncertain months of the pandemic helped protect the most vulnerable. In Japan, this early intervention had little to do with political leadership and top down crisis management. Instead, as this paper demonstrates, it was part of a well-established routine protocol for the prevention and control of communicable diseases in LTCFs. The specific organizational characteristics of the Japanese LTCF sector helped contain viral transmissions into LTCFs during the first months of the pandemic when so little was known. The remarkable success of Japan in limiting fatalities in LTCFs highlights the importance of: (i) the presence of hierarchically organized government agencies whose sole missions are elderly care; (ii) the presence of effective communication channels between LTCFs and the regulatory authorities; and (iii) the well-established routine protocols of prevention and control in LTCFs.

Japan's small death toll

Table 1 shows the number of deaths due to COVID-19 as well as the number of polymerase chain reaction (PCR) tests – the type of test that most countries used in the early days of the pandemic – conducted per one million people in selected East Asian and Western countries. The numbers provide ample evidence both of Japan's small death toll and limited tests.

It is known that COVID-19 causes more severe symptoms in older people. In Europe, people aged 80 years and older constitute more than 50% of the death toll from this virus (World Health Organization, 2020). As the most aged society in the world, Japan has the largest share of vulnerable adults 80 or older (8.5% of the total population in 2017). In Germany and Italy, which are also among the most aged societies, respectively 6.1% and 6.9% of their populations are aged 80 or older. The figure for the United States is a mere 3.8% (Organization for Economic Co-operation and Development, 2019, Figure 11.1). Yet the percentage of those aged 80 and older in the total COVID-19 deaths remained lower in Japan (56%) than in Germany (63%) and Italy (59%) (August 5 update Japan from Ministry of Health, Labour and Welfare, 2020a; August 5 and 4 updates respectively for Germany and Italy from INED (Institut National d'Études Démographiques), 2020). Although the data for the United States use different age breakdowns, the situation is

Table 1. Numbers of COVID-19 deaths and polymerase chain reaction testing (PCR) per one million population by country.

	COVID-19 deaths	Tests/1 million
Taiwan	0.3	3,124
Hong Kong	0.5	36,734
Singapore	4	83,562
South Korea	5	21,568
Japan	7	2,678
Germany	106	56,034
USA	356	75,030
France	451	21,215
Italy	568	76,419
Spain	580	103,232
Britain	614	99,787
Belgium	834	89,435

Data from Worldometer (as of June 16, 2020) https://www.world ometers.info/coronavirus/

similar. In the United States, those aged 75 years and older and those aged 85 and older constitute, respectively, 59% and 32% of the total COVID-19 deaths (Centers for Disease Control and Prevention, 2020).

LTCFs, whose residents are elderly, are particularly high-risk facilities in the event of a viral transmission. An international study reports the following figures for the percentage of nursing home residents among those who died of COVID-19 (by the end of May or June depending on the country data): 34% in Austria, 50% in Belgium, 85% in Canada, 49% in France, 39% in Germany and 45% in the United States (Comas-Herrera, Zalakain et al., 2020). In contrast, Japan recorded relatively few deaths in its LTCFs. As of May 8, only 14% of COVID-19-related deaths in Japan had occurred in LTCFs (Kaigo shisestu de shibou zentai no juyon-pa-sento [Fourteen percent of death by COVID-19 occurs in LTCs], 2020). Less than 0.01% of LTCF residents died of COVID-19 in Japan compared to 0.4% in Germany, 5.3%, in Britain and 6.1% in Spain. A more recent update by the Tokyo Medical Association also confirms a very low incidence rate of cluster infection in LTCFs (0.0017%) as of July 5 (the Tokyo Medical Association, 2020).

These comparative statistics provide an initial indication that LTCFs in Japan did not become a major locus of cluster infections, as they did elsewhere. Statistics on deaths from COVID-19, however, face certain problems of comparability because not all countries count deaths with the same accuracy. In the case of Japan, its low death toll might be an artifact of its extremely small number of tests. For this reason, we compare overall excess death rates. Although the currently available statistics on the number of deaths (the Vital Statistics) only cover the period until the end of March nationally and until the end of April in Tokyo, given that the daily number of confirmed cases peaked during the first week of April in Tokyo, we nonetheless think that they provide us with a confirmation of the Japanese success in containing the first wave of deaths from COVID-19. To ensure comparability, we use the same formula to calculate excess mortality as the Financial Times COVID-19 dataset (Financial Times, 2020). Tokyo's excess mortality rates in March and April were 2.2% and 8.4% respectively. The figures for similarly large Western cities where people use public transportation as in Tokyo were much higher: 8.8% and 192% in London, and 49% and 480% in New York City. Tokyo's numbers are very similar to the numbers for Germany (whole country): 2% and 8.8%. Yet while Germany – a country often upheld as Europe's great COVID-19 success story – controlled the virus by scaling up its COVID-19 testing capacity, Japan never adopted mass testing. Given Tokyo's population density – comparable to London and New York City – and the failure to conduct widespread testing, Japan's low death toll is all the more surprising.

Although Japan's rate of excess mortality has been low, the data also indicate that Japan has experienced an increase in mortality. It is possible that COVID-19 has contributed to this trend. However, Japan's excess deaths are not attributable to clusters of infections in LTCFs as is the case in the United States and many European countries. The Japanese media, which has closely followed the COVID-19 cases in hospitals and LTCFs, reported a small number of clusters of infection. We conducted article searches for the four national newspapers – Asahi, Yomiuri, Mainichi and Nikkei – which cover local news extensively. Our survey of news articles reveals that the majority of cases of infections in Japanese LTCFs tended to be isolated cases of one or two caregivers or residents testing positive. This suggests that most LTCFs successfully contained the spread of the virus, thereby preventing large deadly clusters.

Japan's swift decision to lockdown LTCFs

Japan locked down its LTCFs very early compared to other countries. According to our interviews, some LTCFs were already in full or semi-lockdown modes due to seasonal flu outbreaks in January and February – a routine prevention and control protocol. Early COVID-19 warnings from the Bureau of Health and Welfare for the Elderly within the Ministry of Health, Labor and Welfare (MHLW) effectively shut down the rest of the LTCFs between mid- and late-February. In European countries and the United States, lockdowns of LTCFs came weeks later only after large clusters of infections and deaths had already occurred. Italy, the first European COVID-19 hotspot, waited until early March; the United States until mid-March; and Britain, Germany and many others waited even longer (Comas-Herrera, Ashcroft et al., 2020).

On January 29, the Bureau of Health and Welfare for the Elderly within the MHLW first contacted the departments of LTCFs in local governments. The

Bureau requested that they alert the LTCFs in their jurisdictions about the new corona virus and instruct them to adopt appropriate protocols for prevention and control (MHLW, 2020b). On February 13, MHLW issued another notification to all relevant departments in prefectures and large cities. The Ministry wanted them to ensure that LTC facilities and service providers in their jurisdiction follow the protocols for prevention of communicable diseases (MHLW, 2020c).

On February 24, the MHLW stepped up its warning and issued a notification to all social welfare facilities and LTCFs, which included the following specific guidelines for: (1) how to report COVID-19 incidents to the authorities; (2) cleaning and sterilizing; (3) identification of probable infected residents and staffs; (4) handling of residents and staff suspected of infection; and (5) restrictions of visitors and delivery personnel (MHLW, 2020d). The interviews we conducted with various LTCFs confirmed that the Ministry's notification played an important role in their decision to lock down (see Note 1 for the details of the interviews).

By acting so soon, the MHLW officials in charge of LTCFs got ahead of the virus. At the time, COVID-19 was still thought of by most Japanese people as a distant threat. For most people, the new virus was a problem only for China and a foreign cruise ship – the "Diamond Princess" – quarantined in Yokohama Bay. On February 24, there were still only 141 confirmed cases in Japan. The MHLW's swift actions were the result of a routine institutional response. When the MHLW officials learned that a new virus had entered the country, they automatically raised the alert level as they would with influenza, tuberculosis and other communicable diseases. LTCFs, which were well-practiced in the protocol to isolate their residents, responded immediately. The Prime Minister, his Welfare Minister and even the expert panel advising them on COVID-19 were all largely unaware of the critical steps already taken by mid-level MHLW officials. Ironically, Prime Minister Abe insisted that a new legal framework would be necessary for his government to fight COVID-19. Yet by the time the new legal framework was implemented on March 14, the LTCFs had been under lockdown for three weeks already.

The MHLW's early intervention worked well. In this respect, Japan's response resembled her East Asian neighbors. Hong Kong and South Korea were also very quick to protect the most vulnerable in LTCFs (Lum et al., 2020; Ministry of Health and Welfare, 2020). Some scholars have attributed these swift responses to the lessons learned from the failure to handle the Severe Acute Respiratory Syndrome (SARS) and Middle East Respiratory Syndrome (MERS) (Cho, 2020; Lum et al., 2020). Japan was different. Japan escaped both SARS and MERS, hence there were no bad recent experiences to learn from. The preparedness of Japan's MHLW and LTCFs had to come from elsewhere.

Although Japan had experienced major outbreaks of neither SARS nor MERS, Japan has long suffered from a relatively high incidence of tuberculosis

(World Health Organization, 2019). In addition, in the years following its defeat in the Second World War, Japan also suffered from cholera and typhus. Citizens who returned to Japan from the former colonies and battlefields brought back new parasites and diseases. Space limits prevent us from fully discussing the institutional legacies here. For the purpose of this paper, it suffices to point out that Japan developed community-based public health agencies known as *Hokenjo* (MHLW, 2014, Chapter 1). These agencies function as local centers of disease control and prevention as well each community's preventive care centers. LTCFs and medical facilities report any outbreaks of communicable diseases such as the seasonal flu and gastroenteritis to *Hokenjo*, which, in turn, keep local and national authorities informed about the scope of transmission within the communities.

When Japan introduced its Long-Term Care Insurance in 2000, it also introduced communicable disease control and prevention guidelines for LTCFs. The Bureau of Health and Welfare for the Elderly in MHLW together with disease prevention and control specialists within the same ministry have frequently upgraded these guidelines so that all care workers were up-to-date on the latest prevention protocols. During the annual influenza season, for instance, LTCFs are accustomed to monitoring updates on influenza outbreaks in order to determine the level of prevention and control measures to adopt. The use of face masks is the norm in any flu season.

In order to fully understand how the Japanese LTCFs effectively responded to the pandemic, it is also important to understand the specific features of the Japanese LTCF sector. Before we discuss specific features, a brief overview of Japan's LTCF sector is in order.

Japan's LTCF system

Most of Japan's LTC services are covered by its public long-term care insurance (LTCI) introduced in 2000 (Campbell & Ikegami, 2000). Japan's LTCI – which is administered by municipal governments – is operated independently of the medical insurance system and subsidizes non-medical benefits-in-kind including residential (long-term and short-term) day care services, care services at the users' home as well as home improvements so that elderly citizens can continue to live in their homes safely (Ministry of Health, Labour and Welfare, Government of Japan, 2017). When an insured person requires services, the municipal government evaluates and determines the level of care to be covered by LTCI. Insured persons then contract any service provider of choice within the municipality and pay a 10% co-payment. The remaining 90% of the service cost is reimbursed directly to the service providers by the municipal LTCI. The LTCI, however, does not cover room and board. LTCF residents have to pay for the cost out of pocket. The funding for LTCI takes the following form: 50% from mandatory insurance contributions from all residents aged 40 years and older; 25% from the national government; and 12.5% each from the prefectural and municipal governments. Each municipality sets the insurance rates on the basis of the insured residents' income levels.

While the municipal governments are the administrators of the system, LTCI is a nationally regulated system. The menu of services and pricing is set by the Ministry of Health, Labor and Welfare (MHLW) and hence is standardized across the country. Furthermore, the MHLW sets the rules over who can operate as service providers and imposes specific requirements on the provision of services such as minimum levels of accommodation, care worker/resident ratio, the number of medical and trained care staff, nutritionists and physical therapists. The MHLW also requires municipal and prefectural governments to update their long-term care service plans every three years.

The Japanese national LTC regulatory framework distinguishes five categories of LTCFs as detailed in Table 2. These are facilities that are specifically licensed to provide long-term care to their residents. In contrast to the United States, where for-profit facilities dominate the LTCF sector, nonprofit facilities dominate this sector in Japan. The most vulnerable elderly population – those who require most nursing and medical care and those with the fewest economic means – are in nonprofit facilities. For-profit assisted living facilities have been increasing in number in recent years. Some of these for-profit facilities provide luxury living arrangements for the elderly. Generally speaking, these facilities cater to the more independent and hence less vulnerable population. They cannot provide LTC services to their residents unless they are specially licensed by the respective prefectural government to do so. (This means that residents in such facilities have to contract external LTC service providers should they need nursing care.) The fifth category of LTCFs listed in our table, therefore, refers to those assisted living facilities specifically licensed to operate as LTCFs. They are subject to more stringent staffing regulations than assisted living facilities.

The two types of nonprofit organizations that dominate the Japanese LTCF sector – social welfare corporations and medical corporations – have very little in common with American nonprofit organizations. Let us focus on social welfare corporations to illustrate the difference. Social welfare corporations are a legal category for entities that are specifically created with the purpose of contracting out public welfare services. Just as governmental social welfare agencies do not make profit out of providing public services, social welfare corporations do not make profits on the services covered by the LTCI system. Their activities consist of operating residential and nonresidential LTC services and other social welfare services. Once licensed, social welfare corporations are required by law to submit annual financial statements to the local government officials overseeing the LTCF sector, who audit the LTCFs every few years.

Table 2. Five categories of residential LTCFs in Japan.

Category	Description	Breakdown by provider type	Number of facilities	Number of beds	Number of residents
(i) Special nursing homes	Residential facilities that provide non-medical nursing care for elderly who require highest level of LTC.	Nonprofit social welfare corporations 94.8%	7,891	542,498	485,795
(ii) Long-term care health facilities	Facilities that provide nursing care to elderly who are undergoing rehabilitation with the goal of returning home	Nonprofit medical corporations 75.3% Nonprofit social welfare corporations. 15.0%	4,322	372,679	308,271
(iii) Sanatorium medical facilities	Hospitals that provide medical care to elderly patients requiring nursing care	Nonprofit medical corporations 83.4% Local governments 5.0%	1,196	53,352	45,359
(iv) Social welfare facilities for elderly citizens	Social welfare residential facilities for elderly who find it difficult to live at home due to non-age-related disabilities, lack of economic means and/or family support	Nonprofit social welfare corporations 76.6% Local governments 14.8%	5,293	152,819	140,173
(v) For-profit LTCFs	For-profit elderly assisted living facilities specifically licensed to provide LTC services to their residents	For-profit firms 82.6% Nonprofit medical corporations 7.6% nonprofit social welfare corporations 5.4%	3,789	230,012	204,251

The figures for the numbers of facilities, beds and residents are from 2017. The figures for the first to third categories come from (MHLW, 2018a; the figures for the fourth from (MHLW, 2018b); and the figures for the fifth category from (MHLW, 2018b; Nomura Research Institute, 2018).

For-profit LTCFs – category five in Table 2 – are dominated by for-profit companies, some of which operate multiple facilities. However, Table 2 shows that a small percentage of them are operated by the two types of nonprofit organizations. This is because these nonprofit organizations are allowed to provide for-profit services that are not reimbursable from the LTCI. Every provider of for-profit LTCFs needs to be licensed by the prefectural government.

Three features of the Japanese LTCF sector and pandemic response

Three features of the Japanese LTCF sector explain why they could swiftly and successfully act upon the MHLW guidelines issued in January/February. These features are: (i) the presence of hierarchically organized government agencies whose sole missions are elderly care; (ii) the presence of effective communication channels between LTCFs and the regulatory authorities; and (iii) the well-established routine protocols of prevention and control in LTCFs.

First, the Japanese LTC-related government agencies are organized hierarchically at each level of local governments (i.e., prefectures, specially-designated cities, and other municipalities). These agencies exclusively focus on LTC issues. The command and oversight structure is streamlined in Japan. Contrast this to the US, where numerous agencies – such as county-level and state-level health departments, Veterans' Affairs, Centers for Medicare & Medicaid Services, Centers for Disease Control and Prevention – crowd the regulatory and advisory landscape. At the top of the Japanese hierarchy is the Bureau of Health and Welfare for the Elderly in the MHLW. Local governments have specific departments that liaise with this Bureau. For instance, when the MHLW periodically updates the prevention and control guidelines for the LTCFs, local government officials overseeing LTCFs ensure that the key points are clearly communicated to LTCFs (based on our interviews with Kanagawa prefectural officials). MHLW's various warnings and guidelines for COVID-19 hence trickle down by way of a routine bureaucratic and institutional procedure.

Second, communications between municipal governments and LTCFs are more frequent, because most of Japan's LTCFs are operated by special types of nonprofit organizations that function as governmental partners. Furthermore, given the highly regulated nature of the LTCF sector and the impact of national policies on their revenues and management decisions, trade associations play an important role as intermediaries between government authorities and their members – i.e., LTCFs and providers of in-home-care services. It should be emphasized that the Japanese government authorities also possess important channels of communication with for-profit facilities. As already mentioned, for-profit LTCFs are licensed by prefectural governments. For the purpose of better oversight and communication with for-profit nursing homes, the MHLW grants special powers and imposes obligations on the trade association of for-profit nursing homes as codified in Article 30 of the Act on Social Welfare for the Elderly. This law defines the trade association's mission as an intermediary between the supervisory authorities and the member facilities for the purpose of better oversight. In other words, even the trade association of for-profit corporations closely works with local government regulators. Our interviewees at the Prefectural Government of Kanagawa (a populous prefecture in Greater Metropolitan Tokyo) told us that they had also contacted for-profit nursing homes. In the case of the February 24 MHLW notification, the LTCF personnel we interviewed stated that they had received the notification from the association of LTC facilities.

Some data indicate recent improvements in the governmental oversight of for-profit LTCFs and elderly assisted living facilities. Ever since the MHLW has required prefectural governments to monitor more closely the for-profit sector, the compliance rate with government regulations has jumped from 80.1% in 2011 to 97.1% in 2017 (MHLW, 2018c). The trade association plays an important role in assisting the authorities by contacting its members and soliciting documentation.

Thirdly, Japan's well-established routine protocols for communicable disease prevention and control in LTCFs played an important role. Since 2000 the MHLW guidelines for prevention and control have required that each LTCF set up an internal prevention and control committee. This committee approach is geared toward involving different types of employees, including not only the medical staff but also non-medical care workers. The MHLW commissioned a survey of disease prevention and control practices in the first type of LTCFs, which take care of the most vulnerable. According to this survey, the legally required committees meet frequently (Mitsubishi Research Institute Inc., 2019). Nearly half of the prevention and control committees meet more than bi-monthly and 90% of them meet multiple times per year. The survey also demonstrates the effective compliance of protocol in handling residents infected with common communicable diseases such as the seasonal flu and gastroenteritis.

As noted earlier, Japanese LTCFs are used to handling outbreaks of influenza and gastroenteritis. During any flu season, LTCF workers use face masks, monitor residents' conditions and isolate the sick. When the public health authorities report flu outbreaks in the community, LTCFs activate higher levels of prevention and control protocols, including suspending social events for residents and restricting family visits. Therefore, when the MHLW alerted the LTCFs to lockdown, some had already been isolating their residents and simply extended the lockdown and the rest of the LTCFs followed suit. Certainly, COVID-19 has impacted all five types of LTCFs in Japan. Our survey of newspaper articles indicates that large clusters of infections in LTCFs have been very rare in Japan. This also applies to for-profit LTCFs.

The LTC personnel we interviewed told us that they did not do anything special for COVID-19 but simply adopted the same routine protocols they always follow during any flu season. However, our interviews revealed that there was one extra (unusual) precautionary measure adopted for COVID-19. Some LTCF workers were asked by their employers to limit social interactions in their private lives in order not to contract and bring the virus into their workplace. We speculate that the absence of COVID-19 testing and a shortage of PPE might have been the reason behind such an unusual request.

In support of the explanation offered in this paper, there is some evidence to show that the incidence of healthcare-associated infections might be lower in Japan. One study of LTCFs in the Osaka area reports that the overall frequency of healthcare associated infections was low (0.18 per 1,000 resident days) relative to Western countries (1.8–13.5 per 1,000 resident days) although the authors caution that the numbers are not completely comparable (Kariya et al., 2018).

Conclusion

LTCFs, which house the most vulnerable population, are at the front line of the fight against COVID-19. Countries that succeeded in keeping COVID-19 out of LTCFs were able to reduce the number of deaths by a large margin. Although Japanese political leaders have not been very aggressive in their fight against the pandemic, the Japanese routine protocols of prevention and control of communicable diseases in the LTCF sector resulted in a swift decision to isolate the most vulnerable from viral transmission. The routine institutional response of the LTCF sector proved to be critical in fighting against COVID-19. Compared to Japan, restrictions on family visits for the purpose of prevention and control have not been usual responses to the seasonal flu in Europe and in the United States. We speculate that this may have led Western countries to delay their decision to isolate LTCFs until it was too late.

Counterintuitively, the silent success of Japan's institutional response has resulted in an underappreciation of the massive efforts undertaken by LTCFs to protect their residents. Politicians and the general population are largely ignorant of the role that LTCF workers have played in Japan's fight against COVID-19. If the government fails to properly acknowledge and provide them with the necessary resources to cope with the second and the third waves, the exhausted LTCF workers may not be as effective in the next round. A lockdown of LTCFs is an emergency measure and cannot be a long-term solution. Japan has been fortunate to have effective protocols in place when the pandemic hit. However, without the Japanese government's effective leadership and resource mobilization in scaling up testing of LTCF workers, residents and family members, Japan's LTCFs might not be spared from tragedy in the months to come.

Key points:

- Despite being the most aged society in the world and having a high population density, Japan maintained low rates of deaths from COVID-19.
- Japan locked down LTCFs, during the first months of the pandemic, several weeks earlier than in Europe and the United States.
- The well-established protocols of prevention and control of communicable diseases such as influenza and tuberculosis proved to be important.
- The presence of public authorities exclusively devoted to the oversight of LTCFs contributed to swift institutional responses.
- The presence of effective channels of communication between the public authorities and LTCFs contributed to the swift implementation of government guidelines.

Note

We interviewed government officials and LTCF personnel as a way of supplementing our analysis based on government documents and other sources mentioned in this paper. Our interviews included four interviews of government officials with direct responsibilities to oversee LTCFs—both at the prefectural and national levels—and five interviews of LTCF personnel. We asked LTCF personnel about: (i) the timing of their decision to lockdown the facility; (ii) the role of the MHLW directives in their decisions; (iii) how they were notified of the MHLW directive (either via local governments and had received; and (iv) whether they had adopted any special prevention and control measures to deal with the new virus. We asked the officials about their routine channels of communications with different levels of the government and with individual LTCFs and whether they relied on the same channels of communication during the pandemic or not.

Our interviewees included:

The Ministry of Health, Labour and Welfare (an official with a nursing certification in the special New Corona Virus Taskforce) on May 26, 2020.

Shizuoka Prefectural Government (an official with a nursing certification in charge of COVID-19 consultations), May 29, 2020.

Kanagawa Prefectural Government (two officials at the New Corona Virus Communicable Disease Task Force and two officials at the Elderly Welfare Section) on June 30 and July 9' 2020.

One physician, certified care worker, care managers, facility manager at four LTCFs in Chiba and Kanagawa Prefectures on May 27, 28 and 29, 2020.

Disclosure statement

No potential conflict of interest was reported by the author(s).

ORCID

Margarita Estévez-Abe (iD) http://orcid.org/0000-0001-7353-0289

References

Campbell, J. C., & Ikegami, N. (2000). Long-term care insurance comes to Japan. *Health Affairs, 19*(3), 26–39. https://doi.org/10.1377/hlthaff.19.3.26

Centers for Disease Control and Prevention. (2020). *Weekly updates by select demographic and geographic characteristics.* Retrieved August 30, 2020, from https://www.cdc.gov/nchs/nvss/vsrr/covid_weekly/index.htm#ExcessDeaths

Cho, H.-W. (2020). Effectiveness for the response to COVID-19: The MERS outbreak containment procedures. *Osong Public Health and Research Perspectives, 11*(1), 1–2. https://doi.org/10.24171/j.phrp.2020.11.1.01

Comas-Herrera, A., Ashcroft, E. C., & Lorenz-Dant, K. (2020, May 2). *International examples of measures to prevent and manage COVID-19 outbreaks in residential care and nursing home settings.* International Long-term Care Policy Network. Retrieved June 16, 2020, from https://ltccovid.org/wp-content/uploads/2020/05/International-measures-to-prevent-and-manage-COVID19-infections-in-care-homes-2-May-1.pdf

Comas-Herrera, A., Zalakain, J., Liwtin, C., Hsu, A. T., Lemmon, E., Henderson, D., & Fernandez, J. L. (2020). *Mortality associated with COVID-19 outbreaks in care homes: Early international evidence.* International Long-term Care Policy Network. Retrieved June 30, 2020, from https://ltccovid.org/wp-content/uploads/2020/06/Mortality-associated-with-COVID-among-people-who-use-long-term-care-26-June.pdf

Financial Times. (2020). *Excess mortality during the Covid-19 pandemic. [Data set].* GitHub. The Financial Times, Ltd. Retrieved June 16, 2020, from https://github.com/Financial-Times/coronavirus-excess-mortality-data

Institut National d'Études Démographiques. (2020). *Demographics of COVID-19 death data.* Retrieved August 31, 2020, from. https://dc-covid.site.ined.fr/en/data/

Kaigo shisestu de shibou zentai no juyon-pa-sento [Fourteen percent of death by COVID-19 occurs in LTCs]. (2020, May 13). The Kyodo news service. Retrieved June 16, 2020, from https://www.47news.jp/4808143.html

Kariya, N., Sakon, N., Komano, J., Tomono, K., & Iso, K. (2018). Current prevention and control of health care-associated infections in long-term care facilities for the elderly in Japan. Journal of Infection and Chemotherapy, 24(5), 347–352. https://doi.org/10.1016/j.jiac.2017.12.004

Lum, T., Shi, C., Wong, G., & Wong, K. (2020). COVID-19 and long-term care policy for older people in Hong Kong. *Journal of Aging & Social Policy, 32*(4–5), 373–379. https://doi.org/10.1080/08959420.2020.1773192

Ministry of Health, Labour and Welfare, Government of Japan. (2017). *Annual health, labour and welfare report 2017.* https://www.mhlw.go.jp/english/wp/wp-hw11/dl/10e.pdf

Ministry of Health and Welfare, Government of South Korea. (2020, February 16). *COVID-19 response meeting presided over by the Prime Minister.* http://www.mohw.go.kr/eng/nw/nw0101vw.jsp?PAR_MENU_ID=1007&MENU_ID=100701&page=3&CONT_SEQ=352978

Ministry of Health, Labour and Welfare, Government of Japan. (2014). *Heisei nijyuroku nen kosei rodo hakusho* [Health, welfare and labour white paper 2014]. https://www.mhlw.go.jp/wp/hakusyo/kousei/14/dl/1-01.pdf

Ministry of Health, Labour and Welfare, Government of Japan. (2018a). *Heisei-niju-kyu-nen kaigo sa-bisu shisetsu jigyousho chosa no gaikyo* [Summary of the survey of institutions and establishments for long-term care]. https://www.mhlw.go.jp/toukei/saikin/hw/kaigo/service17/index.html

Ministry of Health, Labour and Welfare, Government of Japan. (2018b). *Heisei-niju-kyu-nen shakaifukushi shisetsu nado chosa no gaikyo* [Summary of the survey of social welfare institutions]. https://www.mhlw.go.jp/toukei/saikin/hw/fukushi/17/index.html

Ministry of Health, Labour and Welfare, Government of Japan. (2018c). *Yuuryo ro-jin-ho-mu ni kansuru saikin no sesaku doukou* [Recent policy trend on for-profit elderly residential facilities]. https://www.yurokyo.or.jp/kakodata/member/sec/info/pdf/20180615_01.pdf

Ministry of Health, Labour and Welfare, Government of Japan. (2020a). *Shingata korona uirusu kansenshou no kokunai hassei doukou, August 5, 2020* [Domestic outbreaks of novel Coronavirus infections, August 5, 2020]. Retrieved August 30, 2020, from https://www.mhlw.go.jp/content/10906000/000657357.pdf

Ministry of Health, Labour and Welfare, Government of Japan. (2020b). *"Shingata korona uirusu ni kansuru Q&A" nado no shuuchi ni tsuite* [Sharing of Q&A on the new corona virus and other information]. Retrieved June 21, 2020, from https://www.fukushihoken.metro.tokyo.lg.jp/kourei/hoken/kaigo_lib/info/saishin/saishin.files/jouhou_756.pdf

Ministry of Health, Labour and Welfare, Government of Japan. (2020c). *Shakaifukushi-shisetsu nado niokeru shingata korona-uirusu eno taiou ni tsuite* [Responses to novel Coronavirus in social welfare facilities]. Retrieved June 16, 2020, from https://www.mhlw.go.jp/content/10900000/000596202.pdf

Ministry of Health, Labour and Welfare, Government of Japan. (2020d). *Shakaifukushi-shisetsu nado niokeru kansen-kakudai-boushi no tameno ryuiten ni tsuite* [Precautions to prevent the epidemic of infection in social welfare facilities]. Retrieved June 16, 2020, from https://www.mhlw.go.jp/content/10900000/000599388.pdf

Mitsubishi Research Institute Inc. (2019). *Koureishashisetsu ni okeru kansenshoutaisaku ni kansuru chousakenkyujigyo houkokuhso* [Report on measures to prevent infectious diseases in long-term care facilities]. Retrieved August 30, 2020, from https://www.mri.co.jp/knowledge/pjt_related/roujinhoken/dia6ou00000204mw-att/H30_098_2_report.pdf

Nomura Research Institute. (2018). Koureisha muke shisetsu ni okeru uneijittai no tayouka ni kansuru jittaichosakenkyuu [Survey research on diversification of management practices in housing for the elderly]. Nomura Research Institute, Ltd. Retrieved May 4, 2021, from. https://www.nri.com/-/media/Corporate/jp/Files/PDF/knowledge/report/cc/social_security/20180420-3_report_1.pdf?la=ja-JP&hash=4885C628FACBBAC4B9AB771D17CED45470B97738

Organization for Economic Cooperation and Development. (2019). Health at a Glance. Organization for Economic Cooperation and Development.

Reynolds, I. (2020, May 28). Masks helped keep Japan's COVID-19 death toll low, says expert panel. *The Japan Times*. https://www.japantimes.co.jp/news/2020/05/28/national/science-health/masks-helped-fight-coronavirus/#.XuZr_y85TyV

Sachs, J. (2020). The East-West. *Divide in COVID-19 Control*. Project Syndicate. Retrieved May 23, 2020, from https://www.project-syndicate.org/commentary/west-must-learn-covid19-control-from-east-asia-by-jeffrey-d-sachs-2020-04?barrier=accesspaylog .

Tokyo Medical Association. (2020). *Koreisha shisetsu ni okeru shingata korona uirusu kansen-jokyo to kongo no taisaku ni tsuite* [The status of the new corona virus infection in elderly facilities and preventive measures going forward]. Tokyo Medical Association. Retrieved August 1, 2020, from https://www.tokyo.med.or.jp/wpcontent/uploads/press_conference/application/pdf/20200730-2.pdf

World Health Organization. (2019). *World tuberculosis report 2019*. https://www.who.int/tb/publications/global_report/en/

World Health Organization. (2020). *Supporting older people during the COVID-19 pandemic is everyone's business.* Retrieved August 30, 2020, from https://www.euro.who.int/en/health-topics/health-emergencies/coronavirus-covid-19/news/news/2020/4/supporting-older-people-during-the-covid-19-pandemic-is-everyones-business

The Impact of COVID-19 on Social Isolation in Long-term Care Homes: Perspectives of Policies and Strategies from Six Countries

Charlene H. Chu (iD), Jing Wang (iD), Chie Fukui (iD),
Sandra Staudacher (iD), Patrick A. Wachholz (iD),
and Bei Wu (iD)

ABSTRACT

Preventing the spread of COVID-19 in long-term care homes is critical for the health of residents who live in these institutions. As a result, broad policies restricting visits to these facilities were put in place internationally. While well meaning, these policies have exacerbated the ongoing social isolation crisis present in long-term care homes prior to the COVID-19 pandemic. This perspective highlights the dominant COVID-19 LTC policies from six countries, and proposes five strategies to address or mitigate social isolation during the COVID-19 pandemic that can also be applied in a post-pandemic world.

Introduction

Residents of long-term care (LTC) homes make up a major proportion of COVID-19 mortality rates internationally within Organization for Economic Co-operation and Development (OECD) countries (Comas-Herrera et al., 2020). During the first wave of COVID-19 between March and August 2020, rates of death were led by Canada, reporting the highest proportion of deaths among all the OECD countries (84%) (Hsu et al., 2020). Throughout the first year of the pandemic, the Unites States of America (U.S.) represented the highest mortality rate in LTC globally, making up 45% of total deaths, including over 100,000 deaths among LTC resident and staff (Chidambaram et al., 2020).

LTC home residents are more susceptible to the virus compared to the general population because they are frailer, have reduced immune function, and multiple comorbidities (L. Wang et al., 2020). This increased vulnerability propelled the implementation of strict public health infection control protocols in LTC homes to control COVID-19 infections and spread in the first wave of the COVID-19 pandemic (Gordon et al., 2020). Most governments primarily focused on acute care and, consequently, did not prepare to mitigate the impact of COVID-19 infections in the LTC sector, resulting in significant resident deaths (Barnett & Grabowski, 2020).

The "failure to plan" (Faghanipour et al., 2020) contributed to a drastic increase in death rates among residents in many countries. Such tragedy led to an overcompensation of paternalistic, broad sweeping, and "overly restrictive reactive policies" (Chu et al., 2020; Faghanipour et al., 2020). The aftermath of these policies has been well documented in media and academic sources: experiences of staff abandoning residents, numerous concerning accounts of residents in solitary confinement for months, barred from family visitations and uncountable residents experiencing their final moments of life alone (Bercovici, 2020; Chu et al., 2020; Levitz & Berger, 2020). Effectively, the ethos of these policies has reprioritized quantity of life over quality of life, physical health over psychological wellbeing, and inadvertently created another competing crisis in LTC homes – a social isolation crisis (Abbasi, 2020; Chu et al., 2020; Wu, 2020).

According to several reports, social isolation and loneliness among older adults have become public health crises (Blazer, 2020; Holt-Lunstad, 2017; National Academies of Sciences, Engineering and Medicine, 2020; Santini et al., 2020). COVID-19 has exacerbated social isolation among LTC residents, a common problem even before the pandemic. Evidence suggests that social isolation increases older adults' risk for anxiety, depression, cognitive impairment, and mortality (Domènech-Abella et al., 2019; Holt-Lundstad et al., 2015; Lara et al., 2019). Isolation may also trigger responsive behaviors from older adults with dementia who are then administered multiple sedation or antipsychotic medications (Oliveira et al., 2021). It is anticipated that social isolation and the COVID-19 countermeasures in LTC homes, including restrictions on social interactions during meals, extracurricular activities, and indoor visitations, will endure at least until the vaccine is widely administered in LTCs (Gordon et al., 2020). (Ireland, 2021) It remains unclear what protocols will be in place in the future to protect residents. (Markowitz, 2021) With this sentiment comes a moral responsibility to incite a realignment of priorities and values to acknowledge residents' quality of life amidst this "new normal".

Despite the strict protocols enacted in the Spring of 2020, and the potential collateral damage to residents and staff from those policies, LTCs continue to be ravaged (Arling et al., 2020; Ioannidis, 2021; The COVID Tracking Project, 2020). There is an urgent need to discuss globally relevant and culturally sensitive strategies to address older residents' sense of social isolation. It is time to critically reflect on the policies and regulations enacted in LTC homes in response to the COVID-19 pandemic. This paper presents an international perspective of LTC home policies that impacted social isolation from Brazil, Canada, China, Japan, Switzerland, and the U.S. We first synthesize the commonalities of dominant policies enacted in the first and second waves of COVID-19, and then we highlight important strategies and efforts to responsibly mitigate social isolation, and reprioritize system policies to consider residents' social and psychological well-being.

A comprehensive international perspective of LTC homes and COVID-19 policies

Given the impact of COVID-19 public health policies on residents, families, staff, and systems, there is a pressing need for a comprehensive international perspective to synthesize these policies and highlight strategies to re-humanize them. The pandemic impacted the six countries represented in this discussion paper very differently; thus, our international perspective represents a wide spectrum of LTC systems drawn from countries with different cultural values and norms, practices, and priorities ranging from collectivism to individualism.

Our international perspective is attuned to our LTC systems that vary in resource allocation, payment systems, development, and integration into the broader healthcare system. For example, Brazil and China are developing their LTC sectors whereas the LTC sectors in Canada, Japan, Switzerland and the U.S are already well established. Correspondingly, the discourse and policies surrounding COVID-19 are very different between these countries. For instance, in the U.S., the act of wearing a mask to reduce transmission of COVID-19 in the general public is mediated by political partisanship and conflated with personal freedom (Makridis & Rothwell, 2020) whereas mask-wearing is considered the norm in China and Japan where there are high compliance rates (Greenhalgh et al., 2020).

Policies and countermeasures in LTC that resulted in social isolation for residents

Several policies have facilitated social isolation of residents by negatively impacting relationships between residents and their family/loved one(s), residents and staff, as well as among residents. Especially striking were the elimination of visitors, elimination of staff and volunteers, and restriction of resident activities and interactions in the home.

Elimination of visitors

Banning all visitors was one of the first policies implemented to prevent the virus's spread. Family members and other private caregivers were prohibited from entering LTC homes despite providing essential care like eating, drinking assistance, and socialization (Anderson & Parmar, 2020). In China, this policy was first implemented in Wuhan and then across the country on January 28, 2020 by the National Health Commission of China along with specific LTC facility COVID-19 prevention and control strategies (National Health Commission of China, 2020). By early April, COVID-19 infections rates in China were low and LTC homes started to allow visitation of immediate family members by appointments (The State Council of the People's Republic of China, 2020b). A similar visitation policy was implemented in the U.S. banning all visitors and non-essential healthcare providers across the country on March 13th, 2020 by the United States Center for Medicare and Medicaid Services (CMS) (Centers for Medicare & Medicaid Services, 2020b). The elimination of visitors was not as clear cut in Brazil, where a major political crisis was occurring, and contradictory public health messages from different levels of government led to significant confusion among the public (Wachholz et al., 2020). Health officials, non-governmental agencies, and Public Prosecutors Offices (PPO) have recommended policies that banned visitors to LTC homes as of March 2020 (Wachholz et al., 2020); however, the Brazilian Health Regulatory Agency contradicted scientific organizations by recommending that the number of visitors and duration of visits simply be reduced.

In comparison, in Canada and Switzerland, healthcare provision falls under provincial or state jurisdiction over healthcare provision, which is reflected in the patchwork quilt of rules, regulations, and health orders as part of the COVID-19 response. Different regions eliminated visitors from LTC at different times during the pandemic. For example, in Canada, the majority of provinces had policies eliminated visitors in early March 2020; however, a few provinces were slow to follow suit (i.e., Alberta banned visits the first week of April). In Switzerland, the Federal Office of Public Health (FOPH) recommended restricting visiting rights until mid-March, by maintaining a distance of 2-meters between visitors and residents. At the beginning of April 2020, it imposed a ban on visits to LTC homes, even if this was legally only a recommendation to the homes (FOPH, 2020c). Legally, it was within the competence of the 26 cantons to decide how visits in LTC homes should be regulated (FOPH, 2020c), but, in practice, the responsibility to decide how to handle visits was mostly delegated to the individual LTC homes with very little guidance.

As the disease burden and number of deaths due to COVID-19 changed over time in different geographical regions across North America, there were significant variations in the relaxation of visitation policies across regions and organizations. In Canada, several provinces began to lift visitor bans after a month while residents in the province of Ontario experienced bans lasting three months (Office of the Premier, 2020). In the U.S., the CMS issued monthly guidance memos and policies starting in the Spring of 2020 on topics such as outdoor visits, compassionate care situations and communal activities, and a recent memo in September stated that individual facilities may still restrict visitation due to the COVID-19 county positivity rate as well as other "relevant factors related to COVID-19" (Centers for Medicare & Medicaid Services, 2020b). As of December 2020, all but three states allowed some form of general visitation (Soergel, 2020). The ending date of this restriction is unknown , leaving residents and their family members wondering when they will be able to visit in-person again. A different approach was taken in Switzerland where they applied a more individualized approach since June 2020, and federal recommendations stated that inside and outside visits should be made possible (FOPH, 2020c). LTC homes needed to carefully plan visits, especially for residents at "particular risk", and follow an authorized precautionary measures plan (e.g., infection control precautions screening visitors, limiting the number of visitors and the duration of visits) (FOPH, 2020c).

Notably, the differences in socio-political climates and cultures between countries drive the policies and corresponding societal reactions within our six countries. In North America and other regions around the world, this was the first time a ban on visitors was ever implemented in LTC sectors. The notable outlier here is Japan, where the societal norm is a deep sense of community safety and the fear of being a vector for the disease outweighs individual freedoms. In Japan, seasonal lockdowns that last 2 to 3 months were typical to prevent the spread of the flu in LTC homes, alongside infection control practices like wearing masks and hand hygiene (Kariya et al., 2018). Families of residents in LTC homes experience visitor restrictions annually during the flu season and consider the lockdowns part of standard care. The use and implementation of a widespread ban on visitors reflect a difference in value systems and daily practice.

Eliminating movement of staff and volunteers to prevent the spread of COVID-19

Staff were the major vectors of the virus and inadvertently spread the virus in and between homes (McMichael et al., 2020). While having low-paying staff is a common problem globally, specifically LTC staff jobs in Brazil, Canada, and the U.S. are often part-time and many LTC staff must work in multiple homes to earn a living wage. During the pandemic, Canada implemented policies to create an "iron ring" or "island" around LTC homes by restricting LTC home staff movement from across multiple healthcare organizations, including hospitals and LTC homes to combat the spread of the virus (National Institute on Ageing, 2020). Consequently, this terminated some longstanding staff-residents' relationships because staff were forced to choose one of multiple employers – leaving some residents without their favorite staff members. Another policy exemplar impacting staff-resident relationships is in Wuhan, China, where LTC staff were prevented from leaving the care homes. The emergency measure, which had staff living in LTC homes, contributed to increased staff social isolation, and negatively impacted the psychological wellbeing of staff, affecting resident well-being as well (H. Wang et al., 2020).

Volunteers were also banned so LTC homes could no longer rely on volunteers to fill crucial gaps in care. In the U.S. and Canada, volunteers provide meaningful one-on-one interactions, social interactions like reading books, playing games, and support recreational staff, necessitating residents to rely on overworked staff members who are short-staffed (Ramesar, 2020). In contrast to North American LTC settings, in Japan and Switzerland, where the LTC sectors are better funded, there is a minimal dependency on volunteers to provide daily activities that keep their residents physically and mentally active.

Restricting resident activities and interactions in the home

In addition to restricting visitors, residents in Canada, Japan, and the U.S. experienced the cancellation of group activities and changes of communal dining, such as staggered dining and dining alone in their rooms, to follow physical distancing rules set out in the respective jurisdiction (Centers for Medicare & Medicaid Services, 2020a; Ministry of Health Labour and Welfare, 2020; Ontario Agency for Health Protection and Promotion (Public Health Ontario), 2020). Further, in North American LTC homes, residents were restricted from exiting the home, and all external activities were canceled, leaving residents to spend the majority of their days in their room for months on end.

In China, indoor communal group activities were restricted, but a small number of LTC homes without confirmed COVID-19 cases and in low-risk areas encouraged outdoor exercise while maintaining physical distancing measures to improve their immune system. The Brazilian Health Regulatory Agency did not prohibit visitors during the pandemic but did cancel group activities or staggered them into smaller groups to ensure physical distancing. Even more flexible was the nuanced way this policy was implemented in Switzerland where social distancing was translated differently in each LTC home. Communal dining was restricted in some care homes and allowed in others (e.g., dining at tables for two residents together). Residents have also been banned from excursions, visits outside the home, and services were prohibited like hairdressers, and podiatrists, but this complete ban was lifted if the home had a protocol in place that was in accordance with national requirements (FOPH, 2020c).

Strategies to responsibly mitigate social isolation for residents

First, we acknowledge that there are differences in LTC sectors between countries with respect to resources, government support, regulations, staffing training and workload; as such, some of the strategies that have worked in some countries may not be applicable in others. While it may not be possible for all homes to implement these strategies, it is important to identify policy objectives that may serve as common ground and viable starting points to refocus on the psychosocial wellbeing of residents. Our suggestions are consistent with other efforts to support a balanced, risk-mitigated approach to reduce residents' physical, functional, cognitive, and mental health declines (Bowers et al., 2021; Stall et al., 2020). In the following section, we suggest several strategies and efforts from an international perspective that can responsibly mitigate social isolation for residents in LTC:

Increased monitoring and resident support to identify and mitigate the negative impacts of visitation restrictions

If policies are creating environments in which residents will be socially isolated for an undetermined length of time, additional monitoring could be integrated into the daily assessments to identify whether residents are experiencing increased anxiety, distress, depression, and other psychological responses. The precedence for this precaution is set in the pediatric population when hospitals were locked down during the SARS pandemic (Chan et al., 2006). Nurses are at the frontlines of health care in LTC and play a significant role in identifying clinical changes and coordinating care in times of crisis (Rosa et al., 2020; Tsay et al., 2020).

Additional monitoring with standardized tools by nurses and other staff members can inform clinicians and stakeholders about declines and when to initiate interventions in a timely manner. Measurement tools should be short and not add to the excessive workload of existing staff, and the selected tool should also be standardized so data can be compared across jurisdictions and over time to identify the downstream effects of different policies. To this end, common data elements are being developed by the WE-THRIVE initiative to measure person-centered care outcomes and may be appropriate to use in the future for cross-comparative work (Corazzini et al., 2019). Staffing issues in LTC is a well-established problem exacerbated by the pandemic; we urge governments to increase the nursing and personal care funding envelopes to support hiring more staff in LTC and improve their work conditions which will enable them to provide high-quality care (Canadian Institute for Health Information, 2020; Estabrooks et al., 2020; Gillese, 2019; Grabowski, 2020).

In lieu of long-term sustainable solutions to address staffing issues in LTC, emergency efforts to rapidly increase staffing levels have been implemented. Some jurisdictions have sought to recruit and train unemployed individuals to act as aides in LTC homes. For example, in Ontario, Canada the provincial government has sought to train newly unemployed individuals as Resident Support Aides (RSAs) (Ministry of Health and Long Term Care, 2020). The RSA assists with activities of daily living including mealtime assistance, recreational activities, or coordinating virtual visits for LTC residents. Such recruitment and training programs can provide persons who have been displaced employment-wise by the pandemic with the opportunity to earn an income, and also engage in valuable and meaningful work that improves the quality of life of LTC residents. Each RSA can be dedicated to a few residents and support them as required (e.g., companionship). These programs can provide additional daily support and may also relieve some of the occupational stressors experienced by LTC staff (Woodhead et al., 2016). While appropriate in the short term, sustainable solutions that address staffing issues are required (Canadian Institute for Health Information, 2020; Gillese, 2019).

Maintaining/supporting safe resident interactions

Many homes have applied a person-centered and creative approach to safeguard relationships by preserving *staff-resident, family-resident, and resident-resident interactions.* One example of this includes safely relocating residents so that they can be next-door or near their friends who they may have only seen in the communal spaces of the home. In situations where a couple is in the same home and located on different floors/units, if desired by the residents, they could be moved to be close to one another. Not all residents can be moved due to clinical needs but in cases where this is possible, relocation is a straightforward way to safeguard relationships while maintaining physical distancing protocols. If a home has space, another option is to rent single rooms to spouses who can provide essential emotional, instrumental, and social care to residents (Mathews, 2020). If staffing allows, homes may be able to maintain resident interactions in small activity groups (e.g., body movement, memory training, etc.) even on isolated wards which as done in Switzerland. Also in Switzerland, several nursing homes installed a "visitors box," a room outside of the LTC facility where residents and relatives could meet in separated spaces while complying to infection control policies (Schweizer Radio und Ferneshen, 2020).

Formation of leadership and management task force

The formation of a small, dedicated interprofessional group of individuals who are responsible for lockdown preparation, collaboration, and communication with families ensures that critical tasks are delegated. The clear delegation of tasks that prioritize residents' quality of life and the prevention of social isolation will prevent oversights and errors and avoids the assumption that all staff are monitoring social isolation. For example, interdisciplinary leadership groups were established in some LTC homes in China (The State Council of the People's Republic of China, 2020a) and Brazil (Frente Nacional de Fortalecimento às ILPIs). Intersectoral working groups are also a strategy identified by the WHO to support the emotional well-being of residents (WHO, 2020).

Use of technologies to connect residents with the outside world

Offering an alternative means of communication for people who would otherwise regularly visit the home, such as virtual communications, is an additional possibility to mitigate social isolation residents with the cognitive or sensory capacity to use such technologies. For example, widely used smart phones and tablets that allow video chatting with family and friends using off-the-shelf commercial devices (Wu, 2020). Tablets and touch screen have had a positive impact in supporting social connections and reducing responsive behaviors of people with dementia in care settings (Hung et al., 2020). Another example is the use of web-enabled cameras that are increasingly being repurposed into "granny cams" by families who want to monitor their loved one through video and audio communication (Berridge et al., 2019; Trager, 2020). Other technologies have also been developed for nursing home residents with varying physical and cognitive impairments (Bedi, 2013).

Clear and timely communication of policies

When government protocols are communicated in a timely manner, to individual homes, their administrators can begin to understand the parameters under which interventions can be implemented. For example, whether the polices have any allowance for creative flexibility or innovation e. visitors' boxes in Switzerland. It is important that there is access to public administrative support to clarify whether individual LTC homes' solutions are in line with infection control regulations to avoid fines or penalties. Moreover, other policies and protocols, such as opening and closing homes, should be communicated to they to ensure family members are prepared and able to follow infection control procedures to maintain the safety of the residents.

Inconsistent messaging can cause confusion and noncompliance (Chan et al., 2006; Wachholz et al., 2020).

Conclusion

This international comparative work highlights the ways in which various well-meaning policies meant to protect LTC home residents from COVID-19 have inadvertently caused a social isolation crisis in LTC homes (Chu et al., 2020). As an international group of researchers, clinicians and experts, our hope is to draw attention to the widespread social isolation of residents, and advocate for an approach that is more holistic and in line with person-centered care. We outlined five strategies and examples from our respective countries that could begin to address social isolation during the COVID-19 pandemic. In the broader context, governments need to address the pervasive staffing and funding issues, and update LTC home infrastructures; until then, LTC home decision makers and administrators need to be more open to innovative person-centered practices that can reduce the trauma experienced by residents caused by social isolation. Implementation of the strategies listed in this article requires LTC leaders who are willing to recognize and address the fact that the psychosocial wellbeing of residents has been tremendously impacted by social isolation.

Key points

- Social distancing guidelines and restrictions meant to protect residents of LTC homes have inadvertently prioritized quantity of life over quality of life, and have worsened the ongoing social isolation crisis among older adults.
- We identified commonalities of dominant policies from Brazil, Canada, China, Japan, Switzerland, and the United States that impacted social isolation in LTC homes during the COVID-19 pandemic.
- We suggest strategies that can be implemented concurrently with broad policies to promote person-centered care and improve residents' social and mental wellbeing.

Acknowledgments

We would like to thank Allison Souter and Amanda My Linh Quan for their contributions to data collection and proofreading the article

Disclosure statement

No potential conflict of interest was reported by the author(s).

ORCID

Charlene H. Chu ⓘ http://orcid.org/0000-0002-0333-7210
Jing Wang ⓘ http://orcid.org/0000-0001-8264-4405
Chie Fukui ⓘ http://orcid.org/0000-0001-9739-9561
Sandra Staudacher ⓘ http://orcid.org/0000-0002-3762-2407
Patrick A. Wachholz ⓘ http://orcid.org/0000-0002-4474-009X
Bei Wu ⓘ http://orcid.org/0000-0002-6891-244X

References

Abbasi, J. (2020). Social isolation - The other COVID-19 threat in nursing homes. *JAMA - Journal of the American Medical Association, 324*(7):619–620. https://doi.org/10.1001/jama. 2020.13484

Anderson, S., & Parmar, J. (2020). *A tale of two solitudes experienced by Alberta family caregivers during the COVID-19 pandemic.* University of Alberta. https://www.chpca.ca/ wp-content/uploads/2020/11/Alberta-Caregivers-Survey-Report-2020-October-13.pdf

Arling, G., Blaser, M., Cailas, M., Canar, J., Cooper, B., Geraci, P., Osiecki, K., & Sambanis, A. (2020). A second wave of COVID-19 in Cook County: What lessons can be applied? *Online Journal of Public Health Informatics, 12*(2). https://doi.org/10.5210/ojphi.v12i2.11506

Barnett, M. L., & Grabowski, D. C. (2020). Nursing homes are ground zero for COVID-19 Pandemic. *JAMA Health Forum, 1*(3), e200369–e200369. https://doi.org/10.1001/ JAMAHEALTHFORUM.2020.0369

Bedi, A. (2013). Gesture technologies & elderly- Overview. *International Journal of Information Systems and Engineering, 1*(2), 51–55. https://doi.org/10.24924/ijise/2013.11/v1.iss2/51.55

Bercovici, V. (2020, June 10). We have failed the elderly during the COVID-19 crisis | National Post. *National Post.* https://nationalpost.com/opinion/vivian-bercovici-we-have-failed-the-elderly-during-the-covid-19-crisis/wcm/e29c7db0-27fa-493b-9381-86539eda0ef9/

Berridge, C., Halpern, J., & Levy, K. (2019). Cameras on beds: The ethics of surveillance in nursing home rooms. *AJOB Empirical Bioethics, 10*(1), 55–62. https://doi.org/10.1080/ 23294515.2019.1568320

Blazer, D. (2020). Social isolation and loneliness in older adults-A mental health/public health challenge. *JAMA Psychiatry, 77*(10), 990. https://doi.org/10.1001/jamapsychiatry.2020.1054

Bowers, B. J., Chu, C. H., Wu, B., Thompson, R. A., Lepore, M. J., Leung, A. Y. M., ... McGilton, K. S. (2021). What COVID-19 Innovations Can Teach Us About Improving Quality of Life in Long-Term Care. Journal of the American Medical Directors Association, 22(5), 929–932. https://doi.org/10.1016/j.jamda.2021.03.018

Canadian Institute for Health Information. (2020). *Pandemic experience in the long-term care sector.* CIHI. Ottawa, ON.

Centers for Medicare & Medicaid Services. (2020a). *CMS announces new measures to protect nursing home residents from COVID-19.* U.S. Centers for Medicare & Medicaid Services. https://www.cms.gov/newsroom/press-releases/cms-announces-new-measures-protect-nursing-home-residents-covid-19

Centers for Medicare & Medicaid Services. (2020b). *Nursing home visitation - COVID-19.* U.S. Centers for Medicare & Medicaid Services. https://www.cms.gov/files/document/qso-20-39-nh.pdf

Chan, S. S. C., Leung, D. Y. K., Wong, E. M. Y., Tiwari, A. F. Y., Wong, D. C. N., Lo, S. L., & Lau, Y. L. (2006). Balancing infection control practices and family-centred care in a cohort of paediatric suspected severe acute respiratory syndrome patients in Hong Kong. *Journal of*

Paediatrics and Child Health, 42(1–2), 20–27. https://doi.org/10.1111/j.1440-1754.2006.00776.x

Chidambaram, P., Garfield, R., & Neuman, T. (2020). *COVID-19 has claimed the lives of 100,000 long-term care residents and staff.* KFF report. https://www.kff.org/policy-watch/covid-19-has-claimed-the-lives-of-100000-long-term-care-residents-and-staff/

Chu, C. H., Donato-Woodger, S., & Dainton, C. J. (2020). Competing crises: COVID-19 countermeasures and social isolation among older adults in long term care. *Journal of Advanced Nursing, 76*(10), 2456-2459. https://doi.org/10.1111/jan.14467

Comas-Herrera, A., Zalakaín, J., Litwin, C., Hsu, A. T., Lane, N., & Fernández, J.-L. (2020). Mortality associated with COVID-19 outbreaks in care homes: early international evidence. Article in LTCcovid.org, International LongTerm Care Policy Network, CPEC-LSE, 26 April 2020

Corazzini, K. N., Anderson, R. A., Bowers, B. J., Chu, C. H., Edvardsson, D., Fagertun, A., Gordon, A. L., Leung, A. Y. M., McGilton, K. S., Meyer, J. E., Siegel, E. O., Thompson, R., Wang, J., Wei, S., Wu, B., & Lepore, M. J. (2019). Toward common data elements for international research in long-term care homes: Advancing person-centered care. *Journal of the American Medical Directors Association, 20*(5), 598–603. https://doi.org/10.1016/j.jamda.2019.01.123

Domènech-Abella, J., Mundó, J., Haro, J. M., & Rubio-Valera, M. (2019). Anxiety, depression, loneliness and social network in the elderly: Longitudinal associations from The Irish Longitudinal Study on Ageing (TILDA). Journal of affective disorders, 246, 82–88

Estabrooks CA, Straus S, Flood, CM, Keefe J, Armstrong P, Donner G, Boscart V, Ducharme F, Silvius J, Wolfson M. (2020). Restoring trust: COVID-19 and the future of long-term care. Royal Society of Canada. https://rsc-src.ca/sites/default/files/LTC%20PB%20%2B%20ES_EN_0.pdf

Faghanipour, S., Monteverde, S., & Peter, E. (2020). COVID-19-related deaths in long-term care: The moral failure to care and prepare. *Nursing Ethics, 27*(5), 1171–1173. https://doi.org/10.1177/0969733020939667

Federal Office of Public Health. (2020a). *COVID-19: Informationen und Empfehlungen für Institutionen wie Alters- und Pflegeheime sowie Einrichtungen für Menschen mit Behinderungen.* Swiss Federation. https://www.infodrog.ch/files/content/schadensminderung_de/2020_covid_19/PHI_200402_Factsheet_Sozialmedizinische%20Institutionen_DE.pdf

Federal Office of Public Health. (2020b). *Ordinance on measures during the special situation to combat the COVID-19 epidemic.* Swiss Confederation. https://www.mediation-ch.org/cms2/fileadmin/dokumente/covid/Erlaeuterungen_zur_Verordnung_2_ueber_die_Bekaempfung_des_Coronavirus-3.pdf [retrieved April 5th 2020]

Federal Office of Public Health. (2020c). *Ordinance on measures to combat the coronavirus (COVID-19).* The Swiss Confederate. https://www.fedlex.admin.ch/eli/cc/2020/496/de

Gillese, E. E. (2019). *Public inquiry into the safety and security of residents in the long-term care homes system.* Queen's Printer for Ontario. http://longtermcareinquiry.ca/wp-content/uploads/LTCI_Final_Report_Volume1_e.pdf

Gordon, A. L., Goodman, C., Achterberg, W., Barker, R. O., Burns, E., Hanratty, B., Martin, F. C., Meyer, J., O'Neill, D., Schols, J., & Spilsbury, K. (2020). Commentary: COVID in care homes—Challenges and dilemmas in healthcare delivery. *Age and Ageing, 49*(5), 701–705. https://doi.org/10.1093/ageing/afaa113

Grabowski, D. C. (2020). Strengthening Nursing Home Policy for the Postpandemic World: How Can We Improve Residents' Health Outcomes and Experiences. New York: Commonwealth Fund. https://www.commonwealthfund.org/sites/default/files/2020 08/Grabowski_strengthening_nursing_home_policy_postpandemic_ib.pdf

Greenhalgh, T., Schmid, M. B., Czypionka, T., Bassler, D., & Gruer, L. (2020). Face masks for the public during the covid-19 crisis. *The BMJ, 369.* https://doi.org/10.1136/bmj.m1435

Holt-Lunstad, J. (2017). The potential public health relevance of social isolation and loneliness: Prevalence, epidemiology, and risk factors. *Public Policy & Aging Report, 27*(4), 127–130. https://doi.org/10.1093/ppar/prx030

Holt-Lunstad, J, Smith, TB, Baker, M, Harris, T, Stephenson, D. (2015). Loneliness and social isolation as risk factors for mortality: a meta-analytic review. Perspect Psychol Sci, 10, 227–237

Hsu, A. T., Lane, N., Sinha, S. K., Dunning, J., Dhuper, M., Kahiel, Z., & Sveistrup, H. (2020). Impact of COVID-19 on residents of Canada's long-term care homes–ongoing challenges and policy response. International Long-Term Care Policy Network, 17. https://ltccovid.org/wp-content/uploads/2020/05/LTCcovid-country-reports_Canada_Hsu-et-al_May-10-2020-2.pdf

Hung, L., Chow, B., Shadarevian, J., O'Neill, R., Berndt, A., Wallsworth, C., Horne, N., Gregorio, M., Mann, J., Son, C., & Chaudhury, H. (2020). Using touchscreen tablets to support social connections and reduce responsive behaviours among people with dementia in care settings: A scoping review. *Dementia (London, England),* 20(3), 1124–1143. https://doi.org/10.1177/1471301220922745

"Iron Ring" for Protecting Older Canadians in Long-Term Care and Congregate Living Settings. (2020).

Ioannidis, J. P., Axfors, C., & Contopoulos-Ioannidis, D. G. (2021). Second versus first wave of COVID-19 deaths: shifts in age distribution and in nursing home fatalities. Environmental research, 195, 110856. https://doi.org/10.1016/j.envres.2021.110856

Ireland, N. (2021). With most long-term care residents vaccinated, restoring their quality of life is urgent, experts sa. CBC News. https://www.cbc.ca/news/canada/toronto/long-term-care-residents-covid-vaccinated-quality-of-life-1.5944683

Kariya, N., Sakon, N., Komano, J., Tomono, K., & Iso, H. (2018). Current prevention and control of health care-associated infections in long-term care facilities for the elderly in Japan. *Journal of Infection and Chemotherapy, 24*(5), 347–352. https://doi.org/10.1016/j.jiac.2017.12.004

Lara, E., Caballero, F. F., Rico-Uribe, L. A., Olaya, B., Haro, J. M., Ayuso-Mateos, J. L., & Miret, M. (2019). Are loneliness and social isolation associated with cognitive decline?. International journal of geriatric psychiatry, 34(11), 1613–1622

Levitz, J., & Berger, P. (2020, April). 'I'm sorry i can't kiss you'—Coronavirus victims are dying alone. *Wall Street Journal.*

Makridis, C., & Rothwell, J. T. (2020). The real cost of political polarization: Evidence from the COVID-19 pandemic. *SSRN Electronic Journal.* https://doi.org/10.2139/ssrn.3638373

Markowitz, A. (2021). When Can Visitors Return to Nursing Homes? (April 30 2020). AARP. https://www.aarp.org/caregiving/health/info-2020/nursing-home-visits-after-coronavirus.html

Mathews, A. W. (2020, August). 'I want to be with her.' When covid closed nursing homes, one husband moved in. *Wall Street Journal.*

McMichael, T. M., Currie, D. W., Clark, S., Pogosjans, S., Kay, M., Schwartz, N. G., Lewis, J., Baer, A., Kawakami, V., Lukoff, M. D., Ferro, J., Brostrom-Smith, C., Rea, T. D., Sayre, M. R., Riedo, F. X., Russell, D., Hiatt, B., Montgomery, P., Rao, A. K., ... Duchin, J. S. (2020). Epidemiology of Covid-19 in a long-term care facility in King County, Washington. *New England Journal of Medicine, 382*(21), 2005–2011. https://doi.org/10.1056/nejmoa2005412

Ministry of Health and Long Term Care. (2020). News Release: *Province launching recruitment program to support long-term care sector.* Queen's Printer for Ontario. https://news.ontario.

ca/en/release/59108/province-launching-recruitment-program-to-support-long-term-care-sector

Ministry of Health Labour and Welfare. (2020). *Points to prevent the spread of infection in social welfare facilities*. Ministry of Health, Labour and Welfare of Japan.

National Academies of Sciences,Engineering, and Medicine. (2020). *Social isolation and loneliness in older adults: Opportunities for the health care system*. Washington, DC: The National Academies Press. https://doi.org/10.17226/25663 .

National Health Commission of China.(2020). *Notice on doing a good job in the prevention and control of the novel coronavirus pneumonia epidemic among the elderly*. [Chinese]. National Health Commission of the People's Republic of China.

National Institute on Ageing.(2020). *The NIA's 'Iron Ring' Guidance for Protecting Older Canadians in Long-Term Care and Congregate Living Settings*.Toronto, ON: National Institute on Ageing Guidance Document.

Office of the Premier. (2020). *Ontario to resume family visits in long-term care homes, retirement homes, and other residential care settings*. Queen's Printer for Ontario. https://news.ontario.ca/en/release/57177/ontario-to-resume-family-visits-in-long-term-care-homes-retirement-homes-and-other-residential-care-settings

Oliveira, L. D. F., Camargos, E. F., Martini, L. L. L., Machado, F. V., & Novaes, M. R. C. G. (2021). Use of psychotropic agents to treat agitation and aggression in Brazilian patients with Alzheimer's disease: A naturalistic and multicenter study. *Psychiatry Research*, *295*, 113591. https://doi.org/10.1016/j.psychres.2020.113591

Ontario Agency for Health Protection and Promotion (Public Health Ontario). (2020). *De-escalation of COVID-19 outbreak control measures in long-term care and retirement homes*. Queen's Printer for Ontario. https://www.publichealthontario.ca/-/media/documents/ncov/ltcrh/2020/06/covid-19-outbreak-de-escalation-ltch.pdf?la=en

Ramesar, V. (2020, August 20). Absence of volunteers creates staffing pressures at N.S. nursing homes | CBC News. *CBCNews*. https://www.cbc.ca/news/canada/nova-scotia/nursing-homes-pandemic-recreation-covid-19-1.5692866

Rosa, W. E., Binagwaho, A., Catton, H., Davis, S., Farmer, P. E., Iro, E., Karanja, V., Khanyola, J., Moreland, P. J., Welch, J. C., & Aiken, L. H. (2020). Rapid Investment in nursing to strengthen the global COVID-19 response. *International Journal of Nursing Studies*, *109*, 103668. https://doi.org/10.1016/j.ijnurstu.2020.103668

Santini, Z. I., Jose, P. E., Cornwell, E. Y., Koyanagi, A., Nielsen, L., Hinrichsen, C., Meilstrup, C., Madsen, K. R., & Koushede, V. (2020). Social disconnectedness, perceived isolation, and symptoms of depression and anxiety among older Americans (NSHAP): A longitudinal mediation analysis. *The Lancet Public Health*, *5*(1), e62–e70. https://doi.org/10.1016/S2468 2667(19)30230-0

Schweizer Radio undFernsehen. (2020). *Coronavirus: Besucherbox im Altersheim[German]*. SRF

Soergel, A. (2020). *Track the status of nursing home visits in your state*. AARP. https://www.aarp.org/caregiving/health/info-2020/nursing-home-visits-by-state.html

Stall, N. M., Johnstone, J., McGeer, A. J., Dhuper, M., Dunning, J., & Sinha, S. K. (2020). Finding the right balance: An evidence-informed guidance document to support the re-opening of Canadian nursing homes to family caregivers and visitors during the coronavirus disease 2019 pandemic. *Journal of the American Medical Directors Association*, *21* (10), 1365–1370.e7. https://doi.org/10.1016/j.jamda.2020.07.038

The COVID Tracking Project. (2020, December). The vaccine is not coming soon enough for nursing homes. *The Atlantic*.

The State Council of the People's Republic of China. (2020a). *Notice of the General Office of the Ministry of Civil Affairs on strengthening the normalization and accurate prevention and control of COVID-19 in long-term care facilities [Chinese].* The State Council Website.

The State Council of the People's Republic of China. (2020b). *Visitation of nursing homes recover: Allowing seven categories of people to access. [Chinese].* The State Council Website. http://www.gov.cn/xinwen/2020-05/17/content_5512461.htm

Trager, L. (2020, May 17). Advocates say COVID-19 outbreak is another reason why there should be cameras in nursing homes [update] | News Headlines | Kmov.com. *KMOV News 4 Investigates.* https://www.kmov.com/news/advocates-say-covid-19-outbreak-is-another-reason-why-there-should-be-cameras-in-nursing/article_8330ecf4-898b-11ea-95c9-3b06f956294f.html

Tsay, S. F., Kao, C. C., Wang, H. H., & Lin, C. C. (2020). Nursing's response to COVID-19: Lessons learned from SARS in Taiwan. *International Journal of Nursing Studies, 108,* 103587. https://doi.org/10.1016/j.ijnurstu.2020.103587

Wachholz, P., Ferri, C., Mateus, E., Da Mata, F., & Oliveira, D. (2020). *COVID-19 situation in Brazilian care homes and actions taken to mitigate infection and reduce mortality.* International Long-Term Care Policy Network.

Wang, H., Li, T., Barbarino, P., Gauthier, S., Brodaty, H., Molinuevo, J. L., Xie, H., Sun, Y., Yu, E., Tang, Y., Weidner, W., & Yu, X. (2020). Dementia care during COVID-19. *The Lancet, 395*(10231), 1190–1191. https://doi.org/10.1016/S0140-6736(20)30755-8

Wang, L., Wang, Y., Ye, D., & Liu, Q. (2020). Review of the 2019 novel coronavirus (SARS-CoV-2) based on current evidence. *International Journal of Antimicrobial Agents, 55*(6). https://doi.org/10.1016/j.ijantimicag.2020.105948

Woodhead, E. L., Northrop, L., & Edelstein, B. (2016). Stress, social support, and burnout among long-term care nursing staff. *Journal of Applied Gerontology, 35*(1), 84–105. https://doi.org/10.1177/0733464814542465

World Health Organization. (2020). *Preventing and managing COVID-19 across long-term care services: web annex (No. WHO/2019-nCoV/Policy_Brief/Long-term_Care/Web_Annex/2020.1).* https://apps.who.int/iris/bitstream/handle/10665/334020/WHO-2019-nCoV-Policy_Brief-Long-term_Care-Web_Annex-2020.1-eng.pdf?sequence=1&isAllowed=y

Wu, B. (2020). Social isolation and loneliness among older adults in the context of COVID-19: A global challenge. *Global Health Research and Policy, 5*(1), 27. https://doi.org/10.1186/s41256-020-00154-3

COVID-19 Pandemic and Resilience of the Transnational Home-Based Elder Care System between Poland and Germany

Magdalena Nowicka, Susanne Bartig, Theresa Schwass, and Kamil Matuszczyk

ABSTRACT

As COVID-19 puts older people in long-term institutional care at the highest risk of infection and death, the need for home-based care has increased. Germany relies largely on migrant caregivers from Poland. Yet the pandemic-related mobility restrictions reveal the deficiencies of this transnational elder care system. This article asks if this system is resilient. In order to answer this question, the research team conducted interviews with 10 experts and randomly selected representatives of brokering and sending agencies in Germany and Poland. We interviewed 13 agencies in Germany and 15 in Poland on the agencies' characteristics, recruitment strategies, challenges of the pandemic, and impact of legal regulations in the sector. The analysis shows that the system could mobilize adaptive capacities and continue to deliver services, but its absorptive capacity is limited. To enhance resilience, policies working toward formalization and legalization of care services across national borders are required.

Introduction

Worldwide, the COVID-19 pandemic has drawn attention to older people and elder care. Measures to protect older adults from infection turned out to be insufficient in most countries, and many nursing homes became COVID-19 hotspots. The recent analyses show that COVID-19 death rates are higher in countries with more long-term care beds, it appears that living in a long-term care facility is a significant risk factor (European Centre for Disease Prevention and Control [ECDC], 2020; Gandal et al., 2020). Given these circumstances, home-based care seems to be a potentially safer alternative for those in need of care services. Due to shortages in supply of domestic elder care workers and high costs of care, households worldwide often rely on immigrant caregivers.

The recent report by the German Internet portal 24h-Pflege-Check.de highlights a sudden increased interest in foreign caregivers in May and in

June 2020, measured by number of internet searches and the frequency with which the terms "24-care" and "foreign caregivers" are mentioned in social media discussions (24h-Pflege Check, 2020, p. 23). However, the severe travel restrictions introduced to contain the spread of the virus affect the system of home-based elder care in Germany. As the demand for home-based care is rising, the resilience of the elder care system between Poland and Germany is of interest and importance both to policymakers regulating the care system and to those in need of care for themselves or their older relatives. The Polish-German case can be instructive for Europe and other world regions where countries become increasingly reliant on migrant carers, for example, in East and Southeast Asia (Peng, 2017) or Canada (Chowdhury & Gutman, 2012).

Resilience is the capacity to cope with difficult situations. System resilience can be defined as the capacity of individual actors, institutions, and the general population to prepare for and effectively respond to crises, maintain core functions when a crisis hits and, informed by lessons learnt during the crisis, reorganize the system if conditions require it (Biddle et al., 2020). Although the concepts of system resilience differ throughout the literature, one of the main conditions for resilience in epidemic crisis is high level of integration of the actors in the system and clear leadership which allows to formulate solutions and initiate actions (Kruk et al., 2015). This condition is not given in the case of a transnational home-based elder care system which is rather loosely organized. Because it spans across nation-state borders, the elder care system in focus here lacks a single regulatory framework or a leading institution. How its resilience could be enhanced by state policies is a major challenge this article addresses.

This article focuses on the system of home-based elder care in Germany that is reliant on transnationally mobile migrant workers, primarily from Poland. It is based on interviews with 28 representatives (owners, directors, heads of departments) of brokering and sending agencies and 10 expert interviews in Poland and Germany. The interviews were conducted between July and October 2020 and aimed at capturing their experiences of service provision during the pandemic, with special focus on restrictions of workers' mobility. In the following, we briefly describe the transnational system of domestic elder care and its main features and introduce readers to the measures in Poland and Germany which were implemented to contain the spread of the virus, focusing on several restrictions to the mobility of workers when crossing borders. We move on to discuss the results of the analysis of the interview material. Firstly, we show how the mobility restrictions challenge the system's absorptive capacity (Blanchet et al., 2017) to deliver the same level of services despite the pandemic; we also focus on the short-term organizational adaptations.

Secondly, we discuss the transformative capacity of the system, thereby distinguishing short-, mid-, and long-term transformations in a larger context of legal and demographic changes. We conclude by discussing the measures for enhancing the system's resilience and the roles of different actors in the medium and long term. We focus the role of the states as regulatory agents. Finally, we argue that the fast-developing scholarship on resilience of health and elder care systems could improve its theoretical basis for studying transnational systems.

Transnational system of home-based elder care

German society, as many other societies in Europe and worldwide, is rapidly advancing in age. Twenty one percent of Germans are older than 65 years, and 6.5% are older than 80 years. In 30 years, one in ten Germans could be over 80 years, and one in four older than 67 years (Statistisches Bundesamt, 2019, 2020a). As more people require care in their final years, meeting their demands is a major short, medium, and long-term challenge for German society and the welfare state.

Germany relies on families as primary care providers. Two-thirds (76%) of Germans in need of care receive it at home (Statistisches Bundesamt, 2018). Yet families in Germany are shrinking. In turn, less than 10% of people aged 60 years or above live in a household with three or more people, for example, with their adult children and their spouses (Statistisches Bundesamt, 2020b). Legally employed care workers and "grey market carers" (Kniejska, 2016) from abroad fill that care gap. An estimated 300.000 households in Germany employ a foreign caregiver (Verband für häusliche Betreuung und Pflege e.V., 2018) who is often provided by a brokering agency (Krawietz, 2014; Leiber et al., 2019). These caregivers, mostly women from Poland (24h-Pflege Check, 2020; Goździak, 2016), commonly work in a live-in and alternating system, which means they reside with the family of the care receiver and take turns working for the same older person with another caregiver. Both caregivers shuttle back-and-forth between Poland and Germany (Kniejska, 2016; Rand, 2011).

The transnational character of this system is inscribed into the specificity of the care work (Lutz, 2011) performed by mostly female caregivers who often have dependents in their country of origin and regularly swap positions with their replacements to be able to return home (comp. Bruquetas-Callejo, 2020; Marchetti, 2013). The usual shifts last 6 to 12 weeks; thereby, a substitution can be agreed informally, and a payment can be unofficial. We refer to this group as "informal care givers" to point to their informal nature of care arrangements not to stigmatize them as "illegal workers". Unlike formal care workers, many of caregivers lack formal training. Also, they support or replace family members in their care activities, thereby entering intimate relationship with care receiving families which places them at the position of "quasi-relatives" (Kałwa, 2007). The brokering agencies also offer contracts for a fixed period of 1 to 3 months, enabling carers to return home, rest, and care for their own families. Geographical proximity of Poland and Germany facilitates the rotation principle but transnational mobile carework is not exclusive to Europe (Makulec, 2014; Peng, 2017).

This transnational care system emerged as early as the 1990s as the result of the informal activities of agents and middlemen brokering jobs for Polish carers in Germany (Elrick & Lewandowska, 2008). Until 2011, when the last restrictions on employment in Germany were removed, caregivers from Poland could work legally as contracted workers (for a maximum of 3 months) or if they registered a company in Germany. Today, informal arrangements between families and migrant carers seem to dominate, but there is no reliable data on the scope of informal care arrangements (Horn et al., 2019). The estimates suggest that up to 80–90% of caregivers from Eastern Europe in Germany are employed informally (Verband für häusliche Betreuung und Pflege e.V., 2018). The German model in which the state pays the elder care insurance to the care recipient only increases the recipient's freedom of choice of the form of care, but it also creates an incentive for informal arrangements (Anderson, 2012). Since the reform in 2017, cash benefits paid for informal home-based care increased by 24% while the state's support for institutional-based care stagnated (Horn et al., 2019). As Lutz and Palenga-Möllenbeck (2010) argue, Germany tolerates undeclared care labor, refraining from work-place inspections in private households (Scheiwe & Krawietz, 2010).

Nevertheless, the share of agencies brokering foreign workers in the market continues to grow dynamically (Horn et al., 2019). These agencies apply different legal models, based on self-employment, posting according to the EU directive or foreign labor law (Leiber et al., 2019). The functions of German and foreign (Polish) agencies are similar but not identical, and they can but do not have to collaborate. Leiber et al. (2019) picture a transnational collaboration model in which local (German) brokerage agencies are responsible for customer relationships (with German older adults or their relatives) and forward open positions to a local (Polish) sending agency; the (Polish) agency recruits and employs (and thus decides on the employment terms and conditions) local labor in Poland and offers potential care worker portfolios to the German counterpart.

Restrictions on cross-border mobility add another dimension to the crisis, next to adapting to new hygiene requirements, which challenge the transnational elder care system. So far, the research focused on resilience of the global health system and its reaction to infectious disease outbreaks, for example, Ebola (Kruk et al., 2015). It pointed to a number of challenges such as access to healthcare, communication between various partners (including central agencies such as the United Nations or WHO), or financing (Meyer et al., 2020). Likewise, researchers also addressed the importance of resilience of workers in terms of their training and availability; yet, the workforce availability has been considered almost exclusively within the states, as a national rather than transnational problem. Collaboration and cooperation between state actors is also a subject of investigation, although the research has taken an international rather than transnational perspective on this challenge so far. The resilience of the health systems in Europe during the ongoing COVID-19 pandemic has already been analyzed and we have learnt from its initial revelations; this includes the challenge of unequal resources in each state, as well as the lack of a transnational approach to health care (Hackenbroich et al., 2020). Yet so far, the attention was dedicated exclusively to healthcare systems. Elder care has either been treated as part of the healthcare system, or as an exclusively national challenge.

We argue that the transnational elder care system's resilience needs to be studied on its own. Care work involves various competences and practices, only some of them related to maintaining someone's good health. Caregivers perform several tasks such as assisting with daily activities at home, help with grocery shopping, cleaning the house, doing the laundry, helping with basic hygiene like washing, tooth cleaning and dressing, but also might be involved in health-related activities as measuring blood pressure. Finally, they also provide emotional support, spending time with their clients, watching television together, reading to them, or simply chatting (Barnes, 2012; Robinson, 1999). Also, the legal framework for home-based elder care and home-based health elder care also differ; in turn, different actors are part of each of the systems (Heintze, 2015).

Restricted mobility as strategy to contain the COVID-19 pandemic

The restrictions introduced by Poland and Germany to contain the COVID-19 pandemic put this transnational system of elder care to the test. The person declared as patient 0, or the first patient, in Poland had arrived in Poland on a bus after a two-week-long stay in Germany which led the Polish government to order health checks on the border from Germany. From March 15th onwards, Poland gradually restricted mobility (comp. Figure 1). Next to border controls, travelers entering Poland were placed under a mandatory 14-

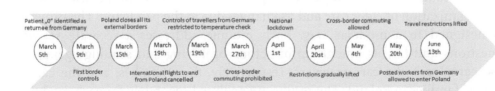

Figure 1. Chronicle of mobility-restricting measures.

day quarantine, which they could spend either at home or in specially designated hostels. International plane and train connections were suspended, and bus traffic was seriously limited. After the intervention of the federal state of Brandenburg (which borders Poland) some measures were lifted to ease the traffic, but professional drivers were subjected to a quick body temperature check at the border.

As a result of the increasing number of COVID-19 cases Poland declared an epidemic on March 21, 2020 and a week later the German-Polish border was closed also for cross-border commuters. From April 1 to April 20 Poland was in lockdown: most shops and service were shut down; parks, boulevards and even forests and beaches were closed to public access as well. Passenger restrictions were implemented for local and trans-local public transport (including private carriers) with passengers only allowed to occupy half of the existing seat capacity of the respective form of transport (a rule which applied to all vehicles with more than 9 seats). While some domestic restrictions were lifted starting April 20, the restrictions on travel, including the 14-day-quarantine requirement, were prolonged. Only on May 4 the cross-border commuters between Germany and Poland were granted exemption from the obligation to a quarantine. Sixteen days later, posted workers from Germany could enter Poland. Finally, on June 13, all the remaining travel restrictions between Poland and Germany were lifted as well.

On the German side, the restrictions on travel were introduced later. Only on April 10, the government decided that European Union (EU) citizens as well as Germans returning from abroad should enter a quarantine, with exception made for job commuters or business travelers without symptoms of the disease who could prove that the travel was essential. The restrictions were canceled mid-June.

Methods

Vis-à-vis the deficits in empirical knowledge on resilience of the transnational elder care system during the pandemic as well as the theoretical interest in transnational arrangements of care, the project "Domestic care for older adults during the pandemic: Impacts of COVID-19 pandemic-related travel restrictions on families in Germany and caregivers from Eastern Europe" asks about the organization of elder care and its changes due to the pandemic. The project is designed in a modular way. Each module addresses a separate set of questions and targets one group of actors: brokering and sending agencies, the caregivers, the care receivers, respectively, their families; and the caregivers' families in Poland. The results are analyzed separately for each module and triangulated toward the end of the project. The first module (Module I) implemented by the project team in Germany and in Poland between June and October 2020 relied on semi-structured interviews with selected experts and representatives of brokering and sending agencies in both countries. This article presents exclusively the results from the Module I of the study.

Sampling strategy

In the first step of sampling, we used existing registers and publicly accessible databases (for example, the German website 24h-Pflege Check.de; Polish portals www.opiekunki24.pl; KRAZ – the register of employment agencies in Poland) and completed the lists of brokering agencies using internet searches. The criteria for selection were 1) that the agency brokers services to private clients (or private and institutional clients), and 2) that the agency offers services by Polish caregivers (or Polish and other nationalities). In this way we identified 206 agencies in Germany and 199 agencies in Poland which – according to their own descriptions at their homepages – fulfil these two criteria.

Out of these agencies, we randomly sampled 27 agencies in Germany and 15 agencies in Poland. In Germany, the population size of the respective federal state was considered by population weights. We chose to interview 15 agencies from the three largest federal states (North Rhine-Westphalia, Bavaria, and Baden-Wuerttemberg) and one from each other state (Saxony-Anhalt was not included because there is no agency offering services by Polish caregivers). For both countries, we also prepared a back-up list (25 agencies in Germany and 10 agencies in Poland) which could be used in case of non-response to achieve the targeted number of 15 interviews in each country.

We also identified five experts in Poland and five experts in Germany. To obtain different points of view, experts from politics, science, welfare organizations, trade unions, and associations working in the field of care migration were chosen for the interviews. We also interviewed lawyers advising agencies and care workers in Poland. Results of the expert interviews helped to specify the interview guide for agencies.

Interview guides

The interviews with agencies included questions divided into five groups. First, we gathered general information about the agency, its size, regional outreach, recruitment strategies, collaborations with other actors, and requirements put on caregivers with respect to their qualifications and language proficiency. The second group of questions related specifically to the COVID-19 pandemic, in particular the travel restrictions and how they affected the work of the agency as well as the situation of the care receivers and caregivers. The third group included questions regarding demands on the side of agencies, for example, with respect to information, support from government, and regional specificities. We also asked the representatives of the agencies for their opinions on the future of the elder-care system with respect to the demand and supply balance, recruitment strategies, qualification needs and standards of care. We specifically addressed (topic 5) the new legal framework. Finally, we granted the opportunity to the agencies to freely express their concerns regarding the domestic elder care in Germany and/or Poland.

Interviews with the experts followed a different script. We asked the experts about their views on the impact of the pandemic and the related travel restrictions on the system of domestic elder care in general, and each group of actors. We were also interested in how they envision the future of the system. We addressed the question of the privatization of the elder care system, and the challenges of the gray market and informal work. Some experts were asked if they collaborate transnationally with other actors. Finally, we gave the experts the possibility to express their expectations toward the scientific research.

Realized interviews

The interview requests were sent to the brokering agencies in Germany by e-mail (two attempts). If necessary, the third contact attempt was by telephone. A total of 52 agencies were contacted for an interview (27 from the first random selection and 25 back-up agencies). Of these, 20 agencies refused an interview due to lack of time or no interest in the study; one agency refused an interview claiming that COVID-19 does not exist. Seventeen agencies did not respond to e-mail invitations or could not be reached by phone; contact details to two agencies turned out to be invalid and no other contact could be established. In turn, we interviewed representatives of 13 agencies in Germany. Of these, 10 interviews were conducted with the director or the founder of the agency; further, three interviews were with a customer consultant, an office manager of a branch, and a person responsible for marketing/cooperation, respectively.

Most of the interviewed agencies have no more than two to eight employees; the largest interviewed agency has approximately 100 employees. Most agencies offer services exclusively in Germany, but four agencies also have clients in other countries (for example, Switzerland, Austria, Luxembourg, and France). The number of clients varies greatly (from 13 to 1.500 clients) and accordingly the number of caregivers the agencies can choose from and refer to German households varies between approximately 30 and 20,000. Only two agencies offer services exclusively by Polish caregivers. In the other agencies, the caregivers come not only from Poland but also Ukraine (6), Bulgaria (6), Lithuania (3), Hungary (2), Romania (2), Slovakia (2), Croatia (1) and Moldova (1).

A similar recruitment strategy was less successful in Poland. Only two out of 15 initially sampled agencies replied to e-mails but rejected an interview for lack of time (1). One agency replied that it no longer sends care-workers to Germany. Telephone requests were more effective, but scheduling of interviews required a lot of effort. The representatives of the agencies were willing to take part in the study, but postponed once meetings had been arranged, sometimes even several times. 15 interviews could be realized. The interviewed agencies have from 40 to couple of hundred care workers on their records. One of them sends workers to older adult's homes in Germany, and one offers workers for the domestic market as well.

Contacting the experts was similar to the procedure with the agencies: the first contact by e-mail included general project information as well as a letter of recommendation and a reminder e-mail was sent in case of non-response within 7 days. Out of 10 requested experts, four canceled due to lack of time or relevance to their work and one person did not respond.

Data analysis

All interviews (agencies and experts) were conducted by telephone/Zoom audio/video call and audio-recorded to avoid misunderstandings. The interviews lasted on average an hour, few exceeded 90 minutes. The interviews were transcribed verbatim. The transcripts were analyzed by the project team (Author 1, 2 in German and author 3 in Polish) using Maxqda software and following the theoretical thematic analysis guidelines (Braun & Clarke, 2006). Initial codes were deductive and followed the interview guide sections as we were interested in explicit knowledge of the experts. For example, we used the code "pandemic" and subcodes "mobility", "border crossing", "transportation," "commuting," or "information sharing." We remained open for new patterns in the data. For example, we added a code "bonus payment", or "requests management". This step aimed at reducing and summarizing the data. All codes were proposed separately by each team member and discussed in team to exclude repeating codes. In the next step, we identified headings and sub-themes to order the preliminary results. Such sub-themes included "transparency" or "quality." This allowed us to find patterns across the interviews. By comparing and abstracting the initial codes we came up with categories of "absorption," "adaptation," and "transformation".

Results

The COVID-19 pandemic and adaptive capacity of the transnational elder care system

Did the pandemic and the related travel restrictions bring the transnational care system to a halt? The answer is no: the system turned out to be capable of delivering the services despite the crisis. The interviewed experts and representatives of the agencies in Germany and in Poland told us that despite all the restrictions, traveling from Poland to Germany was possible throughout the whole period although it was logistically challenging. The care workers were required to present a certificate of employment in Germany to enter the country. Due to the cancellation of the train connections, fewer bus connections, and a smaller number of passengers on the buses all actors – the agencies, care workers and the families of care receivers – needed to find new modes of travel. With the large companies such as Flixbus or Sindbad, popular among caregivers, limiting or suspending their connections between Poland and Germany, Polish caregivers were occasionally forced to use their own private cars. The agencies also reported that caregivers were picked up at the border by their client's family members in their private vehicles. Few representatives of the agencies in Poland reported having driven their care workers themselves. But also new actors entered the system: the commercial bus companies offered minibuses which were not subject to strict passenger limitations. Thereby, the actors tried to avoid the quarantine regulation for the bus drivers by navigating how they split the travel from one place in Poland to another place in Germany: one minibus brought people to the border with Germany, the care workers passed the border as pedestrians, and took another minibus on the German side to their final destination. Such arrangements were time-consuming for all parties involved. Also, less buses were in service which made this solution more expensive. A representative of one of the agencies in Poland estimated that the travel costs doubled at the beginning of the period (it is March and April). These findings are consistent with what Leiblfinger et al. (2020) described in both Austrian and Swiss contexts as well, it is that reestablishing of transnational mobility was a priority for institutional actors despite the fact that traveling was related to the higher risk of contagion.

The owner of a medium-sized agency in Poland recalled the slightly chaotic situation in March 2020 when neither the agencies nor the caregivers could estimate how serious the risks were:

> So the first 2-3 weeks were (...) bumpy. And it was probably on March 20th that we'd heard that the borders will be closing, we had literally just 24 or 48 hours to prepare. And I won't forget it, it was a Friday, we were at work until 1 or 2 in the morning, with our ladies, they all wanted to leave [Germany] before the introduction of the quarantine but everybody was scared, everyone imagined that corpses [of COVID-19 victims] were lying on the streets or so ... it was such a terrible panic, all the bus connections were cancelled. It was hard to organize the transport. And then with the mandatory quarantine we tried to offer our employees and contractors longer stays [in Germany], bonuses to the workers for extending their stay to two months.

This quotation reminds us that the crisis hit an unprepared system, and there were no established measures to assure the system's resilience. Yet, the system proved to be able to mobilize adaptive capacities and continue to deliver services with different, and at times fewer, resources. Organizational adaptations were needed from all actors in the system: the sending and brokering agencies, the care workers, and the German clients as well as transportation companies which made the mobility possible.

Absorptive capacity – assuring the quality of care during the pandemic

The logistics of how to provide the care workers with basic hygiene equipment, including face masks, gloves, disinfection sprays and liquids, was mentioned by the Polish agencies as the second, after transportation, main challenge related to the pandemic. Most representatives we interviewed told us that if at all, they sent such hygiene sets to their German partnering agencies which they forwarded it to the care workers. German agencies reported that the families of care receivers also equipped the caregivers with the masks. One Polish agency decided to send the sets by regular mail to the care workers directly, together with the amended work contracts and hygiene instructions. The amendments to the contracts included a new clause on safety at work. Most of the agencies, though, simply informed the caregivers of the risks related to COVID-19 before they left Poland, or when they were already in Germany. The need to constantly provide correct and updated information was, according to the agencies in Germany, related to a high workload for their employees. Also, some of the German agencies complained that their Polish collaborating agencies did not provide hygiene sets to the caregivers and entrusted it to them. One agency in Germany blamed its Polish partner for doing too little to assure that the caregivers are well informed about the risks. In turn, the care workers from this agency stopped commuting.

The experts we interviewed noticed that prolonged stay in Germany meant additional physical and psychological burdens and the worsening already difficult work conditions for many caregivers. Due to limited capacities of ambulatory care services and daily care activities for older adults, the demand for care during the pandemic could only be met by migrant caregivers. They often worked longer hours and had less breaks, although the agencies stressed that the caregivers negotiated their working time with their clients. Many undertook new tasks, such as shopping for the client, otherwise performed by the client's family members. Also, they were affected by isolation at home, which is commonly their workplace as well (the so-called live-in arrangement). To minimize the risk of infection for themselves and their elder-care receiver, they avoided social contacts outside of the home, refraining from accepting visits from outside. Additionally, the longer periods without return to Poland meant that they were unable to meet their relatives and friends. Some agencies and experts in Poland told us that they received telephone requests from the caregivers seeking further or reliable information on the pandemic. Many were plagued by general fears related to the overwhelming and at times contradictory or false information.

The absorptive capacity of the system, we could summarize, seems limited. The agencies could engage limited staff to deliver necessary equipment and information to the caregivers and care receivers, yet this information and these hygiene sets are essential for assuring the quality of care. Also, the care workers have only limited or no professional training; with ambulant care less or not available, this is a serious limitation to the quality of elder care (see Leiber et al., 2019). The agencies we spoke to had therefore wished for more support from various state actors, and better coordination between the national governments. Furthermore, the resilience of the whole care system relies on the resilience of each actor as well; we only have limited knowledge on the resilience of care workers in the pandemic. Information we obtained indirectly, from the agencies and experts in the field, suggests that the pandemic was a serious burden on the care workers both psychologically and physically, whilst the agencies only had restricted resources to support them.

Transformative capacity of the transnational elder care system in response to the COVID-19 pandemic

With the second wave of the pandemic underway in most countries, and new restrictions introduced by Germany and Poland in October 2020 in order to contain the spread of the virus, it is hardly possible to judge the transformative capacity of the transnational system of elder care. And yet, the representatives of the brokering and sending agencies and the experts we interviewed in both countries agreed that the COVID-19 pandemic highlighted and at times intensified the preexisting problems troubling the transnational system of elder domestic care. Thus, transformation of the system is needed for the system to be resilient, yet the pandemic is just one of the factors imposing the changes.

First, most of the agencies have been facing shortages of care workers prior to the pandemic. These are often aggravated seasonally; for example, when longer holidays (such as Easter or Christmas) approach, fewer caregivers agree to commute to Germany, despite monetary incentives. Polish agencies that are predominantly responsible for recruiting care workers stressed that they had been experiencing serious problems in finding workers who would fulfill the requirements of the German clients, in particular with respect to their professional qualifications.

The increasing care gap (that is the gap between demand and supply of care workers) has led to more competition between the sending agencies in Poland in the last two to three years. Caregivers have started to dictate the conditions of employment and express their preferences for clients in Germany. Also, German agencies and clients are now more likely to accept caregivers with limited language or professional skills and less experience. Increasingly, the central role of the agencies is providing the best possible match between the caregiver and care receiver.

The experts and the agencies estimated that the German market can accommodate much higher number of care workers than Poland (and new sending countries, such as Romania, Bulgaria or Ukraine) could supply. The pandemic increased the already high demand on the side of German families for legal care arrangements rather than for more care workers. Legalizing existing care arrangements was seen by German care receivers as a path to secure continuous care, for informally employed carers were more likely to return or remain in Poland where they have full health insurance. For the same reasons, the families in Germany, according to one of the experts in Poland, showed greater flexibility to meet the demands of Polish caregivers to convince them to stay in Germany. Some told the agencies that they would cover a rent for a caregiver. An interviewed agency owner in Poland said:

> The pandemic certainly increased pay claims from already hired as well as potential care workers. Those who stayed in Germany [during the travel restrictions] received higher salaries or special benefits. We could cover these costs for we saved money on transportation. But also, the German clients now start to understand the importance of this matter [good pay] [...] The wage pressure appeared at the beginning of the pandemic, but we continue to record it. People who earned more over that period will not go below this level now to pre-pandemic rates.

As estimated by the interviewed experts in Poland, the pandemic-related push to legalization and better work and payment conditions may, in the medium and long term, change the system which is still relying mostly on informal care arrangements and strengthen the position of legal actors sending care workers to Germany. The shrinking of the gray market may also give new power to professional networks and associations in Poland which require their members to be transparent about the employment conditions but also drive professionalization of care. So far, associations of care providers in Poland have little power and cannot effectively work toward improving the standards in elder care, both in terms of the quality of the service provision and in terms of fair employment conditions. At the same time, they cannot effectively lobby for legal regulations that would favor the legal actors and effectively eliminate unfair competition and illegal actors.

Also, the pandemic highlighted the need for actors in Germany and in Poland to work more closely in collaboration and coordination of activities. Our interview partners in Germany said that the contact between the agencies and their clients intensified. The agencies in Poland started to regularly exchange information on new hygiene rules or mobility restrictions. Agencies in Poland and in Germany also intensified their collaboration to provide caregivers with hygiene sets, organize transportation or share information. It is unclear if these bottom-up transformations will be durable. The absence of strong coordinating actors such as professional networks and associations in Poland may hinder the transformation and building up of resilience within the existing system.

Discussion

Our interview partners in Poland told us that the COVID-19 pandemic demonstrated that the transnational elder care system is robust: people could do without many other services, but they cannot afford other forms of care for their older relatives. We think that this is true, but we want to point here to the difference between robust and resilient systems. Analyzing the performance of health systems in light of the Ebola epidemic, Kruk et al. (2015) formulated a number of preconditions for resilience as well as features of a resilient healthcare system, which we discuss below in regard to the transnational elder care system.

As the first precondition for resilience, Kruk et al. (2015) indicated the importance of clarity around the roles of all actors at all levels of the system. We see this clarity as emerging but not predefined: the sending and brokering agencies understood their role as central actors in providing information, solving logistical problems, and supporting the care receivers and caregivers in coping with the pandemic. The professional associations could in the future take a leadership role, advance awareness of risks, and create a system to manage them, and in turn enhance the system's resilience. The state can provide active support for such associations.

A second precondition of resilience identified by Kruk et al. (2015) is a strong and committed workforce. The experts we interviewed stress the need for increasing professional qualifications of migrant care workers in general; this includes the German language skills but also training in handling health and care demands of particular groups, such as dementia patients. Social capital matters also in terms of individual psychological resilience of caregivers. The agencies and the experts we interviewed gave us many examples of absence of support networks, supervision instruments, access to information and legal advice for the migrant care workers in general and during the pandemic. As a third precondition of resilience, Kruk et al. (2015) mentioned legal regulations and policy foundation; while we did not assess the legislation and how it shapes resilience of the transnational elder care system, we follow Hackenbroich et al. (2020) in their judgment that health (and we add here elder care) systems in Europe need collaboration within transnational networks which requires regulations that break with an exclusionary national thinking and policy making. For example, Poland faces a shortage of caregivers as much as Germany does; higher earnings for care workers drain the Polish care market. In the medium-term, Poland can fill neither the domestic care gap nor meet the demands of the German society. In turn, elder care systems in both countries become fragile.

Resilient systems are, according to Kruk et al. (2015), diverse, in that they rely on a large number of actors with different roles and characteristics. The elder care system is diverse insofar it encompasses domestic and migrant workers, ambulant care, medical doctors, social workers, physiotherapists and other specialists, families of care receivers, volunteers, local, regional, and national policymakers, and various institutions such as nonprofit organizations, health insurance companies, hospitals, etc. If we take a transnational perspective, we need to consider Polish actors as integral part of this system, and thus must include sending agencies, their professional associations, agents providing training to care workers and so on. Given that the system spans between the countries, it also encompasses these actors which make the mobility possible, such as brokering agencies or transport companies. The complexity of this system makes its integration challenging, but the system integration is considered a characteristic of resilient systems. For the transnational elder care system to become resilient, it seems necessary to create platforms and mechanisms for communication and coordination between the actors.

This puts new responsibility on state actors in Germany and in Poland to build resilience of the elder care system spanning across the state borders. Their regulatory capacities are not limited to shaping the domestic conditions; they also impact the transnational mobility of workers. Germany, for example, signed bilateral agreements with several countries (Philippines, Bosnia and Herzegovina, Tunisia, Serbia, Vietnam) for recruitment of nurses and care workers which may impact the German-Polish mobility of caregivers as well; furthermore, the new Skilled Workers Immigration Act that came into force on March 1, 2020 creates preferable conditions for non-EU citizens who want to work in Germany, also in the health and care system. The implications of these two schemes are so far unclear. The major impact on the transnational home-based elder care is expected by the interviewed experts and agencies from the anticipated new legal regulation of the so-called 24-care in Germany, which requires the care receiver to pay for on-call hours of migrant caregivers in full, which might bring the current practice of live-in and standby arrangements to a halt. The agencies and the experts we interviewed pointed also to the revised EU-directive on posting of workers which imposes that foreign workers are to be employed on the same terms as local workers; for this reason, some interviewed agency owners in Poland predict the end of posted work regime in the medium term.

Limitations

While the pandemic is ongoing and the elder care system continues to adapt to a new situation, our data and the analysis results should be considered a momentary picture. To ensure that the study can be repeated, we prepared detailed documentation of data collection and analysis procedures. We believe that this will increase dependability of our data. Other limitation at this stage is lack of comprehensive data from all actors in the system, in particular care workers and care receivers. While we rely on two sources – the representatives of agencies and the experts – we enhanced credibility of our research by random sampling of agencies, systematic comparison of data between countries and agencies and groups, and standardized coding done by the transnational team of researchers. The transnational comparison of informants' perspectives reduced the researchers' bias, increased their reflexivity and in turn contributed to higher confirmability of our results. Random sampling that we used increases to some degree transferability of our results, but we could not reach informal brokers to obtain their perspectives. The European Union regulative framework as context in which the Polish-German elder care system operates, limits though transferability to other systems and regulatory frameworks. A systematic comparison of Canadian, Southeast Asian, and European contexts would thus be in the future of great benefit.

Conclusions

The COVID-19 pandemic demonstrated the necessity for changes in the system of care. Thereby, the experts and the majority of agencies we interviewed point primarily to the need for greater formalization and legalization of the system while assuring better qualifications and renumeration of careworkers. Legally operating companies could better assist their clients and the care workers in how they provide information, practical help, transportation, equipment but also basic psychological support. Some of the experts we interviewed indicated that the Austrian model of live-in elder care which relies on migrant carers could be adapted by Germany. This model, introduced in 2007, includes a status of "Personal Carers," working conditions, social security, and some minimum standards, training, and competencies for migrant care workers (Schmidt et al., 2016), yet it has also become clear that such regulations are also insufficient to make the system resilient (Leichsenring et al., 2020). Overall, the participating states need to undertake additional and coordinated policy efforts to enhance the resilience of the transnational elder care systems in Europe.

Key points

- Pandemic restrictions were a logistical challenge and burden to all transnational system actors.
- Adaptive capacities were mobilized to deliver services with fewer resources.
- Absorptive capacity of the system needs improvement to secure good quality care.

- Resilient care system reliant on migrant work requires transnational cooperation.
- Legalisation is key for improving quality and enhancing the transnational system's resilience.

Disclosure statement

No potential conflict of interest was reported by the author(s).

References

24h-Pflege Check. (2020). *BRANCHENREPORT 2020. Häusliche 24-Stunden-Pflege und - Betreuung.* 24h-Pflege-Check.de. https://www.24h-pflege-check.de/assets/downloads/Branchenreport-2020.pdf

Anderson, A. (2012). Europe's care regimes and the role of migrant care workers within them. *Journal of Population Ageing, 5*(2), 135–146. https://doi.org/10.1007/s12062-012-9063-y

Barnes, M. (2012). *Care in everyday life: An ethic of care in practice.* Policy Press.

Biddle, L., Wahedi, K., & Bozorgmehr, K. (2020). Health system resilience: A literature review of empirical research. *Health Policy and Planning, 35*(8), 1084–1109. https://doi.org/10.1093/heapol/czaa032

Blanchet, K., Nam, S. L., Ramalingam, B., & Pozo-Martin, F. (2017). Governance and capacity to manage resilience of health systems: Towards a new conceptual framework. *International Journal of Health Policy and Management, 6*(8), 431–435. https://doi.org/10.15171/ijhpm.2017.36

Braun, N., & Clarke, V. (2006). Using thematic analysis in psychology. *Qualitative Research in Psychology, 3*(2), 77–101. https://doi.org/10.1191/1478088706qp063oa

Bruquetas-Callejo, M. (2020). Long-term care crisis in The Netherlands and migration of live-in care workers: Transnational trajectories, coping strategies and motivation mixes. *International Migration, 58*(1), 105–118. https://doi.org/10.1111/imig.12628

Chowdhury, R., & Gutman, G. (2012). Migrant live-in caregivers providing care to Canadian older adults: An exploratory study of workers' life and job satisfaction. *Journal of Population Ageing, 5*(4), 215–240. https://doi.org/10.1007/s12062-012-9073-9

Elrick, T., & Lewandowska, E. (2008). Matching and making labour demand and supply: Agents in Polish migrant networks of domestic elderly care in Germany and Italy. *Journal of Ethnic and Migration Studies, 34*(5), 717–734. https://doi.org/10.1080/13691830802105954

European Centre for Disease Prevention and Control. (2020, May 19). *Surveillance of COVID-19 at long-term care facilities in the EU/EEA.* ECDC (European Centre for Disease Prevention andControl). https://www.ecdc.europa.eu/sites/default/files/documents/COVID-19-long-term-care-facilities-surveillance-guidance.pdf

Gandal, N., Yonas, M., Feldman, M., Pauzner, A., & Tabbach, A. (2020, July 13). *Long-term care facilities as a risk factor in death from COVID-19.* CEPR (Centre for Economic Policy Research). https://voxeu.org/article/long-term-care-facilities-risk-factor-death-COVID-19

Goździak, E. (2016). Biała emigracja: Variegated mobility of Polish care workers. *Social Identities, 22*(1), 26–43. https://doi.org/10.1080/13504630.2015.1110354

Hackenbroich, J., Shapiro, J., & Warma, T. (2020). *Health sovereignty: How to build a resilient European response to pandemics: Policy brief.* European Council on Foreign Relations.

Heintze, C. (2015). *On the Highroad –The Scandinavian Path to a care system for today. A comparison between Five Nordic Countries and Germany.* Friedrich-Ebert-Stiftung.

Horn, V., Schweppe, C., Böcker, A., & Bruquetas-Callejo, M. (2019). Live-in migrant care worker arrangements in Germany and the Netherlands: Motivations and justifications in family decision-making. *International Journal of Ageing and Later Life, 13*(2), 83–113. https://doi.org/10.3384/ijal.1652-8670.18410

Kałwa, D. (2007). „So wie zuhause". Die private Sphäre als Arbeitsplatz polnischer Migrantinnen. In M. Nowicka (Ed.), *Von Polen nach Deutschland und zurück* (pp. 205–225). transcript Verlag.

Kniejska, P. (2016). *Migrant Care Workers aus Polen in der häuslichen Pflege: Zwischen familiärer Nähe und beruflicher Distanz.* Springer.

Krawietz, J. (2014). *Pflege grenzüberschreitend organisieren: Eine Studie zur transnationalen Vermittlung von Care-Arbeit.* Mabuse Verlag.

Kruk, M. E., Myers, M., Varpilah, S. T., & Dahn, B. T. (2015). What is a resilient health system? Lessons from Ebola. *The Lancet, 385*(9980), 1910–1912. https://doi.org/10.1016/S0140-6736(15)60755-3

Leiber, S., Matuszczyk, K., & Rossow, V. (2019). Private labor market intermediaries in the Europeanized live-in care market between Germany and Poland: A typology. *Zeitschrift Für Sozialreform, 65*(3), 365–392. https://doi.org/10.1515/zsr-2019-0014

Leiblfinger, M., Prieler, V., Schwiter, K., Steiner, J., Benazha, A., & Lutz, H. (2020). Impact of COVID-19 Policy responses on live-in care workers in Austria, Germany, and Switzerland. *Journal of Long-Term Care*, 144–150. https://doi.org/10.31389/jltc.51

Leichsenring, K. A. I., Staflinger, H., & Bauer, A. (2020). *Report: The importance of migrant caregivers in the Austrian Long Term Care system highlighted by the COVID-19 outbreak.: Article in LTCCOVID.org,* International Long-Term Care Policy Network, CPEC-LSE. https://ltcCOVID.org/2020/04/01/report-the-importance-of-migrant-caregivers-in-the-austrian-long-term-care-system-highlighted-by-the-COVID-19-outbreak/

Lutz, H. (2011). *The new maids: Transnational women and the care economy.* Zed Books.

Lutz, H., & Palenga-Möllenbeck, E. (2010). Care work migration in Germany: Semi-compliance and complicity. *Social Policy and Society, 9*(3), 419–430. https://doi.org/10.1017/S1474746410000138

Makulec, A. (2014). Philippines' bilateral labour arrangements on health-care professional migration: In search of meaning. *ILO Asia-Pacific Working Paper Series.*

Marchetti, S. (2013). Dreaming circularity? Eastern European women and job sharing in paid home care. *Journal of Immigrant & Refugee Studies, 11*(4), 347–363. https://doi.org/10.1080/15562948.2013.827770

Meyer, D., Bishai, D., Ravi, S. J., Rashid, H., Mahmood, S. S., Toner, E., & Nuzzo, J. B. (2020). A checklist to improve health system resilience to infectious disease outbreaks and natural hazards. *BMJ Global Health, 5*(8), e002429. https://doi.org/10.1136/bmjgh-2020-002429

Peng, I. (2017). *Transnational migration of domestic and care workers in Asia Pacific.* ILO.

Rand, S. (2011). Undeclared labour of Polish women in private households in Germany and Austria. In C. Larsen, R. Hasberg, A. Schmid, M. Bittner, & F. Clément (Eds.), *Measuring geographical mobility in regional labour market monitoring: State of the art and perspectives* (pp. 133–141). Rainer Hampp Verlag.

Robinson, F. (1999). *Globalizing care: Ethics, feminist theory, and international relations.* Perseus.

Scheiwe, K., & Krawietz, J. (Eds.). (2010). *Transnationale Sorgearbeit: Rechtliche Rahmenbedingungen und gesellschaftliche Praxis.* VS Verlag.

Schmidt, A. E., Winkelmann, J., Rodrigues, R., & Leichsenring, K. A. I. (2016). Lessons for regulating informal markets and implications for quality assurance – The case of migrant care workers in Austria. *Ageing and Society, 36*(4), 741–763. https://doi.org/10.1017/S0144686X1500001X

Statistisches Bundesamt. (2018) . *Pflegestatistik 2017. Pflege im Rahmen der Pflegeversicherung. Deutschlandergebnisse.* Destatis.

Statistisches Bundesamt. (2019) . *Bevölkerung im Wandel. Annahmen und Ergebnisse der 14. Koordinierten Bevölkerungsvorausberechnung.* Destatis.

Statistisches Bundesamt. (2020a) . *Bevölkerung und Erwerbstätigkeit. Bevölkerungsfortschreibung auf Grundlage des Zensus 2011: Fachserie 1 Reihe 1.3.* Destatis.

Statistisches Bundesamt. (2020b) . *Entwicklung der Privathaushalte bis 2040. Ergebnisse der Haushaltsvorausberechnung 2020.* Destatis.

Verband für häusliche Betreuung und Pflege e.V. (2018). *Rechtskonformität von Betreuung in häuslicher Gemeinschaft.* Verband für häusliche Betreuung und Pflege e.V.

End-of-Life Care

Rethinking the Role of Advance Care Planning in the Context of Infectious Disease

Sara Moorman (iD), Kathrin Boerner, and Deborah Carr (iD)

ABSTRACT

Advance care planning (ACP) for medical decision-making at the end of life has developed around the expectation of death from long-term, progressive chronic illnesses. We reexamine advance care planning in light of the increased probability of death from COVID-19, an exemplar of death that occurs relatively quickly after disease onset. We draw several conclusions about ACP in the context of infectious diseases: interpersonal and sociostructural barriers to ACP are high; ACP is not well-oriented toward decision-making for treatment of an acute illness; and the U.S. health care system is not well positioned to fulfill patients' end of life preferences in a pandemic. Passing the peak of the crisis will reduce, but not eliminate, these problems.

As social gerontologists who study death, dying, and bereavement in later life, we have based most of our work on the assumption that 21st century death is a product of non-communicable diseases, usually chronic conditions such as cancer and heart disease, or to a lesser extent, injury. Three-quarters of deaths in the U.S. each year occur to older adults and are caused by long-term, progressive, chronic diseases (Boerner et al., 2018; Boerner & Schulz, 2009; Moorman, 2020). The end of life, we have argued, is a prolonged life course stage like infancy or adolescence, and this period – lasting months if not years – provides a time and space to discuss one's treatment preferences, prepare family members for life after loss, and even make preparations for one's own funeral, creating a "post-self" in the process (Carr & Luth, 2019).

But then the COVID-19 pandemic struck, reorienting our attention and forcing us to reevaluate what we thought we knew about how people die, and how they and their families prepare for and adapt to loss. We had overlooked the observation by microbiologists over a decade ago that human infectious diseases have been emerging at the rate of three per year (Woolhouse & Gaunt, 2007). They attribute this rise to the intensifying ways in which humans encroach upon the natural world, such as deforestation, the market for wild game and livestock, urban sprawl, and the exotic animal trade. Although the spread of COVID-19 will eventually taper off, other infectious diseases will inevitably follow. Rising rates of deaths that occur relatively quickly after the onset of illness raise important questions about how dying patients and their families can prepare for the end of life.

Our collaborative work has focused primarily on advance care planning (ACP), the legal and medical process of documenting one's preferences for health care in the final stage of life (Boerner et al., 2013; Carr et al., 2013; Moorman et al., 2014). Although ACP may be most salient to older adults who have one or more illnesses, all adults should complete ACP periodically to be prepared in case of sudden injury, illness, or incapacitation. Adults of any age can complete a living will, which is a document establishing one's values and specific preferences for end-of-life medical care. People can also designate a durable power of attorney for health care (DPAHC), an individual who is empowered to make medical decisions on behalf of an incapacitated patient. These legal mechanisms are most effective when preceded and accompanied by conversations, both with one's health care providers and with loved ones, which helps them to enact a patient's wishes. The premise underlying ACP is that patients and their families, together, will decide whether they desire potentially life-extending interventions like feeding tubes and mechanical ventilation, or whether they lean toward palliation and comfort care. Yet this concept of *choice* – the assumption that treatments are available as needed – has been challenged in the COVID-19 era, as health care providers struggle with shortages of ventilators and hospital beds, and debate whether rationing is necessary (Emanuel et al., 2020).

We maintain that ACP is as essential as ever, yet COVID-19 has forced us to reflect upon and reevaluate the use of ACP, and to speculate about changes in ACP should there be future resurgences of death from infectious disease. We offer four reflections regarding ways that current thinking about ACP poses problems for what we anticipate to be a rising number of infectious disease deaths in the decades to come.

Interpersonal barriers to ACP are high

Interpersonal barriers to ACP are especially high in a time of pandemic. In our studies based on large population-based samples of older adults, we have found that loneliness and social isolation hinder planning because isolated people lack a readily accessible person to assist in these efforts (Boerner et al., 2013; Carr et al., 2013). The social distancing and self-quarantining necessary to stem the spread of COVID-19 has made us more socially isolated than ever before, especially older adults. Our research also shows that supportive family relationships promote ACP, whereas family conflict can prevent it (Moorman

& Boerner, 2018). The added psychosocial and economic stressors of the pandemic, as well as limited personal control over where and with whom one spends one's time, are likely to intensify family tensions which may impede effective ACP. Additionally, living wills and DPAHC appointments ideally follow conversations with loved ones (Carr & Khodyakov, 2007; Moorman, 2011). Simply having legal documents, in the absence of conversations with people who must make the medical decisions, is ineffective. However, the rapid decline many COVID-19 patients experience may cause conversations to occur too late to be meaningful, or prevent conversations entirely.

Sociostructural barriers to ACP are high

Sociostructural barriers to ACP are also especially high in a time of pandemic. Persons with fewer economic resources, with lower levels of education, and of racial and ethnic minority backgrounds tend to be more vulnerable to most major illnesses, and these disparities have been glaringly evident in the COVID-19 era. The coronavirus crisis has cast light on the health risks incurred by nursing home aides, grocery store clerks, prison guards, bus drivers, factory workers, and people in other manual occupations (Baker et al., 2020). Work-at-home is a privilege, one that is frequently unavailable to persons of color, given their clustering in service occupations (Yancy, 2020). Inequalities such as these underscore the importance of promoting discussions and formal ACP among these potentially vulnerable populations, and doing so "early and often" before aggressive infectious disease strikes. Unfortunately, our research shows that race and class disparities extend to ACP, such that persons of color, persons with lower levels of education, and those with fewer economic resources have ACP rates dramatically lower than their more advantaged counterparts (Carr, 2011, 2012a, 2012b, 2016). The low rates of ACP found among Black and Latinx persons, in particular, partly reflect their preferences for aggressive life-sustaining treatment, which is often the standard course of care unless a patient refuses it (Portanova et al., 2017). This desire for treatment is a product of institutional racism and ensuing mistrust of the health care system which have historically deprived people of color of timely and high-quality care (Sanders et al., 2016).

ACP processes are structured for chronic, not infectious, diseases

ACP tools are poorly structured for decisions required when the underlying cause of death occurs quickly or without advanced forewarning. ACP is best approached as an ongoing process that evolves alongside the relatively slow progression of most chronic illnesses like cancer, congestive heart failure, and Alzheimer's disease or related dementias (Sudore & Fried, 2010). COVID-19, by contrast, progresses rapidly from symptoms to death, especially for older adults who have comorbid conditions. Because COVID-19 is an emerging disease, health care providers do not yet have sufficient data to predict how a person's disease will progress in the next days or weeks, making advance decisions difficult. Reports recount patients who are on ventilators mere hours after they were talking with friends (Brown & Beasley, 2020). This is in stark contrast with deaths from chronic illnesses, which generally follow one of three trajectories: terminal disease, major organ failure, and frailty (Lynn, 2004). For this reason, older adults who have already done ACP may need to reassess their plans and preferences because they may have quite different feelings about the treatment they would want for COVID-19. Similarly, older adults who complete ACP during this time of crisis may need to revise their documents later, once the peak of the COVID-19 pandemic has passed. COVID-19 is a stark reminder of a persistent reality: ACP demands continuous engagement to stay current through changing circumstances, at a time when people are already inundated with fears of death.

The health care system lacks capacity

The current overload of the health care system may limit practitioners' capacities to enact patients' advance care plans. Hospitals with a large number of patients and an insufficient supply of resources may be forced to perform triage, and may not be in a position to dedicate ventilator care to every patient who wants it (Emanuel et al., 2020). Likewise, patients who desire palliative care may not have access to it, as palliative care settings are temporarily converted into COVID-19 wards to meet the surge of patients (Arya et al., 2020). These problems are particularly acute in the United States, where health care is a consumer good sold on the private market. In 2013, for example, 55% of hospitals failed to earn a profit (Bai & Anderson, 2016). These businesses respond to market forces, and cannot afford to stockpile extra ventilators or maintain empty beds when no pandemic is in sight. As a result, when a pandemic did occur, the U.S. was poorly prepared to meet the treatment preferences of patients and their families in such large numbers. These capacities may be further undermined in the future. According to some estimates, hospitals' operating revenues dropped by nearly 50% during the pandemic, as revenue-generating outpatient departments closed and elective visits and procedures were postponed or canceled so that facilities could meet the demands of COVID-19 care (Khullar et al., 2020).

Conclusion

The emergence of COVID-19 has strained the efforts of individuals to complete ACP and the efforts of health care professionals to meet the preferences of dying persons and their families. The disease outbreak highlights the ways in which ACP is oriented toward non-communicable chronic disease. We argue that the policy solution is not to simply emphasize the importance of completing ACP. Rather, efforts to increase the rate of ACP need to account for interpersonal and sociostructural barriers to the practice. National organizations including Compassion & Choices (2020) and Respecting Choices (2020) have already begun developing useful tools to adapt ACP for the epidemic. Practitioners will need to develop innovative ways to establish older adults' treatment preferences, and discuss with them whether their preferences might vary based on the particular health condition from which they are suffering. Health care providers also should meet with patients, and ideally a family member or informal caregiver within the short period of time available before death from acute illness or injury.

Key Points:

- Enforced social isolation is a barrier to advance care planning.
- Racial and socioeconomic inequality are barriers to advance care planning.
- Advance care planning is currently designed around death from chronic illness.
- Health care system overload makes patient preferences unlikely to be realized.

Disclosure statement

No potential conflict of interest was reported by the authors.

ORCID

Sara Moorman (iD) http://orcid.org/0000-0002-7555-1769
Deborah Carr (iD) http://orcid.org/0000-0002-8175-5303

References

Arya, A., Buchman, S., Gagnon, B., & Downar, J. (2020). Pandemic palliative care: Beyond ventilators and saving lives. *Canadian Medical Association Journal, 192*(15), E400–E404. https://doi.org/10.1503/cmaj.200465

Bai, G., & Anderson, G. F. (2016). A more detailed understanding of factors associated with hospital profitability.*Health Affairs, 35*(5), 889–897. https://doi.org/10.1377/hlthaff.2015.1193

Baker, M. G., Peckham, T. K., & Seixas, N. S. (2020). Estimating the burden of United States workers exposed to infection or disease: A key factor in containing risk of COVID-19 infection. *MedRxiv.* 2020.03.02.20030288. https://doi.org/10.1101/2020.03.02.20030288

Boerner, K., & Schulz, R. (2009). Caregiving, bereavement and complicated grief. *Bereavement Care, 28*(3), 10–13. https://doi.org/10.1080/02682620903355382

Boerner, K., Kim, K., Kim, Y., Rott, C., & Jopp, D. S. (2018). Centenarians' end-of-life thoughts and plans: Is their social network on the same page? *Journal of the American Geriatrics Society, 66* (7), 1311–1317. https://doi.org/10.1111/jgs.15398

Boerner, K., Carr, D., & Moorman, S. (2013). Family relationships and advance care planning: Do supportive and critical relations encourage or hinder planning? The Journals of Gerontology Series B: Psychological Sciences and Social Sciences, 68(2), 246–256. https://doi.org/10.1093/geronb/gbs161

Brown, N., & Beasley, D. (2020, April 9). From fine to flailing—Rapid health declines in COVID-19 patients jar doctors, nurses. Reuters. https://www.reuters.com/article/us-health-coronavirus-usa-deaths-idUSKCN21Q36V

Carr, D. (2012a). Racial and ethnic differences in advance care planning: Identifying subgroup patterns and obstacles. Journal of Aging and Health, 24(6), 923–947. https://doi.org/10.1177/0898264312449185

Carr, D. (2012b). The social stratification of older adults' preparations for end-of-life health care. Journal of Health and Social Behavior, 53(3), 297–312.https://doi.org/10.1177/0022146512455427

Carr, D. (2016). Is death "the great equalizer"? The social stratification of death quality in the United States. The ANNALS of the American Academy of Political and Social Science, 663(1), 331–354. https://doi.org/10.1177/0002716215596982

Carr, D., & Luth, E. A. (2019). Well-being at the end of life. Annual Review of Sociology, 45(1), 515–534. https://doi.org/10.1146/annurev-soc-073018-022524

Carr, D., Moorman, S. M., & Boerner, K. (2013) End-of-life planning in a family context: Does relationship quality affect whether (and with whom) older adults plan? The Journals of Gerontology: Series B, 68(4), 586–592. https://doi.org/10.1093/geronb/gbt034

Carr, D., & Khodyakov, D. (2007) Health care proxies: Whom do young old adults choose and why? Journal of Health and Social Behavior, 48(2), 180–194. https://doi.org/10.1177/002214650704800206

Carr, D. (2011) Racial differences in end-of-life planning: Why don't Blacks and Latinos prepare for the inevitable?Omega - Journal of Death and Dying, 63(1), 1–20 https://doi.org/10.2190/OM.63.1.a

Emanuel, E. J., Persad, G., Upshur, R., Thome, B., Parker, M., Glickman, A., Zhang, C., Boyle, C., Smith, M., & Phillips, J. P. (2020). Fair allocation of scarce medical resources in the time of COVID-19. New England Journal of Medicine, 382(21), 2049–2055. https://doi.org/10.1056/NEJMsb2005114

Khullar, D., Bond, A. M., & Schpero, W. L. (2020). COVID-19 and the financial health of US hospitals. Journal of the American Medical Association, 323(21), 2127. https://doi.org/10.1001/jama.2020.6269

Lynn, J. (2004). Sick to death and not going to take it anymore! University of California Press. https://www.ucpress.edu/book/9780520243002/sick-to-death-and-not-going-to-take-it-anymore

Moorman, S. M. (2011). The importance of feeling understood in marital conversations about end-of-life health care. Journal of Social and Personal Relationships, 28(1), 100–116. https://doi.org/10.1177/0265407510386137

Moorman, S. M. (2020). Dying in old age: U.S. practice and policy. Routledge. https://www.routledge.com/Dying-in-Old-Age-US-Practice-and-Policy/Moorman/p/book/9781138496934

Moorman, S. M., & Boerner, K. (2018). How social network size and quality affect end-of-life surrogate preferences. The Journals of Gerontology: Series B. https://doi.org/10.1093/geronb/gbx031

Moorman, S. M., Carr, D., & Boerner, K. (2014). The role of relationship biography in advance care planning. Journal of Aging and Health, 26(6), 969–992. https://doi.org/10.1177/0898264314534895

Portanova, J., Ailshire, J., Rahman, A., & Enguidanos, S. (2017). Ethnic differences in advance directive completion and care preferences: What has changed in a decade? *Journal of the American Geriatrics Society, 65*(6), 1352–1357. https://doi.org/10.1111/jgs.14800

Sanders, J. J., Robinson, M. T., & Block, S. D. (2016). Factors impacting advance care planning among African Americans: Results of a systematic integrated review. *Journal of Palliative Medicine, 19*(2), 202–227. https://doi.org/10.1089/jpm.2015.0325

Sudore, R. L., & Fried, T. R. (2010). Redefining the "planning" in advance care planning: Preparing for end-of-life decision making. *Annals of Internal Medicine, 153*(4), 256–261. https://doi.org/10.7326/0003-4819-153-4-201008170-00008

Woolhouse, M., & Gaunt, E. (2007). Ecological origins of novel human pathogens. *Critical Reviews in Microbiology, 33*(4), 231–242. https://doi.org/10.1080/10408410701647560

Yancy, C. W. (2020). COVID-19 and African Americans. *Journal of the American Medical Association, 323*(19), 1891. https://doi.org/10.1001/jama.2020.6548

Palliative Care for Older Adults with Multimorbidity in the Time of COVID 19

Victoria D. Powell ⓘ and Maria J. Silveira

ABSTRACT

Older adults with multimorbidity face difficulty accessing healthcare in the COVID era. Palliative care referral may be appropriate to provide additional support for symptoms, advance care planning, or caregiver distress. Since COVID, many palliative care providers have become more accessible through telehealth; however, older adults may have challenges with technology and require caregiver involvement to use. In the inpatient setting, palliative consult teams have assumed a greater role in daily communication with families who cannot visit the patient and in providing emotional support to front-line colleagues. Busy primary clinicians have embraced these efforts, but challenges remain to sustaining these changes.

Introduction

Older adults with multimorbidity is a group for which early, integrated palliative care is rarely considered (Nicholson et al., 2018). This vulnerable population can have poorly controlled symptoms, functional dependence, poor quality of life and distressed caregivers, but a prolonged life expectancy. Prior to the COVID-19 pandemic, these individuals had established relationships with primary care doctors or subspecialists who could address these needs over a matter of years. When these needs could not be addressed otherwise, patients might have been hospitalized to access the supports needed. In the COVID era, these patients have the same needs, but their access to supports is more challenging. Older adults in general are disproportionately likely to experience severe COVID-19 infection and death, and multimorbidity and frailty greatly increase these risks (Hewitt et al., 2020; Ma et al., 2020). Furthermore, the risk of contracting COVID makes hospitalization less attractive and the need for advance care planning more urgent than ever. In this article, we consider how palliative care specialists can help support this population and review how palliative care can be accessed by outpatients and inpatients during this pandemic.

What is Palliative Care?

Palliative care provides an additional layer of support for patients with multi-morbidity and their families; it supplements, not supplants, existing care. Typical palliative care teams are interdisciplinary and can include a physician, nurse practitioner or physician assistant, case manager, clinical pharmacist, and social worker. While most often recognized for their skill in symptom management, palliative care teams also help with education, communication, coping, caregiver distress, care coordination, and advance care planning.

Palliative care is appropriate for most patients with serious illness(Palliative Care, 2018); "serious illness" is any health condition that carries a high risk of mortality and either negatively impacts the person's daily functioning or quality of life, or excessively strains his or her caregivers (Kelley & Bollens-Lund, 2018). Unlike hospice, which is limited to patients with a prognosis of less than six months, palliative care is appropriate for patients with longer life expectancies if their condition is burdensome; most older patients with multi-morbidity, especially those who require assistance with activities of daily living, are appropriate for palliative care referral.

What palliative care can do for patients with multimorbidity during the COVID-19 pandemic

Among the most important things palliative care teams do is communicate with patients about their condition, prognosis, hopes and fears. Palliative care providers receive training in how to discuss these in a way that minimizes emotional distress and reduces inter-personal conflict. Because their caseload is typically small, palliative care providers have time to learn patients' life stories and understand how their home life and life plan have been impacted by their medical condition. Palliative care specialists are skilled at communicating in a language that patients understand and contextualize the conversation to patients' clinical and social circumstances. Palliative care providers often coordinate with patients' other physicians to ensure an accurate understanding of patients' condition, prognosis, and treatment options. Here we discuss specifically how traditional palliative care services have changed in response to the pandemic.

Goals of care and advance care planning discussions

With a complete picture, palliative care providers help patients and families define "goals of care," or what they are hoping medical care will be able to achieve. They use goals of care, in turn, to assist patients in formulating "advance care plans" for what care should look like moving forward.

The COVID crisis has increased the urgency for goals of care and advance care planning discussions among older adults with multimorbidity and frailty.

This population has been disproportionately affected by this disease; increasing age and frailty are major predictors of hospitalization and death from COVID-19 (Bialek et al., 2020; Coronavirus Disease 2020(COVID-19): Who Is at Increased Risk for Severe Illness?, 2020; Hewitt et al., 2020; Ma et al., 2020). Increasing Clinical Frailty Scale scores are associated with a hazard ratio of death of almost 2.5 times that of non-frail adults (Hewitt et al., 2020). However, hospitalization can lead to a cascade of consequences, which many older adults with multimorbidity may want to consider before deciding to come to the hospital. These consequences are worth discussing in advance, especially for older adults who lack decisional capacity at baseline or are at risk of losing it from complications of COVID. Palliative care clinicians can have COVID-specific goals of care discussions to help older adults with multimorbidity and their families prepare in the event the patient contracts COVID, or in the event that they are hospitalized for other reasons during this unusual period.

Advance care planning and goals of care conversations with older adults in the COVID era need to take a variety of unique issues into account. COVID can cause respiratory failure that necessitates intubation and prolonged ventilation; however, few older adults who are intubated survive (Zhou et al., 2020). Patients can develop renal failure and require dialysis, which has a greater chance of becoming permanent for older adults with preexisting conditions. Hospitalizations for COVID can be long and older adults can experience significant physical debility and mental decline, leaving those who were once independent in a state of permanent dependency post discharge. Discharge options after hospitalization can be limited due to COVID fears and outbreaks in post-acute facilities. Lastly, admission to facilities (acute and post-acute) during this time can be a very lonely experience as most have severely limited visitor access; indeed, there is a significant chance that patients dying in such institutions may do so without family at the bedside. Using a structured framework, palliative care providers can discuss these considerations with patients and families in a skillful and efficient manner without having them feel pressured or frightened. Moreover, they know how to document patients' preferences so that they are available to other providers when patients access the healthcare system.

Surrogate decision-making

Additionally, palliative care providers are skilled at helping patients work through their social supports to identify and document a surrogate decision maker. It is particularly important that patients complete a formal Durable Power of Attorney for Healthcare (DPAHC), especially if the surrogate is different from the person who would be appointed by default. During the pandemic, inability to contact surrogates who are not allowed at the bedside has caused extreme difficulty for gravely ill patients whose life-sustaining treatment decisions were not planned or documented and medical teams caring for them (Friedman et al., 2020). Thus, particular attention needs to be given to obtaining and maintaining multiple lines of contact for at least two surrogate decision makers. Palliative care clinicians are familiar with the legal requirements for DPAHCs, as well as those for living wills and orders for life-sustaining treatment. They can help ensure that patients' wishes are properly documented and disseminated.

Complex symptom management

Patients with multimorbidity frequently have pain, fatigue, and dyspnea, and experience depressed mood and anxiety (Boockvar et al., 2006; Gould et al., 2016; Read et al., 2017). Palliative care providers are skilled at symptom management, particularly the management of pain. When indicated, they prescribe opioids; changes in Federal DEA requirements for providing controlled substances during the COVID era allow them to do so with a virtual visit. (How to Prescribe Controlled Substances to Patients During the COVID-19 Public Health Emergency, 2020). Palliative care providers try to limit polypharmacy and are knowledgeable of non-pharmacologic and complementary options for symptom management. They can support caregivers with advice for medication management as well as teach techniques for non-pharmacologic management of symptoms, including physical positioning, diet, activity pacing, and sleep hygiene. Palliative care teams can identify maladaptive coping and either counsel patients and families or refer them to grief counselors and psychotherapists that can provide formal therapy.

Supporting caregivers

Caregivers of patients with multimorbidity and frailty who live at home are experiencing increased burden and anxiety and need additional support in the COVID era (Cohen et al., 2020; Selman et al., 2020). These struggles include reduced access to in-home paid caregivers and fear that leaving the home for routine errands such as shopping will infect their loved ones (Cohen et al., 2020; Rowe et al., 2020). Palliative care teams are skilled at identifying caregiver burden, counseling caregivers, and locating formal supports for patients at home. They know how to determine the level of support necessary to keep someone at home, and are familiar with the resources in the community to meet those needs (of note, the availability of resources in the community is highly variable lately due to limited staffing). Many palliative care practices have social workers to help with disposition and specialized nurses who can provide case management. For those who do not qualify for hospice and who wish to stay at home, these supports can be the defining factor in meeting this goal.

Outpatient palliative care adaptations to the COVID-19 pandemic

During the pandemic, seriously ill patients have expressed worry about contracting COVID-19 while seeking health care services in person. The changing times have encouraged palliative care providers to open their practices to patients and caregivers by phone and video. The palliative care provider community has been quick to issue guidance and recommendations for best-practice use of telemedicine from the initial wave of the pandemic (CAPC COVID-19 Response Resources: Using Telehealth, n.d.). The best way to find a palliative care provider in the community is by searching the Center to Advance Palliative Care (CAPC) directory at https://getpalliativecare.org/pro vider-directory. Programs should be contacted directly about their ability to provide virtual services.

In our experience with tele-palliative care as practicing palliative care physicians, we have been pleasantly surprised by the amount we can accomplish virtually. While it may take longer to establish rapport this way, we rarely fail to meet our goals for the visit. Moreover, patients and families who might have once bristled at the idea of discussing difficult topics by phone have expressed gratitude for the opportunity and convenience.

Admittedly, older adults with multimorbidity or frailty are a group for whom tele-palliative care may be challenging. Many have difficulties with technology (Dewar et al., 2020). Others have issues with hearing and vision that make it nearly impossible to communicate this way. Still others have enough cognitive impairment to make it impossible to obtain a good history or assure proper uptake of clinical advice. For these individuals, caregiver involvement in the virtual consultation is essential. Providers referring patients to palliative care can improve the first visit's success by recommending that caregivers be present during the appointment. Including the caregiver's contact information in the referral helps the palliative care team coordinate technical support for the patient and caregiver on the day of the appointment. Other palliative care teams' experiences during the pandemic supports the idea of providing anticipatory guidance regarding the limitations of technology (ie., limited video resolution and sound quality, etc.) and establishing back-up plans for communication (Ritchey et al., 2020). Delegating support staff to provide templated instructions for platform access in advance of the appointment can be helpful (Calton et al., 2020).

Expanding and integrated roles for inpatient palliative care as the COVID-19 pandemic evolves

Palliative care continues to be available in most hospitals through consultation to address symptoms, goals of care, advance care planning, and caregiver distress. For older adults with multimorbidity who are COVID negative, palliative care teams can provide traditional consultation in a face to face fashion, with masks donned. Their services remain mostly unchanged during this new era, with one very important exception: palliative care teams have become liaisons and advocates for family who cannot visit patients who are hospitalized. Perhaps no other change has created as much distress for older patients and families than the COVID-era limitations on visitors to the hospital. Older adults, especially those with cognitive impairment, feel vulnerable without their family at the bedside and families feel guilty for leaving them alone. Moreover, inability to be at the bedside cuts families off from the most common vehicle for receiving updates on the patient's status – bedside rounds. In many health systems, including ours, palliative care teams have been providing daily updates to families, as well as helping to facilitate regular video conferences between them and the patient (even when the patient is unconscious) (Calton et al., 2020; Ritchey et al., 2020). Anecdotally, this has helped both patients and families feel more connected with each other as well as to the medical team.

COVID has also impacted the kinds of conversations that palliative care teams are having with older inpatients around disposition. Stringent COVID screening criteria and reduced availability of post-acute rehabilitation beds can mean patients must either wait or travel long distances after discharge before starting rehabilitation; these considerations can impact the benefit-burden calculus in favor of returning home prematurely or going into a long-term care facility instead. Palliative care teams can help patients and families adjust when the options for discharge do not match their expectations.

When older inpatients are COVID-positive, palliative care teams have been avoiding face to face interactions in order to protect the health of their small teams. Despite this, the frequency and intensity of their conversations with these highly distressed and at-risk patients and families has not waivered. They will call patients in their rooms to assess symptoms, discuss COVID-specific goals of care, and elicit treatment preferences. They will call families to provide daily updates and emotional support; their continuity with families helps families prepare for the moment when patients fail to recover. In order to ensure communication is coordinated and accurate, palliative care teams have found it necessary to have regular check-ins with hospitalist and ICU teams caring for shared COVID patients.

Most older adults with COVID who die do so in the hospital, given the reduced options for discharge. Some institutions allow palliative care teams to assume full responsibility for managing these patients at the end of life; this can help facilitate patients and families have a peaceful transition. Other institutions have closed their palliative care units or hospice beds during COVID, and require that end-of-life patients be managed by their original inpatient providers. In these institutions, palliative care works closely with the primary team and nursing to ensure symptom management recommendations are adopted and families are given special permission to visit the patient.

Throughout hospitals, palliative care teams have been providing emotional support and guidance for colleagues on the frontlines who have become stressed by their clinical burden and distressed by the mortality that surrounds them (Alford & Chester, 2020). This includes providing empathetic listening, at-the-elbow communication coaching, as well as guidance for where to access wellness resources at their institutions.

Conclusion

Now more than ever, palliative care can be a valuable resource for older adults with multimorbidity, their families, and their primary providers. The services that palliative care teams provide can help patients and families navigate the new challenges that they face due to COVID's impact on the healthcare system, including fewer supports in the community, restrictive hospital visitation policies and limited access to post-acute care. Recognizing the expanded spectrum of what palliative care can do can give primary providers opportunities for involving palliative care earlier in the care of their older adult patients with multimorbidity. This, in turn, can allow providers who are under pressure to see more patients in less time to devote their time to disease management.

Key Points

• Palliative care can provide an additional layer of support for adults with multimorbidity

• Adoption of telehealth by palliative clinics during the COVID-19 pandemic has increased access

• Visitor limitations place additional stress on inpatients, families, and primary teams

• Inpatient palliative care consult teams can provide daily updates to families to reduce their distress

Disclosure Statement

No potential conflict of interest was reported by the authors.

Funding

Silveira's time was funded by the Geriatric Research Education and Clinical Center; Dr. Powell's time was funded by the VA Advanced Fellowship in Geriatrics and NIA under training grant AG062043.

ORCID

Victoria D. Powell ⓘ http://orcid.org/0000-0002-7108-5449

References

Alford, G. W., & Chester, R. (2020). *Providing soul care in the COVID-19 era*. Center to Advance Palliative Care. Retrieved September 9, 2020, from https://www.capc.org/blog/providing-soul-care-covid-19-era/

Bialek, S., Boundy, E., Bowen, V., Chow, N., Cohn, A., Dowling, N., ... Sauber-Schatz, E. (2020). Severe outcomes among patients with coronavirus disease 2019 (COVID-19) — United States, February 12–March 16, 2020. *MMWR. Morbidity and Mortality Weekly Report, 69*(12), 343–346. https://doi.org/10.15585/mmwr.mm6912e2

Boockvar, K. S., & Meier, D. E. (2006). Palliative care for frail older adults: "there are things I can't do anymore that I wish I could". *JAMA, 296*(18), 2245–2253. PMID: 17090771. https://doi.org/10.1001/jama.296.18.2245

Calton, B., Abedini, N., & Fratkin, M. (2020). Telemedicine in the time of coronavirus. *Journal of Pain and Symptom Management, 60*(1), e12–e14. https://doi.org/10.1016/j.jpainsymman.2020.03.019

CAPC COVID-19 Response Resources: Using Telehealth. (n.d.). *COVID-19 Response Resources Hub*. Center to Advance Palliative Care. Retrieved September 9, 2020, from https://www.capc.org/toolkits/covid-19-response-resources/

Cohen, G., Russo, M. J., Campos, J. A., & Allegri, R. F. (2020). Living with dementia: Increased level of caregiver stress in times of COVID-19. *International Psychogeriatrics*, 1–11. https://doi.org/10.1017/S1041610220001593

Coronavirus Disease 2019 (COVID-19): Who Is at Increased Risk for Severe Illness? (2020). Centers for Disease Control. Retrieved June 26, 2020, from https://www.cdc.gov/coronavirus/2019-ncov/need-extra-precautions/people-at-increased-risk.html?CDC_AA_refVal=https%3A%2F%2Fwww.cdc.gov%2Fcoronavirus%2F2019-ncov%2Fneed-extra-precautions%2Fpeople-at-higher-risk.html

Dewar, S., Lee, P. G., Suh, T. T., & Min, L. (2020). Uptake of virtual visits in a geriatric primary care clinic during the COVID-19 pandemic. *Journal of the American Geriatrics Society, 68*(7), 1392–1394. https://doi.org/10.1111/jgs.16534

Friedman, D. N., Blackler, L., Alici, Y., Scharf, A. E., Chin, M., Chawla, S., ... Voigt, L. P. (2020). COVID-19-related ethics consultations at a cancer center in New York City: A content review of ethics consultations during the early stages of the pandemic. *JCO Oncology Practice*, OP2000440. https://doi.org/10.1200/OP.20.00440

Gould, C. E., O'Hara, R., Goldstein, M. K., & Beaudreau, S. A. (2016). Multimorbidity is associated with anxiety in older adults in the health and retirement study. *International Journal of Geriatric Psychiatry, 31*(10), 1105–1115. https://doi.org/10.1002/gps.4532

Hewitt, J., Carter, B., Vilches-Moraga, A., Quinn, T. J., Braude, P., Verduri, A., ... Guaraldi, G. (2020). The effect of frailty on survival in patients with COVID-19 (COPE): A multicentre, European, observational cohort study. *The Lancet Public Health, 5*(8), e444–e451. https://doi.org/10.1016/S2468-2667(20)30146-8

How to Prescribe Controlled Substances to Patients During the COVID-19 Public Health Emergency. (2020). Drug Enforcement Administration/Diversion Control Division. Retrieved June 26, 2020, from https://www.deadiversion.usdoj.gov/GDP/(DEA-DC-023)(DEA075)Decision_Tree_(Final)_33120_2007.pdf

Kelley, A. S., & Bollens-Lund, E. (2018). Identifying the population with serious illness: The "denominator" challenge. *Journal of Palliative Medicine, 21*(S2), S-7-S-16. https://doi.org/10.1089/jpm.2017.0548

Ma, Y., Hou, L., Yang, X., Huang, Z., Yang, X., Zhao, N., ... Wu, C. (2020). The association between frailty and severe disease among COVID-19 patients aged over 60 years in China: A prospective cohort study. *BMC Medicine, 18*(1), 274. https://doi.org/10.1186/s12916-020-01761-0

Nicholson, C., Davies, J. M., George, R., Smith, B., Pace, V., Harris, L., ... Murtagh, F. E. M. (2018). What are the main palliative care symptoms and concerns of older people with multimorbidity?—A comparative cross-sectional study using routinely collected phase of illness, Australia-modified karnofsky performance status and integrated palliative care out. *Annals of Palliative Medicine, 7*(Suppl 3), S164–S175. https://doi.org/10.21037/apm.2018.06.07

Palliative Care. (2018). World Health Organization. Retrieved June 26, 2020, from https://www.who.int/news-room/fact-sheets/detail/palliative-care

Read, J. R., Sharpe, L., Modini, M., & Dear, B. F. (2017). Multimorbidity and depression: A systematic review and meta-analysis. *Journal of Affective Disorders, 221*, 36–46. https://doi.org/10.1016/j.jad.2017.06.009

Ritchey, K. C., Foy, A., McArdel, E., & Gruenewald, D. A. (2020). Reinventing palliative care delivery in the era of COVID-19: How telemedicine can support end of life care. *American Journal of Hospice and Palliative Medicine, 37*(11), 992–997. https://doi.org/10.1177/1049909120948235

Rowe, T. A., Patel, M., O'Conor, R., McMackin, S., Hoak, V., & Lindquist, L. A. (2020). COVID-19 exposures and infection control among home care agencies. *Archives of Gerontology and Geriatrics, 91*(July), 104214. https://doi.org/10.1016/j.archger.2020.104214

Selman, L. E., Chao, D., Sowden, R., Marshall, S., Chamberlain, C., & Koffman, J. (2020). Bereavement support on the frontline of COVID-19: Recommendations for hospital clinicians. *Journal of Pain and Symptom Management, 60*(2), e81–e86. https://doi.org/10.1016/j.jpainsymman.2020.04.024

Zhou, F., Yu, T., Du, R., Fan, G., Liu, Y., Liu, Z., ... Cao, B. (2020). Clinical course and risk factors for mortality of adult inpatients with COVID-19 in Wuhan, China: A retrospective cohort study. *The Lancet, 395*(10229), 1054–1062. https://doi.org/10.1016/S0140-6736(20)30566-3

Technology and Innovation

Cross-Border Medical Services for Hong Kong's Older Adults in Mainland China: The Implications of COVID-19 for the Future of Telemedicine

Genghua Huang, Yin Ma, and Zhaiwen Peng ⓘD

ABSTRACT
Cross-border services and support are becoming an increasingly important part of Hong Kong's social policy because an increasing number of its older citizens are choosing to live in mainland China. Unfortunately, with the recent outbreak of COVID-19, medical services for cross-border older adults have been blocked due to strict immigration controls. This article examines the effects of COVID-19 on these older adults, with a specific focus on the interruption of medical services and the remedial measures taken by the government and non-governmental organizations. It also discusses the prospect of delivering care for cross-border older people using telemedicine, which is considered one of the most important methods for overcoming space-distance and reducing the risk of cross-contamination caused by close contact.

Introduction

Hong Kong is one of the most crowded cities in the world. Its population density was about 6,880 per km² in 2018 (The Government of Hong Kong Special Administrative Region [GovHK], 2020), and the median per capita floor area of accommodation was only 15 m² in 2016 (Commissioner for Census and Statistics [CSD], 2016). Hong Kong is also an aging society, and older adults – aged 65 and over – accounted for more than 17% of its total population in 2019 (Commissioner for Census and Statistics [CSD], 2020). In recent years, a growing cohort of older adults in Hong Kong have chosen to live in mainland China for the lower cost of living and larger houses (Wang, 2011). To respond to the increasing demand for social welfare and services from such a significant cross-border group, the Hong Kong government has extended some of its social policies beyond Hong Kong, breaking its traditional principle of "welfare could only be provided for residents within the borders" (Cao & Fang, 2019; Seui, 2014; Wang, 2011). For example,

Hong Kong's older adults who have chosen to live in Guangdong or Fujian provinces have become entitled to the old-age allowance that was designed for those living in Hong Kong, and the Hong Kong government also subsidizes its older citizens who choose to live in residential care homes in Guangdong (The Government of Hong Kong Special Administrative Region [GovHK], 2014). In this context, cross-border services and support are becoming an increasingly important part of Hong Kong's social policy.

However, medical services in Hong Kong still cannot be provided beyond its borders because of the limitations of space-distance and technology. Given that most of Hong Kong's older adults living in mainland China have chronic diseases, such as high blood pressure and diabetes, they must return to Hong Kong frequently for medical matters (Wang, 2011). Unfortunately, with the recent outbreak of COVID-19, medical services for cross-border older adults have been blocked due to strict immigration controls. Against this background, the current article examines changing policies around cross-border services and supports in Hong Kong and summarizes the effects of COVID-19 on cross-border older adults, with a specific focus on the interruption of medical and the remedial measures taken by the government and non-governmental organizations (NGO) (The Government of Hong Kong Special Administrative Region [GovHK], 2020a). It also discusses the prospect of delivering care for cross-border older people using telemedicine, which is considered one of the most important methods for overcoming space-distance and reducing the risk of cross-contamination caused by close contact (Hollander & Carr, 2020; Mallineni et al., 2020).

Cross-border social policy for Hong Kong's older adults in mainland China

Hong Kong is an immigrant society, and a significant proportion of its population is descended from migrants from mainland China (Chou et al., 2004; Law & Lee, 2006). The influx of mainland migrants continued long after its establishment as a British colony in 1841, and, in the 1960s and 1970s, a massive wave of migrants fled to Hong Kong to seek refuge because of the famine and political unrest caused by the Great Leap Forward and the Cultural Revolution in mainland China (Chan & Chou, 2016). Representing a plentiful supply of cheap labor, these migrants were essential to Hong Kong's economic miracle (Chan & Chou, 2016; Law & Lee, 2006). However, with the rapid development of the Chinese economy and society, an increasing number of older adults in Hong Kong in recent years have chosen to enjoy their retirement in mainland China. In addition to sharing a similar culture and living habits, a key reason for older adults deciding to retire on the mainland is the lower cost of living, and the ability to buy larger houses or move to residential care homes with better environments (Wang, 2011). In 2013, figures from the Hong Kong government showed that about 67,600 of Hong Kong's older adults (aged 65 and over), accounting for about 7% of its aging population, were living in Guangdong, a mainland province bordering Hong Kong (Commissioner for Census and Statistics [CSD], 2014, 2020a).

This new situation and trend have presented a big challenge to the traditional social policy in Hong Kong and prompted calls for the portability of welfare benefits, which allows Hong Kong citizens to maintain acquired benefits when moving to mainland China (Cao & Fang, 2019; Mok et al., 2017; Seui, 2014; Wang, 2011). Old Age Allowance (OAA) and Old Age Living Allowance (OALA), colloquially known as fruit money, are important components of Hong Kong's welfare system for older adults. Financed by the government, they supplement the income of older adults in different ways: OAA provides recipients aged 70 and above with universal allowances, while OALA offers means-tested monthly allowances to residents who are aged 65 and above and fall below certain income and asset thresholds (Bai, 2019; Yu, 2008). However, OAA and OALA recipients were originally required to stay in Hong Kong, which meant that a large number of Hong Kong's older adults living in mainland China were excluded from these benefits. To respond to the increasing demand for social welfare from such a huge cross-border group, the Hong Kong government has extended some of its social policies beyond Hong Kong. Since 2013 and 2018, the Hong Kong government has launched the Guangdong Scheme and Fujian Scheme to make Hong Kong's older adults living in Guangdong and Fujian provinces, respectively, entitled to the OAA and OALA. In addition, Hong Kong has a severe shortage of care facilities and nursing home places, and older adults who need long-term care are always subject to long waiting times for residential care services – 41 months on average for government-funded care facilities and nursing homes (Social Welfare Department, 2020). For this reason, some older people also want to move to the mainland for residential care services. In another move toward welfare portability, in 2014, the Hong Kong government introduced the Pilot Residential Care Services Scheme in Guangdong, which subsidizes those who choose to live in residential care homes in Guangdong operated by two Hong Kong NGOs – The Hong Kong Society for Rehabilitation and Helping Hand (GovHK, 2014).

The establishment of the Guangdong–Hong Kong–Macao Greater Bay Area was initiated by the central government of China in 2016 (China State Council, 2016), aiming to facilitate in-depth regional integration and develop a world-class city cluster ideal for living in the Pearl River Delta (Hui et al., 2018). With this national strategy as a catalyst, the mainland's high-speed railway was extended to Hong Kong in 2018. Convenient transportation has further encouraged Hong Kong's older adults to consider moving to the mainland, especially Guangdong province. In 2019, the number of Hong Kong's older adults (aged 65 and over) living in Guangdong increased to about 90,200 (CSD, 2020a), which was 33% higher than in 2013. These people are becoming increasingly important targets in the context of Hong Kong's social policy; more attention needs to be given to the question of how to efficiently deliver services and support to this population.

The challenge posed to medical services by COVID-19

Although Hong Kong has traditionally been labeled as a residual welfare state (Chan, 1998), the government does intervene to a large extent in the health-care system (Ramesh, 2004). Public hospitals provide tax-funded medical services for every Hong Kong resident, making them universally accessible (Wong, 2008). In other words, as a welfare benefit, both older adults in general and those with long-term care needs can be offered quality medical services with a high rate of subsidy in Hong Kong.

Among cross-border services and supports, medical services have borne the brunt of the COVID-19 pandemic. Most of Hong Kong's older adults living in mainland China have chronic diseases, such as high blood pressure and diabetes, and medical services are essential for them. On the one hand, medical services in Hong Kong still cannot be provided beyond the borders because of limitations in space-distance and technology; on the other hand, it could be very expensive if these older adults chose to go to local hospitals, as few of them are covered by the requisite social medical insurance needed to obtain care on the mainland. Consequently, cross-border older adults must return to Hong Kong frequently for medical reasons. Even those living in subsidized residential care homes in Guangdong usually need to be escorted back to Hong Kong for medical follow-up, as the services provided in the care homes themselves are just basic nursing and personal care.

Existing cross-border medical practices have been disrupted by the COVID-19 pandemic. On January 23, 2020, the first case in Hong Kong was confirmed, and it became one of the first places to experience the COVID-19 outbreak outside mainland China. As of November 27, 2020, the overall number of infections had reached 6,040, while 108 deaths had been confirmed (The Government of Hong Kong Special Administrative Region [GovHK], 2020b). According to a study by The Chinese University of Hong Kong (2020), the case fatality rate for older adults – aged 60 or above – in Hong Kong was about 6.27%, which was almost 105 times that of the other group – below 60. Similarly, older adults have a higher case fatality rate in mainland China. Wu and McGoogan (2020) analyzed 44,672 confirmed cases in mainland China, and they found that the case fatality rate for people aged between 70 and 79 was about 8%. To prevent imported coronavirus infections, the Hong Kong government has imposed immigration controls since February 2020. Although Hong Kong residents are still allowed to enter from the mainland, they are required to be placed under mandatory quarantine for 14 days. This stringent measure has undoubtedly created difficulties for medical follow-up in Hong Kong. Far worse, most of the older adults with chronic diseases have begun facing drug shortages. Although they may seek help from their family members or friends to collect medications from medical institutions in Hong Kong, the drugs are not allowed to be mailed out of Hong Kong by individuals according to present legal regulations (GovHK, 2020a).

To deal with this tricky problem, the Hong Kong government introduced a special scheme for delivering prescription medications to Hong Kong residents in Guangdong and Fujian (GovHK, 2020a). The government commissioned the Hong Kong Federation of Trade Unions (FTU) to provide the relevant services, since it has many offices and a well-established service network on the mainland. The FTU helps those with an urgent need for medications to collect them in Hong Kong and then sends them by express delivery to its offices on the mainland; the government bears all the delivery costs (GovHK, 2020a). These special arrangements have received a warm response, and more than 7,600 Hong Kong residents – mostly older adults – had received their prescription medications under the scheme by the end of April 2020 (The Government of Hong Kong Special Administrative Region [GovHK], 2020c).

The future of telemedicine

While the special scheme with the FTU targets the immediate need for medications, it leaves unaddressed the problem that most in-person medical treatment and follow-up will continue to be delayed. In fact, only patients in stable conditions can benefit from the cross-border medication delivery service, and for patients with new symptoms or in unstable conditions, in-person medical treatment and follow-up are necessary, which cannot be provided under the special scheme (GovHK, 2020a). Given continued COVID-19 infections, both in Hong Kong and globally, there is no indication that the immigration controls will be relaxed in the near future (Kissler et al., 2020). It is thus worth accelerating the development of telemedicine, since it has great potential to address cross-border medical services challenges posed by COVID-19 and beyond (Hollander & Carr, 2020; Mallineni et al., 2020).

The term "telemedicine" was originally coined in 1948 and was used to describe the transmission of radiological images by telephone (Field, 1996). However, with advances in information technology, it has now come to refer to a new mode of medical service delivery, with doctors and patients connected by interactive video (Weinstein et al., 2014). A great advantage of telemedicine is that it enables physicians to provide clinical services at a distance, and there is hence a recognition that telemedicine – more simply, medicine at a distance – is ideal for the management of communicable diseases as it can reduce the risk of cross-contamination caused by close contact (Smith et al., 2020). It could also play a critical role in the global response to the COVID-19 pandemic because it is an effective way to deliver medical services to cross-border patients (Hollander & Carr, 2020; Mallineni et al., 2020).

Another advantage of telemedicine is that it can lead to cost savings for patients. A study by the University of Arkansas shows that, compared with those without telemedicine, more than 90% of patients with telemedicine would travel less than 70 miles for medical care; more than 80% of patients with telemedicine would save one missed day at work; and more than 70% of patients with telemedicine would save 75 USD-$150 in expenses (Bynum et al., 2003). After analyzing the data from the Houston Fire Department, Langabeer et al. (2017) found telemedicine was a more cost-effective alternative in pre-hospital care, since its use could lead to a 6.7% reduction in unnecessary medical emergency department visits and a 44-minute reduction in ambulance back-in-service times. In addition, Batsis et al. (2019) systematically reviewed the English-language literature on telemedicine (January 2012 to July 2018), and their findings demonstrate that it is feasible and acceptable to deliver care to older adults by telemedicine, and it achieves similar outcomes to usual, in-person care.

In fact, the current pandemic is not the first time we have turned to telemedicine to enhance health care responses in emergency situations. In 2000, the North Atlantic Treaty Organization (NATO) developed a multinational telemedicine system to enable soldiers to receive medical services from doctors located in other countries during various crises (Doarn et al., 2018). During the SARS pandemic in 2003, China began exploring telemedicine to enable medical experts to provide health support for clients remotely during infectious disease outbreaks (Zhao et al., 2010).

However, outside of emergency situations, little has been achieved to promote the application of telemedicine in routine medical activities. The main reasons behind this are multifold. First, telemedicine adoption in the healthcare system is a systematic project, requiring a strategy to mobilize and coordinate multiple actors and resources, such as policy makers, clinics, and manufacturers. Unfortunately, there is no corresponding overall planning in many countries, and the applications of telemedicine have been temporary and fragmented (Peddle, 2007; Smith & Gray, 2009). Second, legal/regulatory issues are always claimed to be constraining factors to telemedicine application (Whitten & Sypher, 2006), which include hospital credentialing (Weinstein et al., 2014), credentialing bureaucracy (Rockwell & Gilroy,, 2020), clinical governance (Cooke & Holmes, 2000), multijurisdictional licensure (Hunter et al., 2015), medical ethics (Chaet et al., 2017), and so on. Many studies suggest that unified legislation is a necessary condition for more widespread application of telemedicine (Nittari et al., 2020; Weinstein et al., 2014). Third, the lack of universal reimbursement for telemedicine services is another major barrier to its expansion. Private medical companies are often pioneers in telemedicine, but to date, reimbursement for telemedicine services from third-party payers has been delayed and confused in many countries (Weinstein et al., 2014; Whitten & Buis, 2007). Furthermore, reimbursement is usually limited to certain geographical locations and service types. For example, in Australia, telemedicine reimbursement is predominantly for medical consultations for patients in rural and remote locations (Smith et al., 2020). Fourth, some studies also reveal that local culture can affect the use and adoption of telemedicine. Alajlani and Clarke (2013) conducted case studies in Jordan and Syria, and they found that the slow development of telemedicine in Middle Eastern countries might be attributed to cultural factors, since local patients "feel uncomfortable with the way the doctor is diagnosing them" (Alajlani & Clarke, 2013, p. 310). Fifth, most clinicians are not knowledgeable about or skilled at operating telemedicine because there is a lack of corresponding training and preregistration curricula, which hampers their acceptance of it (Smith et al., 2020).

In fact, Hong Kong had already established a video conferencing system to provide limited medical consultation services for older adults at 18 long-term care facilities in the 2000s. This could have been seen as a prototype of a telemedicine system in Hong Kong. Regretfully, little effort went into scaling up the project and it ultimately foundered, even though a study supported by the community geriatric assessment team of the Hospital Authority of Hong Kong suggested that video conferencing was a feasible means of care delivery. They found it could lead to a 9% reduction in visits to the hospital emergency department and 11% fewer hospital bed-days (Hui & Woo, 2002). The COVID-19 pandemic provides a good opportunity for the overall uptake of telemedicine in Hong Kong and other places around the world. In the context of COVID-19, telemedicine is an effective tool to avoid overcrowding and prevent human exposure while delivering high-quality care (Rockwell & Gilroy, 2020). More importantly, telemedicine is useful to conduct "forward triage" – the sorting of patients before they arrive in the emergency department, which is a central strategy for managing public health emergencies (Hollander & Carr, 2020). Besides, there is a growing number of studies suggest that telemedicine is helpful to address the delivery of medical care to older adults in the context of COVID-19 (Sekhon et al., 2020; Vergara et al., 2020), especially those with chronic diseases living in remote areas (Sekhon et al., 2020).

Given the pandemic will likely last a long time, it is necessary for governments to reconsider the integration of telemedicine into current medical systems (Hollander & Carr, 2020; Portnoy et al., 2020; Rockwell & Gilroy, 2020). Specifically, there have been some conditions favoring telemedicine applications in Hong Kong. First, The Medical Council of Hong Kong (2019) issued *Ethical Guidelines on the Practice of Telemedicine* in 2019. It fills the gaps in the regulation of telemedicine services by clarifying the rights and obligations of clinicians and patients. Second, the COVID-19 pandemic has made the Hong Kong government aware of the importance of telemedicine, and the Chief Executive of Hong Kong has expressly stated that the government would further promote the broader application of telemedicine service in the *2020 Policy Address* (The Government of Hong Kong Special Administrative Region [GovHK], 2020d, p. 28). Third, some surveys during the COVID-19 pandemic have shown that Hong Kong residents have a high acceptance of telemedicine (Lingnan University, 2020). Certainly, as in many other parts of the world, some barriers against wide implementation of telemedicine also exist in Hong Kong, particularly limited knowledge of clinicians on telemedicine, lack of policies for reimbursement, and patients' concern about their privacy. In response, to push the development of telemedicine in Hong Kong, telemedicine-related training should be included in the training for medical staff to ensure they are telehealth-ready, and specific policies for reimbursement for private payers and regulations on electronic medical records should be formulated as soon as possible.

Cross-border older adults need telemedicine services more than those living in Hong Kong. In fact, the most urgent task of Hong Kong's telemedicine system is to provide cross-border medical services in the context of COVID-19. In this regard, specific recommendations include the following: First, the telemedicine terminal for patients should be set up in the offices of the FTU in Guangdong and Fujian, and the two residential care homes that have been included in the Pilot Residential Care Services Scheme in Guangdong, and then expanded to other locations and even personal portable electronics. Second, as telemedicine is new to older adults, on-site support teams are necessary in the early stages. Selected staff from the FTU and the residential care homes can be trained as telemedicine assistants, and then they can provide technical support for elderly patients. Third, for the telemedicine system, it is important to have close cooperation with local hospitals in mainland China. After remote diagnostics, some patients might be advised to have further physical examinations, and in this case, an institutional arrangement for the referral of these patients to a local hospital would be very useful.

In recent years, "telehealth" – a more inclusive term – has been brought forward as a proposal for extending telemedicine into a variety of nonphysician services, including tele-nursing, tele-care, and tele-pharmacy (Weinstein et al., 2014). Furthermore, with the advent of 5 G and the popularization of smart phones, mobile health is another important trend in telemedicine that allows the public easy access to health care services via personal portable electronics, leaving a great deal of imagination space for the application of telemedicine in cross-border care.

Given the growing international mobility of people (International Organization for Migration [IOM], 2020), telemedicine or telehealth will be widely applied to deliver cross-border medical services. Thus, cross-border telemedicine licensure, cross-border medication delivery or cross-border pharmacy, and referral arrangements between cross-border telehealth and local hospitals should be the research emphases in the future.

Conclusion

It is tricky to provide medical services for cross-border group – especially older adults with chronic diseases – during the COVID-19 pandemic, as most countries have imposed immigration controls. The experience of Hong Kong shows that a special scheme for delivering prescription medications introduced by the government can temporarily address the immediate needs for medications, but this does not address the in-person treatment and follow-up. Given that the pandemic will likely last a long time, it is worth accelerating the development of telemedicine, as it has great potential to offer a permanent solution for cross-border medical services. As a new trend, telemedicine is also extending into a variety of nonphysician services, and there are good prospects for integrating telemedicine into traditional care systems and delivering care for cross-border people.

Key Points

• More and more of Hong Kong's older adults have chosen to live in mainland China.
  • Many of them have to return to Hong Kong frequently for medical reasons.
  • Existing cross-border medical practices have been disrupted by the COVID-19 pandemic due to strict immigration control measures.
  • Telemedicine is a promising solution for delivering cross-border medical services.

Disclosure statement

No potential conflict of interest was reported by the author(s).

Funding

This work was supported by Lingnan University Innovation and Impact Fund (IIF) (Project Number: KT19A6).

ORCID

Zhaiwen Peng (iD) http://orcid.org/0000-0003-2093-0582

References

Alajlani, M., & Clarke, M. (2013). Effect of culture on acceptance of telemedicine in Middle Eastern countries: Case study of Jordan and Syria. *Telemedicine and e-Health*, *19*(4), 305–311. https://doi.org/10.1089/tmj.2012.0106

Bai, X. (2019). Hong Kong Chinese aging adults voice financial care expectations in changing family and sociocultural contexts: Implications for policy and services. *Journal of Aging & Social Policy*, *31*(5), 415–444. https://doi.org/10.1080/08959420.2018.1471308

Batsis, J. A., DiMilia, P. R., Seo, L. M., Fortuna, K. L., Kennedy, M. A., Blunt, H. B., Bagley, P. J., Brooks, J., Brooks, E., Kim, J. Y., Masutani, R. K., Bruce, M. L., & Bartels, S. J. (2019). Effectiveness of ambulatory telemedicine care in older adults: A systematic review. *Journal of the American Geriatrics Society*, *67*(8), 1737–1749. https://doi.org/10.1111/jgs.15959

Bynum, A. B., Irwin, C. A., Cranford, C. O., & Denny, G. S. (2003). The impact of telemedicine on patients' cost savings: Some preliminary findings. *Telemedicine Journal and e-Health*, *9*(4), 361–367. https://doi.org/10.1089/153056203772744680

Cao, J., & Fang, H. (2019, July). *Study on the welfare portability of cross-border eldercare services in Guangdong-Hong Kong-Macao Greater Bay Area*. 16th International Conference on Service Systems and Service Management (ICSSSM) (pp. 1–6), Shenzhen, China: IEEE.

Chaet, D., Clearfield, R., Sabin, J. E., & Skimming, K. (2017). Ethical practice in telehealth and telemedicine. *Journal of General Internal Medicine*, *32*(10), 1136–1140. https://doi.org/10.1007/s11606-017-4082-2

Chan, C. K. (1998). Welfare policies and the construction of welfare relations in a residual welfare state: The case of Hong Kong. *Social Policy & Administration*, *32*(3), 278–291. https://doi.org/10.1111/1467-9515.00103

Chan, L. S., & Chou, K. L. (2016). Immigration, living arrangement and the poverty risk of older adults in Hong Kong. *International Journal of Social Welfare*, *25*(3), 247–258. https://doi.org/10.1111/ijsw.12187

China State Council. (2016). *The 13th five-year plan for national economic and social development of the People's Republic of China*. http://www.enaea.edu.cn/uploadfiles/wysztsg/1458281224.pdf

The Chinese University of Hong Kong. (2020). *Most deaths from COVID-19 in Hong Kong are of 60 years old or above. CUHK initiated international efforts in devising strategies to protect older people with dementia amid COVID-19 pandemic* [Press release]. https://www.cpr.cuhk.edu.hk/en/press_detail.php?1=1&1=1&id=3346&t

Chou, K. L., Chow, N. W., & Chi, I. (2004). Preventing economic hardship among Chinese elderly in Hong Kong. *Journal of Aging & Social Policy*, *16*(4), 79–97. https://doi.org/10.1300/J031v16n04_05

Commissioner for Census and Statistics. (2014). *Hong Kong annual digest of statistics*. https://www.statistics.gov.hk/pub/B10100032014AN14B0100.pdf

Commissioner for Census and Statistics. (2016). *Population by-census: Main results*. https://www.bycensus2016.gov.hk/data/16bc-main-results.pdf

Commissioner for Census and Statistics. (2020). *Hong Kong annual digest of statistics 2020*. https://www.statistics.gov.hk/pub/B10100032020AN20B0100.pdf

Commissioner for Census and Statistics. (2020a). *Government of the Hong Kong special administrative region. Statistics on Hong Kong residents usually staying in Guangdong* [Data set]. https://www.censtatd.gov.hk/hkstat/sub/sp150.jsp?productCode=D5320188

Cooke, F. J., & Holmes, A. (2000). E-mail consultations in international health. *The Lancet, 356* (9224), 138. https://doi.org/10.1016/S0140-6736(00)02454-5

Doarn, C. R., Latifi, R., Poropatich, R. K., Sokolovich, N., Kosiak, D., Hostiuc, F., Zoicas, C., Buciu, A., & Arafat, R. (2018). Development and validation of telemedicine for disaster response: The North Atlantic Treaty Organization multinational system. *Telemedicine and e-Health, 24*(9), 657–668. https://doi.org/10.1089/tmj.2017.0237

Field, M. J. (1996). *Telemedicine: A guide to assessing telecommunications in health care.* National Academy Press.

The Government of Hong Kong Special Administrative Region. (2014, June 26). *Eligible elderly persons to be invited to join pilot residential care services scheme in Guangdong* [Press release]. https://www.info.gov.hk/gia/general/201406/26/P201406260335.htm

The Government of Hong Kong Special Administrative Region. (2020). *Hong Kong – The facts.* https://www.gov.hk/en/about/abouthk/facts.htm

The Government of Hong Kong Special Administrative Region. (2020a, February 24). *Special scheme introduced for delivering prescription medications to Hong Kong people in Guangdong and Fujian with urgent need for medications* [Press release]. https://www.info.gov.hk/gia/general/202002/24/P2020022400501.htm?fontSize=1

The Government of Hong Kong Special Administrative Region. (2020b, November 27). *Latest situation of Coronavirus disease (COVID-19) in Hong Kong* [Data set]. https://chp-dashboard.geodata.gov.hk/covid-19/zh.html

The Government of Hong Kong Special Administrative Region. (2020c, May 4). *Drug delivery scheme examined.* https://www.news.gov.hk/eng/2020/05/20200504/20200504_224547_645.html

The Government of Hong Kong Special Administrative Region. (2020d). *The chief executive's 2020 policy address* [Government document]. https://www.policyaddress.gov.hk/2020/eng/index.html

Hollander, J. E., & Carr, B. G. (2020). Virtually perfect? Telemedicine for COVID-19. *New England Journal of Medicine, 382*(18), 1679–1681. https://doi.org/10.1056/NEJMp2003539

Hui, E., & Woo, J. (2002). Telehealth for older patients: The Hong Kong experience. *Journal of Telemedicine and Telecare, 8*(3_suppl), 39–41. https://doi.org/10.1258/13576330260440808

Hui, E. C., Li, X., Chen, T., & Lang, W. (2018). Deciphering the spatial structure of China's megacity region: A new bay area—The Guangdong-Hong Kong-Macao Greater Bay Area in the making. *Cities, 105*(9), 102168. https://doi.org/10.1016/j.cities.2018.10.011

Hunter, T. B., Weinstein, R. S., & Krupinski, E. A. (2015). State medical licensure for telemedicine and teleradiology. *Telemedicine and e-Health, 21*(4), 315–318. https://doi.org/10.1089/tmj.2015.9997

International Organization for Migration. (2020). *World migration report 2020* [Report]. https://publications.iom.int/system/files/pdf/wmr_2020.pdf

Kissler, S. M., Tedijanto, C., Goldstein, E., Grad, Y. H., & Lipsitch, M. (2020). Projecting the transmission dynamics of SARS-CoV-2 through the postpandemic period. *Science, 368* (6493), 860–868. https://doi.org/10.1126/science.abb5793

Langabeer, J. R., Champagne-Langabeer, T., Alqusairi, D., Kim, J., Jackson, A., Persse, D., & Gonzalez, M. (2017). Cost–benefit analysis of telehealth in pre-hospital care. *Journal of Telemedicine and Telecare, 23*(8), 747–751. https://doi.org/10.1177/1357633X16680541

Law, K. Y., & Lee, K. M. (2006). Citizenship, economy and social exclusion of mainland Chinese immigrants in Hong Kong. *Journal of Contemporary Asia, 36*(2), 217–242. https://doi.org/10.1080/00472330680000131

Lingnan University. (2020, June 19). *Survey finds over 60% of senior citizens are willing to try online medical consultations* [Press release]. https://www.ln.edu.hk/sgs/cn/news/survey-findings-on-video-medical-consultation-for-elderly

Mallineni, S. K., Innes, N. P., Raggio, D. P., Araujo, M. P., Robertson, M. D., & Jayaraman, J. (2020). Coronavirus disease (COVID-19): Characteristics in children and considerations for dentists providing their care. *International Journal of Paediatric Dentistry, 30*(3), 245–250. https://doi.org/10.1111/ipd.12653

The Medical Council of Hong Kong. (2019). *Ethical guidelines on practice of telemedicine* [Regulation]. https://www.mchk.org.hk/files/PDF_File_Ethical_Guidelines_on_Telemedicine.pdf

Mok, K. H., Kühner, S., & Huang, G. (2017). The productivist construction of selective welfare pragmatism in China. *Social Policy & Administration, 51*(6), 876–897. https://doi.org/10.1111/spol.12337

Nittari, G., Khuman, R., Baldoni, S., Pallotta, G., Battineni, G., Sirignano, A., Amenta, F., & Ricci, G. (2020). Telemedicine practice: Review of the current ethical and legal challenges. *Telemedicine and e-Health, 26*(12), 1427–1437. https://doi.org/10.1089/tmj.2019.0158

Peddle, K. (2007). Telehealth in context: Socio-technical barriers to telehealth use in Labrador, Canada. *Computer Supported Cooperative Work (CSCW), 16*(6), 595–614. https://doi.org/10.1007/s10606-006-9030-3

Portnoy, J., Waller, M., & Elliott, T. (2020). Telemedicine in the Era of COVID-19. *The Journal of Allergy and Clinical Immunology: In Practice, 8*(5), 1489–1491. https://doi.org/10.1016/j.jaip.2020.03.008

Ramesh, M. (2004). *Social policy in East and Southeast Asia.* Routledge.

Rockwell, K. L., & Gilroy, A. S. (2020). Incorporating telemedicine as part of COVID-19 outbreak response systems. *The American Journal of Managed Care, 26*(4), 147–148. http://ajmc.s3.amazonaws.com/_media/_pdf/AJMC_04_2020_Rockwell.pdf

Sekhon, H., Sekhon, K., Launay, C., Afililo, M., Innocente, N., Vahia, I., Rej, S., & Beauchet, O. (2020). Telemedicine and the rural dementia population: A systematic review. *Maturitas, 143*(1), 105–114. https://doi.org/10.1016/j.maturitas.2020.09.001

Seui, S. (2014, November 15). *That welfare could not be provided for Hong Kong's older adults in Guangzhou makes life difficult for them* [Press release]. http://paper.wenweipo.com/2014/11/15/YO1411150011.htm

Smith, A. C., & Gray, L. C. (2009). Telemedicine across the ages. *Medical Journal of Australia, 190*(1), 15–19. https://doi.org/10.5694/j.1326-5377.2009.tb02255.x

Smith, A. C., Thomas, E., Snoswell, C. L., Haydon, H., Mehrotra, A., Clemensen, J., & Caffery, L. J. (2020). Telehealth for global emergencies: Implications for coronavirus disease 2019 (COVID-19). *Journal of Telemedicine and Telecare, 26*(5), 309–313. https://doi.org/10.1177/1357633X20916567

Social Welfare Department. (2020). *Statistics on "Waiting time for residential care services".* https://www.swd.gov.hk/storage/asset/section/632/en/LTC_statistics_HP-Eng(202010).pdf

Vergara, J., Parish, A., & Smallheer, B. (2020). Telehealth: Opportunities in geriatric patient care during COVID-19. *Geriatric Nursing, 41*(5), 657–658. https://doi.org/10.1016/j.gerinurse.2020.08.013

Wang, N. (2011). *Hong Kong elderly people retiring in the mainland* [Report]. https://www.pico.gov.hk/doc/en/research_reports/hong_kong_elderly_people_retiring_in_the_mainland.pdf

Weinstein, R. S., Lopez, A. M., Joseph, B. A., Erps, K. A., Holcomb, M., Barker, G. P., & Krupinski, E. A. (2014). Telemedicine, telehealth, and mobile health applications that work: Opportunities and barriers. *The American Journal of Medicine, 127*(3), 183–187. https://doi.org/10.1016/j.amjmed.2013.09.032

Whitten, P., & Buis, L. (2007). Private payer reimbursement for telemedicine services in the United States. *Telemedicine and e-Health*, *13*(1), 15–24. https://doi.org/10.1089/tmj.2006.0028

Whitten, P., & Sypher, B. D. (2006). Evolution of telemedicine from an applied communication perspective in the United States. *Telemedicine Journal & e-Health*, *12*(5), 590–600. https://doi.org/10.1089/tmj.2006.12.590

Wong, L. (2008, November 3–4). *Hong Kong's welfare model reconsidered – —What model? What traits? And What Function?* [Paper presented]. East Asian Social Policy Network conference, Taipei, Taiwan. http://www.welfareasia.org/5thconference/papers/Wong%20L_Hong%20Kong%20Welfare%20Model.pdf

Wu, Z., & McGoogan, J. M. (2020). Characteristics of and important lessons from the coronavirus disease 2019 (COVID-19) outbreak in China: Summary of a report of 72 314 cases from the Chinese Center for Disease Control and Prevention. *Jama*, *323*(13), 1239–1242. https://doi.org/10.1001/jama.2020.2648

Yu, S. W. K. (2008). Pension reforms in Hong Kong: Using residual and collaborative strategies to deal with the government's financial responsibility in providing retirement protection. *Journal of Aging & Social Policy*, *20*(4), 493–510. https://doi.org/10.1080/08959420802191704

Zhao, J., Zhang, Z., Guo, H., Li, Y., Xue, W., Ren, L., Chen, Y., Chen, S., & Zhang, X. (2010). E-health in China: Challenges, initial directions, and experience. *Telemedicine and e-Health*, *16*(3), 344–349. https://doi.org/10.1089/tmj.2009.0076

Telephone-Based Emotional Support for Older Adults during the COVID-19 Pandemic

Liora Bar-Tur, Michal Inbal-Jacobson, Sharon Brik-Deshen, Yael Zilbershlag, Sigal Pearl Naim, and Yitzhak Brick

ABSTRACT
Isolation and lockdowns stemming from the COVID-19 pandemic exacerbate older adults' vulnerability to emotional harm. This paper stresses the importance of establishing an ongoing system of distant emotional care by experienced gerontologists as a routine practice, parallel to physical healthcare services. It introduces a tele-based emotional support program for older adults operated by the Israel Gerontological Society during COVID-19. Experience with the telephone-support initiative suggests it to be an effective and meaningful means of providing emotional support to older adults and their families and assisting community caregiving agencies. Policymakers and gerontologists should address older adults' needs for emotional support and develop effective tele-support solutions in routine times as a promising relief for homebound, frail, or lonely older adults. Tele-based emotional support can substitute for in-person meetings and easily and quickly reach out to many older adults who otherwise would not receive support.

Key points

• COVID-19 has had a negative effect on frail and needy older adults' mental health.

• Online and telephone support to older adults is essential to address their mental and emotional needs.

• Experience with a telephone-based initiative suggests an effective and efficient means of providing emotional support by gerontologists.

• New avenues must be found to reach out to older adults at risk for isolation and loneliness.

Introduction

The COVID-19 pandemic continues to be a serious threat to older adults' physical and mental health. In response to the growing number of infected individuals in Israel, public health measures were taken to mitigate the virus's spread. Restrictions and lockdown were imposed, particularly among the older population in the community and in sheltered homes, to protect them from COVID-19. All home services, such as caregivers from the National Insurance Institute, were discontinued. These protective physical health measures exacerbated the risk for increased social isolation, loneliness, health deterioration, and ageism. Social contact and emotional support for isolated and stay-at-home populations are crucial to combat loneliness and anxiety.

As isolation requirements continue and other lockdowns are operated, a corresponding increase in the risk of emotional harm has become evident (Brooks et al., 2020), including suicide risk (Applegate & Ouslander, 2020; Levi-Belz & Aisenberg, 2020; Vahia et al., 2020; Yip et al., 2010). In lockdown conditions, establishing remote emotional support systems is essential, parallel to physical healthcare services (Steinman et al., 2020). Emotional support is needed primarily for the oldest-old (80 years and over), especially the physically frail and homebound who are at risk for poor physical and emotional deterioration. During routine times, these older adults are likely to receive regular home services and visits from various health professionals, caregivers, and volunteers. During the pandemic, all of these contacts came to a halt or were dramatically reduced. The oldest-old typically have relatively less access to digital communication than the general population (e.g., Dobransky & Hargittai, 2016), leaving the telephone as their primary contact medium. The provision of emotional support is a critical resource not only for the frail and needy but also for primary caregivers, spouses, and children undertaking the care of their loved ones (Czeisler et al., 2020). Providing emotional support has also proven valuable for widows and widowers of any age who need to talk and share their difficulties.

Prior to the COVID-19 outbreak, loneliness was recognized as a major public health concern for older adults (Gerst-Emerson & Jayawardhana, 2015). The implications of the COVID-19-related stay-at-home order and social distancing measures for the older adult population can increase the risk of adverse consequences associated with social isolation (Morrow-Howell et al., 2020) and should therefore be addressed by public health professionals, community service providers, and policymakers. Novel approaches to increase support and services are required to supplement reduced caregiving and social interactions (Hoffman et al., 2020). We propose an accessible and quick tele-support intervention of gerontologist volunteers to help combat loneliness and distress of older adults and their families. This service's unique contribution lines in adopting a pro-active approach to older adults needing emotional support but are unlikely to initiate contact as they would for medical consultations. This reluctance stems from a range of factors, including ageism and a lack of awareness, stigma, or reduced energy due to depression.

This paper introduces the proposed tele-support program that can substitute for in-person meetings and easily and quickly reach out to many older adults who otherwise would not receive emotional support. The tele-support operated in Israel successfully during the first, second, and third lockdowns. Given the encouraging responses from the older adult clients and their families, we suggest that this service continue in routine times as a promising relief for homebound, frail, or lonely older adults. Before introducing the program, however, we review isolation, loneliness, and the mental well-being of older adults during the COVID-19 pandemic, focusing specifically on the role of ageism.

Isolation and the sense of loneliness in older adults

The sense of loneliness – defined as the perceived disparity between the individual's desired social relationships and those available – is considered today to be one of the many scourges of the 21st century (Killeen, 2002). Experiencing loneliness can impair individuals' emotional and cognitive well-being and lead to a high degree of suicidal ideation, even resulting in mortality (Barth et al., 2010; Cacioppo et al., 2006; Holt-Lunstad et al., 2015; National Institute on Aging, 2019; Santini et al., 2020; Shankar et al., 2017; Tanskanen & Anttila, 2016). About one-third of older adults (aged 65 and over) have been reported to regularly suffer from loneliness due to diminished or loss of social contact when the resources available to them are limited (Cohen-Mansfield et al., 2016; Jansson et al., 2018).

Recent surveys have indicated that loneliness has negatively affected the health of older adults in the current COVID-19 pandemic (Berg-Weger & Morley, 2020; Gaeta & Brydges, 2020; Steinman et al., 2020), with ramifications of loneliness particularly felt among the oldest population. Unlike younger people, older adults face more restrictions and are less likely to be "connected" digitally (Dobransky & Hargittai, 2016; Lev-On et al., 2019); thus, they are less likely to benefit from online digital support and mental stimulation during a period of lockdown and reduced family gatherings and social activities. Moreover, for some older adults, lack of physical activity due to home isolation may exacerbate physical decline with its attendant weakness and risk of falling. Having limited access to the cognitive stimulation that accompanies regular socializing and general engagement with the outside world may intensify the cognitive and behavioral symptoms of dementia (Steinman et al., 2020).

Additionally, Older adults with medical, cognitive, or social frailty have less reserve to compensate when their homeostasis is threatened. When facing social isolation challenges, these individuals are particularly vulnerable to rapid decline (Steinman et al., 2020). During emergencies such as the pandemic crisis, frail older adults with cognitive or physical impairments face greater risks for having their autonomy compromised and their human rights infringed. Masi et al. (2011) found that addressing maladaptive social cognition was the most successful intervention, better than improving social skills, enhancing social support, and increasing opportunities for social contact. In a systematic review and analysis (Cohen-Mansfield & Perachm, 2015) examining the utility of loneliness alleviation interventions among older persons, findings suggested that loneliness can be reduced by enhancing social support, increasing opportunities for social contact, and network enhancement. These interventions can be discharged directly in face-to-face meetings, including group psychoeducation encounters. During the COVID-19 pandemic and other restrictions and limitations to leave home, tele-support online emotional interventions should be implemented to support older adults in need of interventions to alleviate loneliness.

The COVID-19 pandemic impact on the mental well-being of older adults in Israel

A survey in Israel found the incidence of loneliness among individuals aged 65 years and above ranging from 24% to 47% (Rotem, 2014; Shiovitz-Ezra, 2012). The spread of the Coronavirus in Israel has had significant health, economic, and social consequences, exacerbating the prevalence of loneliness among the 1.1 million people (12% of the population) aged 65 and over in Israel. A study conducted in Israel in May 2020 among the 65+ population (Shnoore, 2020) revealed that 85% of this population experienced emotional difficulties arising from being physically disconnected from support systems, anxiety for the future of family members, uncertainty, and fear of contracting the disease. Those over age 74 years, particularly the physically frail, were at especially high risk for poor emotional state. The study further revealed that those living with an incapacitated spouse were in considerably greater danger of decline in all types of pathology relative to the decline experienced by those not in their situation. The emotional and functional decline among older adults seemed to be impervious to the extent of family assistance, as 80% of the sample reported being "satisfied" or "very satisfied" with family support.

A second survey conducted by Joint-Eshel and the ERI- Research for Social Impact Institute (Israel Psychological Association, 2020) in December 2020 showed continuing deterioration in 65 and older adults' physical and mental health. The survey revealed that 51% of older adults experienced increased frailty, and 32% were suffering from impairment in their daily functioning. Over 47% of the older adults reported experiencing a poor mental state, including loneliness, depression, or a feeling that "life has no meaning." Whereas in the first wave, conducted in May, these feelings did not differ from pre-pandemic measures, the protraction of the COVID crisis over many long months has led to a significant spike. Of the sample, 31% reported depression (compared with 24% in the first wave), 36% reported that loneliness (compared with 32%), and 15% contended that life had no meaning (compared with 10%).

The second Israeli survey demonstrates the continuing threat of the COVID-19 pandemic to older adults' emotional condition. Indeed, 75% of the frail were in poor emotional condition during the lockdown, while only 23% of the independent older adults were in a similar state. Data analysis suggests that 40% of the older adults were at high risk for multifactorial decline, including physical health, financial condition, and psychological state.

An additional survey among family members assisting relatives revealed that their assistance was twice as burdensome to them during the pandemic than routine times (Resnizki & Izhaak, 2020). Whereas 40% of the family members reported feelings of gloom, depression, and hopelessness, some reported a sense of competence due to the situation. A study conducted by Shrira et al. (2020) found that loneliness at the time of the crisis was associated with an increase in psychiatric symptoms, particularly among those perceiving themselves as older than their chronological age compared with those reporting feeling younger than their biological age. The impact of the lockdown was manifested most severely in institutional settings and assisted-living facilities. Some older adults, primarily Holocaust survivors and others who had endured previous trauma (Bar-Tur, 2020; Pau, 2020), suffered emotional flooding related to earlier posttraumatic experiences (Ayalon & Avidor, 2020).

In summary, the ongoing isolation, uncertainty about the future, reduction or discontinuation of social and familial contacts, and the sense of loneliness have significantly impaired the emotional resilience of older adults, their families, and their caregivers. Family networks provided critical stabilizing support. Moreover, a third of older adults reported feeling fine and could leverage the crisis, enabling online learning, meaningful activity, and strengthening family ties. Others, however, have struggled. Thus, even from a distance, communities should provide opportunities for more emotional support for older adults, especially for the frail and oldest-old, to foster their well-being and resilience.

Ageism and the implications on mental well-being during the coronavirus crisis

Alongside the limited attention paid to older adults' mental health, ageism has pervaded the public and media discourse, and it also had adverse implications for older adults' well-being. Policymakers, the media, and even senior medical professionals relate to older adults with prejudice, paternalism, and the exercise of power, without distinguishing between healthy, independent older adults and the frail and ill (Ayalon, 2021; Doron, 2020). Whereas sheltered housing has confined their residences to safeguard their physical health, inadequate concern has been paid to the accompanying risk to their mental health. To ensure social distancing and avoid contagion, there was a call to impose lockdown on all older adults, aged 65 and older, following the lockdown that was already imposed on older adults living in sheltered homes, which prohibited the residents from any outside face-to-face contact, including family members, and exacerbated the risk of emotional problems. This policy failed to address older adults' need for autonomy and their right to choose to be or not to be in full isolation. The media has emphasized the extent to which older adults are weak and vulnerable, requiring the protection of and ties with family for food and medicine, but without offering a fuller picture by including the independent and functional older adult population in their reports. However, classification by age alone is a manifestation of ageism. Thus, these policy deliberations produced an outcry among many advocates of aging populations and among many seniors in the community.

Position papers issued by the Israel Gerontological Society (Israel Psychological Association, 2020), the Israel Psychological Association (2020), and Tel-Aviv University's Faculty of Health Studies University (Israel Psychological Association, 2020) all cautioned against the dangers inherent in the government plans to classify everyone over a certain age as old and thus, by definition, at high risk and isolated. Whereas this proposal would have enabled easing restrictions on younger populations, applying this single age criterion while disregarding other factors (e.g., high mobility, living with a partner, lack of severe underlying conditions) was said to jeopardize the mental well-being and autonomy of high-functioning older adults.

Some prominent active Israeli academics, artists, writers, and philosophers, all over 80 years old, also called on the media to eschew regulations based on ageism, to avoid judging older adults according to their chronological age, and to distinguish between the sick and the frail older adults and the healthy independent ones. In response to these vigorous calls, the Council for National Security and the Ministry of Health acceded to the principle that policy should not be determined based on chronological age alone and that older adults can and should determine their own behavior. This development drew attention to two different groups among the older adult population who experienced ageism and distress and could benefit from emotional support. The first group comprised functioning older adults, who felt mostly angry and distressed as they could not meet their friends and families and were not allowed to pursue their routine outdoor activities; some of them felt very lonely, anxious, and depressed. The second group comprised the high-risk, frail, and sick older adults who were disconnected, locked in sheltered homes, and helpless; they were kept from receiving the minimal daily support they enjoyed before the COVID-19 crisis and were unable to engage and communicate with others digitally.

Some scholars underscored the importance of providing regular emotional and social support for the at-risk older population during the current crisis (Ayalon et al., 2020; Brooks et al., 2020), among them many gerontologists, members of the Israel Gerontological society who were very concerned and decided to be more active in their support of older adults.

Establishing the telephone-support initiative

The Israel Gerontological Society responded to this call to action and established a telephone-based emotional support service, initiating substantive online conversations to ascertain that the emotional and mental needs of older adults who are at risk were being met. Older adults in need of support were referred to the service by welfare agencies or family members. They were encouraged to talk and share their difficulties with a professional volunteer under the Israel Gerontological Society's auspices. These online conversations helped mitigate feelings of loneliness and isolation that are acknowledged to accompany long-term lockdowns.

The Israel Gerontological Society is an association of professionals in the field of aging whose principal goals are to advance knowledge in the field, protect older adults' rights, establish the discipline of gerontology in Israel, and influence policy regarding aging and the aged. Following the pandemic outbreak, the Society's leadership decided to directly assist the older adult population and enlist the members' professionally diverse resources. The need to provide direct services to the older adult population was triggered by the closure of all senior day-care centers, thus suspending older adults' community activities. Even the volunteers who had regularly conducted home visits to shut-ins were compelled to curtail their support. Since all the professionals who regularly provided social services to older adults in the community were under lockdown, it appeared that older adults needed a tie with a professional who could provide emotional support beyond the basic provision of food and medications, a task generally taken up by the municipalities, the government, as well as by the family and community volunteers.

The goal of the telephone-based emotional support service was to address the mental health needs of older adults suffering from various forms of emotional distress and tension due to the lockdown at home. Its guiding principle was that a professional volunteer's telephone call would contribute to the older adult––most of whom had never initiated a call for emotional support––to combat fear, loneliness, or other mental health needs. As opposed to other hotlines and community support, the tele-support is a proactive approach to older adults who need emotional support but are not likely to initiate contact as they would for medical consultations

(Gum et al., 2014; Gur-Yaish et al., 2016). These calls would contribute to the older adult's sense of not being alone and that someone is showing an interest in their situation and is prepared to attend to them as they contend with a challenging reality

Program development

A steering committee was established to plan and direct the volunteer-based telephone initiative. Volunteers were recruited through an online question-naire distributed to the Society's members and academic institutions involved in aging. The volunteers represented a broad spectrum of disciplines and experience in the field: gerontologists, academics, psychologists, social work-ers, occupational therapists, nurses, bibliotherapists, retirees, and heads of organizations providing services to older adults in Israel.

To locate older adults in need of emotional support, the Society distributed a letter explaining the initiative's goals and the referral procedure to the various organizations and agencies providing community-based services to older adults. The initiative was also publicized in the media. Representatives of 31 agencies completed referral forms requesting basic information about each referral (name, telephone number, whether living alone) along with back-ground information (level of care received, the extent of cognitive decline, hearing loss, language level, and distress level). Older adult participants also affirmed their willingness to receive phone calls from the initiative volunteers.

The second source of older adult referrals was through the Ministry for Social Equality's hotline that received thousands of calls daily at the crisis's peak. Country-wide calls to the hotline that dealt with older adults' emotional difficulties were referred, among other services, to the Society's initiative. Additional community-dwelling older adult referrals were received privately from their family members.

Program implementation

More than 200 volunteers provided services to more than 300 older adults and their families over the first three months of the lockdown and during the continuing restrictions. An additional 98 referrals received support in the subsequent second and third lockdowns into the beginning of 2021. About 10% (29) people of those approached declined to schedule a second call with the volunteer. The primary reasons for their rejection were that they felt that they did not need support. Some older adults refused to speak with an unknown caller.

Sixty-five percent of the tele-support service referrals were aged 80 and older, and about 70% were women. However, some younger older adults, in their 60s and 70s, benefited from the tele-support. These were widows, primary caregivers of a cognitively impaired spouse, or lonely people who needed to talk and share their loneliness and difficulties. Many of the clientele lived alone, whereas others lived with a partner or a foreign worker caretaker. The telephone relationships formed between the volunteers and the participants were varied and appeared to meet the older adults' needs. The conversations' duration ranged from 15–60 minutes, with their frequency varying from single-session calls to continuing conversations over the full months of the lockdown. Approximately half of the dyads spoke more than four times, and meaningful relationships were established. The length and frequency of the calls were determined jointly by the conversation partners. In some cases, daily contact early in the crisis dissipated as the situation improved. The relationship continued as long as the participants needed support. Due to the volunteers' professional status as gerontologists, the ongoing relationships facilitated trust and a meaningful connection.

The unique features of the telephone-support initiative

Several factors facilitated the initiative's positive outcomes. First, the initiative based its service on volunteers, all experts in the field of aging. Recruited volunteers represented a broad range of trained therapists, such as psychologists, social workers, art therapists, occupational therapists, and other professionals with experience in working with the older population. The professional steering team paired the referrals and volunteers according to the information received concerning the referrals. The tele-support was primarily targeted to alleviate loneliness, anxieties, and poor mood. When the persons' needs went beyond emotional support, they were referred to senior therapists who could offer short-term interventions or focused problem-solving interventions. An experienced senior clinical psychologist gave supervision to volunteers who needed more guidance. The variety of specialties among the volunteers enabled effective matching between the person's needs and the suitable volunteer.

Second, the telephone encounter was initiated by the volunteer, who proactively established contact with the older person. This procedure differs from traditional mental health hotlines, which rely on the consumer's initiative to contact the service. In most hotlines, the staff are not permanent, are typically available only in certain time slots, and the connection between the counselor and client is most often limited to that single encounter. Moreover, many older adults who need assistance are not proactive in asking for help and are unlikely to call hotline services.

Third, the relationship continued for as long as there was a need for support during the lockdown period. Similarly, the duration and scope of the support were mutually determined. Some volunteers remained in close touch with their clients over several weeks, with several conducting daily conversations. Fourth, the leadership team fully monitored the volunteers' activity and provided an attentive ear for the volunteers dealing with professional issues. When confronting complex circumstances, the volunteers received advice, counsel, and supervision, as needed.

Type of support provided by the telephone support initiative

Over the three months of the project's operation, the volunteers provided support to older adults and their families for a variety of issues that arose or were exacerbated due to the lockdown. Most of these issues involved feelings of isolation and loneliness. Among those receiving telephone support were widows and widowers and cases concerning housebound individuals whose weekly visits by volunteers and physical and occupational therapists were frozen during the lockdown period. The volunteer assisted them in planning a daily routine, initiating telephone conversations, and were available in some cases several times a week for brief calls.

Many issues dealt with emotional difficulties resulting from the absence of family visits, social activities, and social contacts. Family relationship difficulties with family members or partners who felt "imprisoned" together in the house were also common. A few adult children of older adults requested emotional support for their parents who have dementia.

The level of support provided was varied. Low-intensity support included brief regular telephone calls to keep in touch and provide a respite from loneliness. In other relationships, volunteers provided guidance in dealing with a partner who was not well, dispelling tension, and devising a suitable daily routine. Higher-intensity intervention levels involved responding to an anxiety attack or depression that required short-term treatment or focused psychiatric or medical treatment. The volunteers also dealt with suicide threats that required the intervention of family members, medical personnel, and social workers in the community.

In some cases, a family member made the referral, such as with 75-year-old Mrs. T. She expressed considerable distress and difficulty coping with her husband, who had Alzheimer's and was agitated from the onset of the pandemic. He did not understand why he could not leave the house and why the children did not visit. He followed the TV evening news, and the experts' dire predictions frightened and confused him. Mrs. T. felt trapped at home with her husband, with whom communication was difficult. His agitated state exacerbated her anxiety. The volunteer psychologist assisted her over six weeks with weekly phone calls and e-mail correspondence. She also spoke with family members, children, and grandchildren, whom she drafted for support from a distance.

Other interventions dealt with support for widows whose husbands had passed away shortly before or during the Coronavirus period. This was the case of Mrs. A., who was in acute mourning since her husband's death two months before the onset of the pandemic. She found it difficult to return to normal functioning and developed a strong dependency on her children. When the lockdown began, she remained at home alone, disconnected from family members, who were also required to remain at home. The volunteer conducted a focused short-term grief intervention with Mrs. A and her children. She was subsequently referred to the local mental health clinic to continue psychological treatment.

Additional benefits of the initiative

The Society's initiative reduced the burden on other organizations and agencies serving older adults in the community. During the closure, professionals had been placed on temporary leave and found it difficult to maintain contact with their older clientele. The Society's volunteers facilitated providing ongoing support, especially for the physically and mentally infirm, who comprised most of the referrals. The agencies praised the immediacy of the connection established between volunteers and older adults and stressed the importance of professional (rather than well-meaning) volunteers, as many referrals required addressing complex family and social circumstances.

The volunteers reported that they also gained from the relationships. They felt professionally and personally productive, that their knowledge was beneficial to others, and that they were a part of an important social cause. They reported feeling a sense of satisfaction at being able to do something of significance at a time when they too experienced isolation and helplessness.

The tele-support was initially designed to operate only as long as there was a need for emotional support during the lockdown due to the cutback of community services. This time constraint was noted to the clients and to the volunteers. However, some volunteers maintained their contact and support for many months after the initial lockdown. Moreover, as the crisis continues, including two further lockdowns, we resumed our tele-support, and it continues to operate successfully. We currently have 80 volunteers that provide support to almost 100 older adults in the form of "crisis routine."

Discussion

This paper highlights the importance of establishing a remote emotional care system to combat social isolation and foster older adults' well-being. Government policy actions that were taken to mitigate the pandemic and protect the health of the Israeli population––particularly the older adults–– had an adverse effect on their well-being, challenged their mental health, and spotlighted inherent ageism. In particular, government policy imperiled the frail, their caregivers, and those residing in homes for the aged. Restrictions imposed on Israeli society followed by the first lockdown resulted in increased social isolation, difficulties in adapting to physical distancing, reduced social and health-promoting activities, and reduced support offered traditionally by community caregiving agencies.

To mitigate these threats to the older population, professionals in the field of aging under the auspices of the Israel Gerontological Society initiated the telephone-support. This initiative proved to be an effective, immediate, accessible, and meaningful means of providing emotional support to older adults and their families and easing the burden on other community caregiving agencies. It also contributed to the volunteers' sense of purpose and meaning, especially in times characterized by helplessness and personal stress. The initiative answered the call to action by Brooke and Jackson (2020), Brooks et al. (2020), Greenberg et al. (2020), Morrow-Howell et al. (2020), Ouslander (2020), and Steinman et al. (2020), who stressed the need to maintain and increase contact with older adults through social media, phone calls, or video-based calls. Ongoing online social support for the older population is critical, particularly for those unable to seek out emotional support or human contact for themselves.

The initiative highlights the importance of establishing a system of distant emotional care, comparable to that implemented for physical healthcare (Cohen & Tavares, 2020; Hoffman et al., 2020; Hollander & Carr, 2020; Vahia et al., 2020). Since the beginning of the pandemic, many older adults have continued to stay away from adult day healthcare and other community-based programs. Family and friends who have served as caregivers may be fearful or unable to visit. Whereas it has been heartening to see volunteer networks spring up to help older adults purchase groceries, pharmaceuticals, and the like, other basic needs, such as assistance with bathing, basic home cleaning, and dementia supports, may remain unmet (Steinman et al., 2020).

Alongside the pandemic's deleterious effects on older adults, it is gratifying to note that some positive change has emerged in its wake. Aging rose much higher on the public agenda due to the pandemic. It became a major challenge for the decision-makers; the media dealt with it regularly, and older adults have received more attention and support from their communities than ever before. Family members are more involved in their older members' lives and communicate more frequently, albeit remotely. Many volunteers assist isolated older adults with shopping, food, medications, technological support, and even supply computer tablets for better communication. Technological start-ups are being introduced since the pandemic's outbreak to help older adults function at home and promote their wellness remotely. In line with these positive changes, an advisory committee to the Israeli government was recently established to draft an enlightened policy to provide for older adults' mental health needs.

Although the telephone-based emotional support service for older adults proved to be an effective and efficient intervention, older adults with hearing loss or cognitive decline would not likely benefit from it. A further limitation is reflected in some lonely older adults' reluctance to receive emotional support over the phone due to their general caution and suspicion of outsiders (Segel-Karpas & Ayalon, 2020). These constraints highlight a need for close coordination between the community's referring agents, the older adult's client, and the volunteer. In some cases, personal encouragement and reassurance are critical in persuading older adults to consent to tele-support. At times, at the request of family members or the referring agency, volunteers may need to persevere in the relationships and provide the tele-based emotional support in the face of clients' objections and initial rejection. A rigorous, systematic evaluation of the service's various components (e.g., recruiting volunteers, the referral process, establishing the client-volunteer relationships, and follow-up) should be carried out in future studies.

Conclusion

The COVID-19 pandemic continues to comprise a serious threat to older adults' physical and mental health. Social contact and emotional support for older adults who are isolated and stay at home are crucial to combat loneliness and anxiety. Loneliness has been acknowledged as a major public health concern for older adults prior to the COVID-19 outbreak and will continue long after. Many lonely older adults struggle with losses and stressful events. Whereas many older adults do not suffer from psychiatric disorders and are not necessarily frail and isolated, they need emotional support to cope with the challenges of aging.

The telephone and video substitutes for in-person meetings pose a great challenge and an opportunity to reach out to many older adults who otherwise would not receive emotional support. Providing emotional support can help older adults continue living at home and avoid referral to a hospital, residential care, or a long-term care facility. Thus, it is critical to devise effective solutions to reach out to those in need. With the increase in life expectancy, it is vital to advance any intervention that can help people grow old respectfully and gracefully. Community support for older adults has eroded over the past months and should improve and upgrade their services.

The tele-support supplemented other digital and technological services for the older population initiated by the Israel Gerontological Society. These included online meetings with the Society's professionals to ask questions and discuss physical and mental health issues and view public lectures on loneliness, mental health, nutrition, and physical activity. Monthly newsletters were also sent out. In many domains, the pandemic has accelerated developments that may have been in the works but only rarely implemented. For instance, telehealth services have grown during the pandemic and will continue to grow, with medical consultations by telephone serving as a substitute for a high proportion of in-person physician visits. We call on other gerontologist associations and social services for the geriatric population to follow our initiative and use their professionals' vast knowledge on aging and mental health to provide older adults in their communities with remote or online professional and emotional support.

Disclosure of statement

No potential conflict of interest was reported by the author(s).

References

Applegate, W. B., & Ouslander, J. G. (2020). COVID-19 presents high risk to older persons. *Journal of the American Geriatrics Society*, 68(4), 681. https://doi.org/10.1111/jgs.16426 .

Ayalon, L., & Avidor, L. (2020). "We have become prisoners of our own age": From a continuing care retirement community to a total institution in the midst of the COVID-19 outbreak [Manuscript under review].

Ayalon, L, Avidor, S. 'We have become prisoners of our own age': from a continuing care retirement community to a total institution in the midst of the COVID-19 outbreak, Age and Ageing, 2021;, afab013, https://doi.org/10.1093/ageing/afab013

Ayalon, L., Chasteen, A., Diehl, M., Levy, B. R., Neupert, S. D., Rothermund, K., Tesch-Römer, C., & Wahl, H.-W. (2020). Aging in times of the COVID-19 pandemic: Avoiding ageism and fostering intergenerational solidarity. *J Gerontol B Psychol Sci Soc Sci*, 1–4. https://doi.org/10.1093/geronb/gbaa051

Barth, J., Schneider, S., & Von Känel, R. (2010). Lack of social support in the etiology and the prognosis of coronary heart disease: A systematic review and meta-analysis. . *Psychosomatic Medicine, 72*(3), 229–238. https://doi.org/10.1097/PSY.0b013e3181d01611

Bar-Tur, L. (2020, 21 June). *Working with a posttraumatic elderly widow during the lockdown in the COVID-19 pandemic* [Paper presentation in Hebrew]. *Coping with loss and trauma in aging: How strong are our lives*, Ruppin Academic Center.

Berg-Weger, M., & Morley, J. E. (2020). Loneliness in old age: An unaddressed health problem. *The Journal of Nutrition, Health & Aging, 24*(3), 243–245. https://doi.org/10.1007/s12603-020-1323-6

Brooke, J., & Jackson, D. (2020). Older people and COVID-19: Isolation, risk and ageism. *Journal of Clinical Nursing*, 2044–2045. https://doi.org/10.1111/jocn.15274

Brooks, A. K., Webster, R. K., Smith, L. E., Woodland, L., Wessely, S., Greenberg, N., & Rubin, G. J. (2020). The psychological impact of quarantine and how to reduce it: Rapid review of the evidence. *The Lancet, 395*(10227), 912–920. https://doi.org/10.1016/S0140-6736(20)30460-8

Cacioppo, J. T., Hughes, M. E., Waite, L. J., Hawkley, L. C., & Thisted, R. A. (2006). Loneliness as a specific risk factor for depressive symptoms: Cross-sectional and longitudinal analyses. . *Psychology and Aging, 21* (1), 140–151. DOI: 10.1037/0882-7974.21.1.140

Cohen, M. A., & Tavares, J. (2020). Who are the most at-risk older adults in the COVID-19 era? It's not just those in nursing homes. *Journal of Aging & Social Policy, 32*(4–5), 380–386. https://doi.org/10.1080/08959420.2020.1764310

Cohen-Mansfield, J., Hazan, H., Lerman, Y., & Shalom, V. (2016). Correlates and predictors of loneliness in older adults: A review of quantitative results informed by qualitative insights. *International Psychogeriatrics, 28*(4), 557–576. https://doi.org/10.1017/S1041610215001532

Cohen-Mansfield, J., & Perachm, R. (2015). Interventions for alleviating loneliness among older persons: A critical review. *American Journal of Health Promotion, 29*(3), 109–125. https://doi.org/10.4278/ajhp.130418-LIT-182 .

Czeisler, M. É., Lane, R. I., Petrosky, E., Wiley, J. F., Christensen, A., Njaji, R., Weaver, M. D., Robbins, R., Facer-Childs, E. R., Barger, L. K., Czeisler, C. A., Howard, M. E., & Rajaratnam, S. M. W. (2020). Mental health, substance use, and suicidal ideation during the COVID-19 pandemic — United States. *Morbidity and Mortality Weekly Report, 69*(32), 1049–1057. https://doi.org/10.15585/mmwr.mm6932a1

Dobransky, K., & Hargittai, E. (2016). Unrealized potential: Exploring the digital disability divide. *Poetics, 58*, 18–28. https://doi.org/10.1016/j.poetic.2016.08.003

Doron, I. (2020). Is 70 is the new 50? https://www.haaretz.co.il/gallery/lifestyle/.premium-MAGAZINE-1.8740907

Gaeta, L., & Brydges, C. R. (2020). Coronavirus-related anxiety, social isolation, and loneliness in older adults in northern California during the stay-at-home order. *Journal of Aging & Social Policy*. https://doi.org/10.1080/08959420.2020.1824541

Gerst-Emerson, K., & Jayawardhana, J. (2015). Loneliness as a public health issue: The impact of loneliness on health care utilization among older adults. *American Journal of Public Health, 105*(5), 1013–1019. https://doi.org/10.2105/AJPH.2014.302427

Greenberg, N., Docherty, M., Gnanapragasam, S., & Wessely, S. (2020). Managing mental health challenges faced by healthcare workers during COVID-19 pandemic. *The BMJ, 368* (1211). https://doi.org/10.1136/bmj.m1211 .

Gum, A. M., Hirsch, A., Dautovich, N. D., Ferrante, S., & Schonfeld, L. (2014). Six-month utilization of psychotherapy by older adults with depressive symptoms. *Community Mental Health Journal, 50*(7), 759–764. https://doi.org/10.1007/s10597-014-9704-0

Gur-Yaish, N., Prilutzky, D., & Palgi, Y. (2016). Predictors of psychotherapy use among community-dwelling older adults with depressive symptoms. *Clinical Gerontologist*, *39*(2), 127–138. https://doi.org/10.1080/07317115.2015.1124957

Hoffman, G. S., Webster, N. J., & Bynum, J. P. W. (2020). A framework for aging-friendly services and supports in the age of COVID-19. *Journal of Aging & Social Policy*, *32*(4–5), 450–459. https://doi.org/10.1080/08959420.2020.1771239

Hollander, J. E., & Carr, B. G. (2020). Virtually perfect? Telemedicine for COVID-19. *New England Journal of Medicine*, *382*(18), 1679–1681. https://doi.org/10.1056/NEJMp2003539

Holt-Lunstad, J., Smith, T. B., Baker, M., Harris, T., & Stephenson, D. (2015). Loneliness and social isolation as risk factors for mortality: A meta-analytic review. *Perspectives on Psychological Science*, *10*(2), 227–237. https://doi.org/10.1177/1745691614568352

Israel Psychological Association. (2020). *A call to urgently provide mental health services to older adults*. https://www.psychology.org.il/sites/psycho/UserContent/files/%D7%A0%D7%99%D7%A8%20%D7%A2%D7%9E%D7%93%D7%94%20%D7%9E%D7%A7%D7%95%D7%A6%D7%A8%20%D7%9C%D7%9E%D7%A9%D7%A8%D7%93%D7%99%20%D7%9E%D7%9E%D7%A9%D7%9C%D7%94%20-%20%D7%A1%D7%95%D7%A4%D7%99(1).pdf

Jansson, A. H., Savikko, N. M., & Pitkälä, K. H. (2018). Training professionals to implement a group model for alleviating loneliness among older people–10-year follow-up study. *Educational Gerontology*, *44*(2–3), 119–127. https://doi.org/10.1080/03601277.2017.1420005

Killeen, C. (2002). Loneliness: An epidemic in modern society. *Journal of Advanced Nursing*, *28* (4), 762–770. https://doi.org/10.1046/j.1365-2648.1998.00703.x

Levi-Belz, Y., & Aisenberg, D. (2020). Together we stand: Suicide risk and suicide prevention among Israeli older adults during and after the COVID-19 world crisis. *Psychological Trauma: Theory, Research, Practice, and Policy*, *12*(S1), S123–S125. http://dx.doi.org/10.1037/tra0000667

Lev-On, A., Brainin, E., Abu-Kishk, H., Zilberstein, T., Steinfeld, N., & Naim, S. P. (2019). *Narrowing the gap: Characterization of participants, short and long-term effects of participation in LEHAVA program (Narrowing the digital gap in Israeli society)*. Ariel University. https://www.researchgate.net/profile/Azi_Lev-On/publication/334958331_mzmzmym_t_hpr_pywn_hmsttpym_whspwt_btwwh_hqzr_whrwk_sl_hhsttpwt_btwknyt_lhbh_lzmzwm_hpr_hdygytly_bhbrh_hysrlyt/links/5d46bda2a6fdcc370a7a1193/mzmzmym-t-hpr-pywn-hmsttpym-whspwt-btwwh-hqzr-whrwk-sl-hhsttpwt-btwknyt-lhbh-lzmzwm-hpr-hdygytly-bhbrh-hysrlyt.pdf

Masi, C. M., Chen, H. Y., Hawkley, L. C., & Cacioppo, J. T. (2011). A meta-analysis of interventions to reduce loneliness. *Personality and Social Psychology Review*, *15*(3), 219–266. https://doi.org/10.1177/1088868310377394

Morrow-Howell, N., Galucia, N., & Swinford, E. (2020). Recovering from the COVID-19 pandemic: A focus on older adults. *Journal of Aging & Social Policy*, *32*(4–5), 526–535. https://doi.org/10.1080/08959420.2020.1759758

National Institute on Aging. (2019). *Social isolation, loneliness in older people pose health risks*. https://www.nia.nih.gov/news/social-isolation-loneliness-older-people-pose-health-risks

Ouslander, J. G. (2020). Coronavirus-19 in geriatrics and long-term care: An update. *Journal of the American Geriatrics Society*, *68*(5), 918–921. https://doi.org/10.1111/jgs.16464

Pau, S. (2020, 21 June). *Appling logotherapy and existentialism treating older adults suffering from posttrauma* [Paper presentation in Hebrew]. *Coping with loss and trauma in Aging: How strong are our lives*, Ruppin Academic Center.

Resnizki, S., & Izhaak, L. (2020). *Family members as caregivers during the severe lockdown in the pandemic-19: First evidence*. Myers JDC–Brookdale. [Hebrew].

Rotem, D. (2014). *Report on loneliness.* JDC-Israel-Eshel [Hebrew]. https://www.eshelnet.org. il/DochVaadatBdidut

Santini, Z., Jose, P., Cornwell, E., Koyanagi, A., Nielsen, L., Hinrichsen, C., Meilstrup, C., Madsen, K. R., & Koushede, V. (2020). Social disconnectedness, perceived isolation, and symptoms of depression and anxiety among older Americans (NSHAP): A longitudinal mediation analysis. *The Lancet Public Health, 5*(1), e62–e70. https://doi.org/10.1016/S2468-2667(19)30230-0

Segel-Karpas, D., & Ayalon, L. (2020). Loneliness and hostility in older adults: A cross-lagged model. *Psychology and Aging, 35*(2), 169–176. https://doi.org/10.1037/pag0000417

Shankar, A., McMunn, A., Demakakos, P., Hamer, M., & Steptoe, A. (2017). Social isolation and loneliness: Prospective associations with functional status in older adults. *Health Psychology, 36*(2), 179–187. https://doi.org/10.1037/hea0000437

Shiovitz-Ezra, S. (2012). Locating and assessing the lonely elderly. In D. Rotem (Ed.), *Report on loneliness,* 14-15. JDC- Israel–Eshel [Hebrew]. https://www.eshelnet.org.il/ DochVaadatBdidut

Shnoore, J. (2020). *Corona -COVID-19 and the elderly in Israel [Hebrew].* Myers-Joint-Brookdale.

Shrira, A., Hoffman, Y., Bodner, E., & Palgi, Y. (2020). COVID-19-related loneliness and psychiatric symptoms among older adults: The buffering role of subjective age. *American Journal of Geriatric Psychiatry, 28*(11), 1200–1204. https://doi.org/10.1016/j.jagp.2020.05. 018

Steinman, M. A., Perry, L., & Perissinotto, C. M. (2020). Meeting the care needs of older adults isolated at home during the COVID-19 pandemic. *JAMA, International Medicine, 180*(6), 819–820. https://doi.org/10.1001/jamainternmed.2020.1661

Tanskanen, J., & Anttila, T. (2016). A prospective study of social isolation, loneliness, and mortality in Finland. *American Journal of Public Health, 106*(11), 2042–2048. https://doi. org/10.2105/AJPH.2016.303431

Vahia, I. V., Blazer, D. G., Smith, G. S., Karp, J. F., Steffens, D. C., Forester, B. P., Tampi, R., Agronin, M., Jeste, D. V., & Reynolds, C. F., III. (2020). COVID-19, mental health and aging: A need for new knowledge to bridge science and service. *The American Journal of Geriatric Psychiatry, 28*(7), 691–694. https://doi.org/10.1016/j.jagp.2020.05.029

Yip, P. S., Cheung, Y. T., Chau, P. H., & Law, Y. W. (2010). The impact of epidemic outbreak: The case of severe acute respiratory syndrome (SARS) and suicide among older adults in Hong Kong. *Crisis: The Journal of Crisis Intervention and Suicide Prevention, 31*(2), 86–92. https://doi.org/10.1027/0227-5910/a000015

Technology Recommendations to Support Person-Centered Care in Long-Term Care Homes during the COVID-19 Pandemic and Beyond

Charlene H. Chu (iD), Charlene Ronquillo (iD),
Shehroz Khan (iD), Lillian Hung (iD), and Veronique Boscart (iD)

ABSTRACT

The COVID-19 pandemic has exposed persistent inequities in the long-term care sector and brought strict social/physical distancing distancing and public health quarantine guidelines that inadvertently put long-term care residents at risk for social isolation and loneliness. Virtual communication and technologies have come to the forefront as the primary mode for residents to maintain connections with their loved ones and the outside world; yet, many long-term care homes do not have the technological capabilities to support modern day technologies. There is an urgent need to replace antiquated technological infrastructures to enable person-centered care and prevent potentially irreversible cognitive and psychological declines by ensuring residents are able to maintain important relationships with their family and friends. To this end, we provide five technological recommendations to support the ethos of person-centered care in residential long-term care homes during the pandemic and in a post-COVID-19 pandemic world.

Introduction

The long-term care (LTC) sector is being profoundly shaken by the COVID-19 crisis, with reports from residents, families and staff revealing long-standing vulnerabilities and incidences of neglect in some LTC homes (Orecchio-Egresitz, 2020). LTC homes (also known as care homes or nursing homes) provide around-the-clock complex care to residents who require frequent assistance with activities of daily living (i.e., eating, bathing, toileting etc.), personal support, and monitoring for safety or well-being, residents are also often physically frail, with multiple chronic conditions (Michalik et al., 2013; Moore et al., 2014; Zhang et al., 2019). The congregate care nature of LTC puts residents as high risk of COVID-19. As the virus spreads throughout communities, LTC homes have become "ground zero" of the pandemic (Barnett & Grabowski, 2020), and have been referred to as "a moral failure" (Faghanipour et al., 2020), and a "tragedy" (Holroyd-Leduc & Laupacis, 2020) of and among our healthcare systems and societies. The highest proportion of COVID-19 deaths in Canada, U.S., and Europe are in LTC homes (Chidambaram, 2020; Comas-Herrera et al., 2020; Orecchio-Egresitz, 2020; World Health Organization, 2020), and the highest proportion of healthcare staff COVID-19 deaths are in those working in LTC homes (Yourish et al., 2020).

With increased scrutiny of how the virus continues to ravage LTC homes, evidence suggests that for-profit status, chain ownership, and outdated building design are associated with a greater extent of outbreaks and resident deaths (Stall et al., 2020; White et al., 2020). Some LTC homes have up to four residents sharing a small bathroom, narrow or cramped hallways, with no air conditioning or poor ventilation – a "disaster" when it comes to infection control (Sinha, 2020). Updating LTC home design standards (e.g., reducing the number of shared rooms) and modernizing buildings has been identified as a primary focus to improve infection control practices as a directive (Stall et al., 2020). To this end, governments have pledged to redesign, rebuild, and update the physical LTC homes. For instance, in Canada the Ontario government in Canada plans to invest 1.75 USD billion into the physical redesign of LTC homes (*Ontario Accelerating the Development of Long-Term Care Homes*, 2020) which will modernize approximately 300 homes (Ontario Long Term Care Association, n.d.), and the British Columbia provincial government is increasing capacity by 450 residents and committing 240 USD million over the next three years to increasing staffing levels in LTC homes (Britten, 2020). Inherent in these outdated physical spaces is antiquated technological infrastructure and obsolete technologies that prevent the application of multifaceted modern technologies to promote resident's quality of life, maintain relationships, and support staff. The lack of basic internet access among other technological deficits has been identified by residents and their families (Ontario Association of Residents' Councils, 2020) and health authorities (Saskatchewan Health Authority, 2019).

Alongside governments addressing structural deficiencies and building new LTC homes to prevent overcrowding, we argue that governments and companies concurrently need to prioritize updating the technological capabilities these new LTC homes need to include modern technological capabilities to support residents' opportunities to pursue life-enhancing relationships with family and friends and participate in activities. Technology is a key enabling factor to providing person-centered care (PCC) which is underpinned by values of respect for persons, individual right to self-determination, mutual respect, empowerment, and understanding (Mccormack et al., 2015). This is especially important for residents of LTC homes who were unable to receive visits from family caregivers/loved ones, go outdoors, or leave their rooms during the pandemic (Seifert et al., 2020; Winstead et al., 2013). This meant that residents were confined and isolated in their rooms for months and months on end (Chu et al., 2021a). This perspective piece starts by highlighting how technology has been leveraged by residents to maintain connections, and by staff to access support, collaborate, and improve practice in LTC. Next, we provide five technological recommendations to support the ethos of PCC in LTC during the COVID-19 pandemic and beyond in a post- COVID-19 pandemic world. These recommendations are intended to be feasible and realistic first steps to build a foundation of technological capabilities in high- and middle-income countries.

Technology enables connections and relationships during the pandemic

Restrictive public health countermeasures were put in place in LTC homes internationally (Chu et al., 2021a). These policies effectively placed LTC residents in solitary confinement for several months in Canada (Bercovici, 2020), and in some U.S. states, these visitation restrictions continued for over 5 months (Champagne, 2020). The banning of visitors, and also the preclusion of family members as essential caregivers, has led to significant physical, social, and psychological harm to residents (Abbasi, 2020; Blazer, 2020). Data from the U.K. show that thousands of excess deaths in LTC homes, especially in residents with dementia, are potentially related to changes in care, services, and engagement due to COVID-19 (Office for National Statistics, 2020; Marcello et al., 2020). A survey of 128 care homes reveals that 79% have seen a deterioration in the health of their residents due to lack of social contact (Alzheimer's Society, 2020). The sudden termination of valuable physical and social connections between residents and their family and loved ones not only has deleterious effects but is the antithesis of a PCC ethos (Chu et al., 2020).

During the pandemic, it has become evident that technologies can be the lifeline between residents and their loved ones outside the LTC home, in addition to supporting overworked LTC staff (Eghtesadi, 2020; Flint et al., 2020). For example, the use of wireless devices to support video conferencing has been used for e-visits with residents, as well as telehealth applications that allow LTC staff to virtually connect with physicians and increase the frequency of medical contact (Edelman et al., 2020; Eghtesadi, 2020; Ramesar, 2020). The significance of technologies has been featured prominently in local and national news outlets highlighting the stories of residents and families connecting via technology during the pandemic (Centers for Medicare & Medicaid Services, 2020; Ramesar, 2020). This is being done despite the fact that the majority of residents have physical, cognitive, and/or sensory impairments that impede their ability to use technology independently and require physical assistance. Despite these challenges, there has been extensive utility of various technologies in LTC during the pandemic to overcome spatial and environmental barriers. For the benefit of residents and their families, LTC homes need to be outfitted with a basic technology infrastructure to enable modern-day technologies which can provide opportunities to engage in social connections and PCC during current and future lockdowns.

We urge decisionmakers in the LTC sector to begin addressing the inequities between LTC homes by upgrading antiquated technologies and replacing them with essential technological infrastructure that is needed, with respect to the hardware, software, internet connectivity, and user capacity, to enable PCC and support the empowerment of residents and staff. This is a critical period of time where healthcare professionals, administrators, and advocates must leverage the opportunities afforded by government's rethinking of LTC design – moving beyond reactionary responses and toward proactive and thoughtful consideration of how PCC and LTC can be best supported in the future. For this reason, the authors have proposed technology recommendations that should be part of all future LTC homes.

Technology recommendations to enhance person-centeredness in LTC

Five recommendations are proposed to comprise the technological infrastructure for LTC homes in the 21st century. These recommendations are informed by the needs and capacities of residents and care partners and by the workflow of staff in LTC, as well as the promising evidence on technologies used in LTC, and person-centered approaches to technology design and implementation.

Stable and reliable Wi-Fi access in every room and/or space in the LTC home

Internet access is essential to support social connectedness and engagement to enhance residents' quality of life and well-being. Widespread adoption of various technologies in LTC has been largely impeded by limited wireless access (Eghtesadi, 2020). The absence of internet access disadvantages and socially excludes LTC residents, and furthermore, is in stark contrast to the belief that internet access is a human right and is in stark related to the right to freedom of expression, development, and assembly (La Rue, 2011). Such beliefs are reflected in country-level commitments to ensure connectivity for populations ("Trudeau promises to connect 98% of Canadians to high-speed internet by 2026" reported by the CBC News in 2020). Social connectedness technologies that help maintain and enhance relationships that older adults have with their loved ones rely on internet access, for instance, live streaming, video calls, messaging platforms, social media platforms, e-mails, and texts.

The expanded use of technology beyond the pandemic could widen a resident's social circle, for example, including geographically distant relatives who are unable to visit, virtually "attend" important family events (e.g. birthdays, weddings) that might otherwise be impossible (Bowers et al., 2021). The internet can also provide a plethora of interactive and entertainment opportunities such as exercise or yoga sessions, book clubs, interest groups, libraries, church services, museum tours, and support groups.

Additionally, many sites and apps offer real-time video and chat capabilities enhancing the speed and quality of social interactions (Teo et al., 2019; Zamir et al., 2018). A systematic review of the effects of communication technology on reducing social isolation in older adults revealed a significant reduction of loneliness when consistently using information communication technologies (i.e., smartphones, iPads, emailing, and online chat rooms or forums), and use of high-technology apps (e.g., Wii, the TV gaming system, virtual pet companions) to alleviate loneliness (Chen & Schulz, 2016). Unfortunately, internet access in LTC is limited, leaving some areas of the building and residents' rooms without Wi-fi (Moyle et al., 2018; Saskatchewan Health Authority, 2019; Tak et al., 2007), and many homes only offer a limited number of desktop computers in a communal area available for resident use (Powell et al., 2019; Seifert et al., 2017). Access to and use of technological innovations, such as stable and reliable Wi-Fi access for communication technology, fosters greater independence (Christophorou et al., 2016), and helps address residents' psychosocial needs by enabling them to communicate and remain connected with friends and family. Given what is known about the effects of social isolation, including increased risk of mortality (Holt-Lunstad et al., 2010), poorer quality of life (Hawton et al., 2011), depression (Cacioppo et al., 2010), and suicidal thoughts (Goldsmith et al., 2002), the use of technologies to mitigate its effects represents a relatively small investment.

Software and peripheral accessories that support residents' independent use

Strategic investments must be made to not only procure the technology but also the software and hardware that increase accessibility so that residents are able to confidently use the technology independently. Common barriers for older adults in using technology include inaccessible interfaces and software, lack of instructions or guidance, design that does not accommodate physical or sensory impairments, and lack of knowledge Gitlow (2014) and Vaportzis et al. (2017). From a usability perspective, these barriers could be addressed with software or well-designed simple interfaces that are easy to use, for example, pre-configured links to call family members (e.g., pre-set video call button that requires press to call, using voice recognition by preloading contact information "call x"). Communication programs with auto-pick up may be beneficial for residents with dementia or physical impairments, which allows the family to video conference the resident with zero effort from the resident (e.g., Skype), and with no additional workload for staff. From a physical perspective, functional capacity of residents (affected by vision and/or hearing loss or difficulty using fine motor skills) may limit their ability to use mobile technologies (Barnard et al., 2013; L. Damodaran et al., 2014). Peripheral tools or supports or assistive devices, such as non-slip cases that can be propped beside the resident on bedside tables, flexible tablet mounts with C-clamps that can attach onto wheelchairs or bed railings for those with physical impairments; magnifying glasses, or a larger screen, may be required for those with visual impairment. For those living with hearing impairment, software on tablets can be customized to ensure the correct volume and tones to optimize hearing, for example, lowering the bass and increasing the treble for those with high-frequency hearing loss (Dereby & Luxford, 2010). Providing adaptive interfaces for technology may encourage its use and increase user satisfaction (Gonçalves et al., 2017). Accessible software and technologies for older adults with dementia can be found on public websites such as AcTo Dementia, and reviews of technology to reduce social isolation in residents in LTC (Leigh-Ann, 2020). Accessible devices and accessories will empower residents and support residents to participate in priority relationships to the fullest extent possible while minimizing staff burden.

Technology to support staff's clinical decision making

Given the rapidly increasing volume of resident data, electronic medical records (EMRs) with intuitive interfaces with demonstrated clinical decision-making support systems(CDS) (Pollack & Pratt, 2020 ; Barber et al., 2016; Dowding et al., 2015). CDS technologies have been purported as necessary tools for healthcare staff to deliver evidence-based care, evaluate care and track quality improvement metrics, and complete performance management (Bright et al., 2012; Dagliati et al., 2018; Hitt & Tambe, 2016; Radionova et al., 2020). EMRs with data visualization capabilities have the potential to transform patient data into actionable knowledge using intuitive color coded displays (Dowding et al., 2015), and could be improved to better support prediction and monitoring of patient health outcomes (Rostamzadeh et al., 2020). To fill this need, CDS technologies have leveraged machine learning and A.I. to mine longitudinal patient data and inform their care (Sloane & Silva, 2020). While such technologies have the potential to drive evidence-based, person-centered decisions in LTC, ethical issues related to accountability, transparency, permission and privacy currently exist around the use of A.I. in healthcare have been noted in the literature (Davenport & Kalakota, 2019). This may be especially concerning given the vulnerability of residents who may not be able to consent to providing data. As health technologies to support CDS become more sophisticated and prevalent in health care we must be conscientious about their design and implementation to ensure resident safety, needs and trust are met, which can be done by including caregivers and residents in in-depth and meaningful engagement (e.g., risks, benefits) when introducing technologies, and in some cases to co-create the technology, and the policies about how new technologies can be used.

The use of social technologies

Technologies that encourage social engagement, physical activity, and provide interactive gaming or exergaming have all demonstrated positive impact on residents' quality of life (Bobillier Chaumon et al., 2014; Jung et al., 2009). The value of social and leisure technologies is obvious especially when all group activities are canceled to maintain physical distance, and residents are isolated in their rooms. In these lockdown circumstances, these technology applications and devices can support PCC by meeting residents' needs and values of social connection (Hung et al., 2020). For example, digital resources such as music playlist, meditation apps, or sports games can be selected to fit the resident's interests. Other technologies for leisure that are in their nascent stages include music technology (Creech, 2019), exergaming systems that encourage physical activity designed for LTC residents (Chu et al., 2021b) and virtual reality (Dermody et al., 2020).

Intelligent assistive technologies (IATs) to control the environment

Environmental adaptations such as IATs (e.g., Echo dot, Google Home) can help staff and residents to manage the LTC home environment by turning on/off lights, TV, or music, control room temperature, open/close blinds, via voice activation (Deen, 2015; Lee & Kim, 2020). These widely used technologies can give residents increased independence, while simultaneously reducing staff burden (Mortenson et al., 2013; O'Brien et al., 2020) during periods of extreme short-staffing during the pandemic. Many residents may be fully dependent on staff for small tasks such as turning the lights on/off in their room and may be waiting for long periods of time. Voice activated technology can empower residents with physical impairments and allow them to modify their space to make it more comfortable. The use of IATs has been used and suggested to support people living with dementia (A. Astell et al., 2019; A. J. Astell et al., 2019; Zanwar et al., 2018); while it may be appropriate for some residents, these types of assistive technologies can pose some challenges to older adults with visual, hearing and cognitive impairments (European Parliamentary Research Service, 2018; Vollmer Dahlke & Ory, 2020). Further research is needed to develop new IATs or to understand which currently available IATs would be most acceptable for use among the hetero-geneous LTC resident population.

Discussion

The COVID-19 pandemic has highlighted longstanding inequities and issues in LTC related to staffing, resources and support, and old buildings that lack the infrastructure to support today's modern technologies. We acknowledge the historical deficits of the LTC system and are aware that access to technology alone will not solve these issues – a greater focus needs to be allotted to healthcare policy and reform to improve the LTC infrastructures (including technological capabilities) to address recognized care gaps and invest in staffing. Our suggestions to prioritize an infrastructure that supports various technologies to facilitate PCC in LTC redesign is consistent with the recommendations from the World Economic Forum (Whitman, 2020), the Long-Term Care Financing Collaborative (Long-Term Care Financing Collaborative, 2015) and others who encourage the use of technologies to support PCC (Goh et al., 2017; Wildevuur & Simonse, 2015). We argue that in a world that is increasingly depends on digital technologies, building LTC homes that do not support modern day technologies is an injustice to individuals who reside in these homes. This deprivation of technology based on the place of residence counters the basic principles outlined in the Declaration of Human Rights promoting equality and the right to an adequate standard of living to promote health and well-being (Seifert et al., 2020). Moreover, researchers have acknowledged the ageist approach in which countermeasures have been implemented to the detriment of LTC residents around the world (Aronson, 2020; Badone, 2021; Cesari & Proietti, 2020; Chang et al., 2020; Chu et al., 2020; Colenda et al., 2020; Faghanipour et al., 2020). Residents in LTC have been disproportionately impacted by COVID-19 policies and have been further socially and digitally excluded from our connected society. Future work should focus on how to meaningfully include the voices of older adults, their families and staff in order to reduce inequalities while building a more inclusive and resilient LTC sector.

The recommendations presented here are not a complete list of potential technologies but only serve as a starting point and a brief overview of feasible tools available in most middle- and high-income countries where the redesign of LTC homes is being addressed in public discourse. We focused on ubiquitous technologies that are commercially available and commonly used, have been implemented to support care, and used to meet the needs of the residents, their families, and staff in LTC.

Barriers and challenges to implementing technology infrastructure in LTC include the lack of financial resources to develop and purchase technologies, LTC staff's lack of time and experience implementing and overseeing technological changes (The Conference Board of Canada & Ontario Long Term Care Association, 2011; U.S. Department of Health and Human Services & Office of Disability, A. and L.-T. C. P., 2005), as well as failure of regulatory bodies to keep up with technological innovation (MacNeil et al., 2019; Vincent et al., 2015). Continued research is needed to parse the costs of technology infrastructure implementation, generate evidence around the cost-effectiveness of technology-based interventions in LTC as well as their benefits and risks to staff and LTC residents. Technology developers, and researchers should work collaboratively with residents and stakeholders to develop technologies and innovations that meet the needs of LTC residents, their families, and staff. Robust collaborations with residents and family partners focused on the needs of the residents in LTC will not only enhance PCC but promote digital inclusion of LTC home residents (Leela Damodaran et al., 2015), for example, projects that include co-creation of technology with residents and stakeholders.

The COVID-19 pandemic has profoundly impacted residents, families and LTC staff. We argue that a foundational technological infrastructure is required in all LTC homes as a preemptive measure to enable technology use and PCC in future lockdown situations. Given that a hallmark of this pandemic is the uncertainty of when strict visitation policies will be lifted, reinstated, or what the "new normal" will look like in LTC, there is a moral urgency to address the digital exclusion of LTC homes. National standards should include that LTC homes are outfitted with basic technological infrastructure including stable internet connectivity with appropriate software, hardware and peripheral accessories to enable residents to overcome physical and sensory impairments and spatial barriers, as well as support staff in their delivery of safe, and high quality care. Such an infrastructure allows residents to meet their human need for connections with loved ones and can also empower residents by increasing their autonomy.

Conclusion

We provide five recommendations to update the technology infrastructure in LTC homes. Such changes will enable the social and digital inclusion of LTC residents, thus facilitating social connections and PCC during current and future pandemics. While we recognize that this list is subject to change based on emerging technologies over time, the proposed technological infrastructure is positioned as a building block for further dialog about the resources necessary to enable PCC in LTC and to reduce inequality to technology access in the 21st century.

Key Points:
- Outdated building designs with crowded spaces have been associated with a greater extent of LTC outbreaks and resident deaths. With the increased attention and impetus to rebuild and update these settings, there is an

opportunity to ensure all residential LTC homes are equipped with the appropriate technological infrastucture.

- Residents living in LTC have been disproportionately impacted by COVID-19 public health "lock down" policies and are consequently, further socially excluded from our digitally connected society without access to modern technologies
- We provide five core recommendations to update and modernize the technological infrastructure for LTC homes in the 21st century.

Acknowledgments

We acknowledge Dr. Chu's Research Associates (Allison Souter and Amanda My Linh Quan) who provided assistance and proofreading of the paper.

Disclosure statement

No potential conflict of interest was reported by the author(s).

Funding

Dr. Chu is supported by the Alzheimer Society of Canada New Investigator Award; Alzheimer Society Research Program; Canadian Institutes of Health Research; Social Sciences and Humanities Research Council of Canada.

ORCID

Charlene H. Chu (iD) http://orcid.org/0000-0002-0333-7210
Charlene Ronquillo (iD) http://orcid.org/0000-0002-6520-1765
Shehroz Khan (iD) http://orcid.org/0000-0002-1195-4999
Lillian Hung (iD) http://orcid.org/0000-0002-7916-2939
Veronique Boscart (iD) http://orcid.org/0000-0002-7420-1978

References

Abbasi, J. (2020). social isolation - The other COVID-19 threat in nursing homes. *JAMA - Journal of the American Medical Association. 324*(7), 619–620. https://doi.org/10.1001/jama.2020.13484

Alzheimer's Society. (2020, June). *Thousands of people with dementia dying or deteriorating – Not just from coronavirus as isolation takes its toll | Alzheimer's Society.* https://www.alzheimers.org.uk/news/2020-06-05/thousands-people-dementia-dying-or-deteriorating-not-just-coronavirus-isolation

Aronson, L. (2020). *ageism is making the coronavirus pandemic worse - The Atlantic.* https://www.theatlantic.com/culture/archive/2020/03/americas-ageism-crisis-is-helping-the-coronavirus/608905/

Astell, A., Dove, E., & Hernandez, A. (2019). An introduction to technology for dementia. In *Using technology in dementia care: A guide to technology solutions for everyday living* (pp. 11). Karger Open access.

Astell, A. J., Bouranis, N., Hoey, J., Lindauer, A., Mihailidis, A., Nugent, C., & Robillard, J. M. (2019). Technology and dementia: The future is now. *Dementia and Geriatric Cognitive Disorders*, 47(3), 131–139. https://doi.org/10.1159/000497800

Badone, E. (2021). From Cruddiness to Catastrophe: COVID-19 and Long-term Care in Ontario. *Medical Anthropology*, 1–15. https://doi.org/10.1080/01459740.2021

Bowers, B. J., Chu, C. H., Wu, B., Thompson, R., Mihailidis, A., Lepore, M. J., Leung, A. Y. Leung, A. Y., & McGilton, K. S. (2021). What COVID-19 Innovations Can Teach Us About Improving Quality of Life in Long-Term Care. *Journal of the American Medical Directors Association*, 22(5), 929–932.

Barber, D., Morkem, R., Queenan, J. A., & Barber, K. H. (2016). Harnessing the power of longitudinal data. *Canadian Family Physician Medecin De Famille Canadien*, 62(4), 355–356. https://pubmed.ncbi.nlm.nih.gov/27076548/

Barnard, Y., Bradley, M. D., Hodgson, F., & Lloyd, A. D. (2013). Learning to use new technologies by older adults: Perceived difficulties, experimentation behaviour and usability. *Computers in Human Behavior*, 29(4), 1715–1724. https://doi.org/10.1016/j.chb.2013.02.006

Barnett, M. L., & Grabowski, D. C. (2020). Nursing homes are ground zero for COVID-19 pandemic. *JAMA Health Forum*, 1(3), e200369–e200369. https://doi.org/10.1001/JAMAHEALTHFORUM.2020.0369

Bercovici, V. (2020, June). We have failed the elderly during the COVID-19 crisis | National Post. *National Post*.

Blazer, D. (2020). Social isolation and loneliness in older adults-A mental health/public health challenge. *JAMA Psychiatry*, 77(10), 990. https://doi.org/10.1001/jamapsychiatry.2020.1054

Bobillier Chaumon, M.-E., Michel, C., Tarpin Bernard, F., & Croisile, B. (2014). Can ICT improve the quality of life of elderly adults living in residential home care units? From actual impacts to hidden artefacts. *Behaviour & Information Technology*, 33(6), 574–590. https://doi.org/10.1080/0144929X.2013.832382

Bright, T. J., Wong, A., Dhurjati, R., Bristow, E., Bastian, L., Coeytaux, R. R., ... Lobach, D. (2012). Effect of clinical decision-support systems: A systematic review. *Annals of Internal Medicine*, 157(1), 29. https://doi.org/10.7326/0003-4819-157-1-201207030-00450

Britten, L. (2020, July). Province announces 495 long-term care beds for seniors in Interior Health Region. *CBC News*.

Cacioppo, J. T., Hawkley, L. C., & Thisted, R. A. (2010). Perceived social isolation makes me sad: 5-year cross-lagged analyses of loneliness and depressive symptomatology in the Chicago health, aging, and social relations study. *Psychology and Aging*, 25(2), 453. https://doi.org/10.1037/a0017216

Centers for Medicare & Medicaid Services. (2020). *CMS announces new measures to protect nursing home residents from COVID-19*. CMS.gov. https://www.cms.gov/newsroom/press-releases/cms-announces-new-measures-protect-nursing-home-residents-covid-19#:~:text=It%20directs%20nursing%20homes%20to,for%20complications%20from%20COVID%2D19

Cesari, M., & Proietti, M. (2020). COVID-19 in Italy: Ageism and decision making in a pandemic. *Journal of the American Medical Directors Association*, 21(5), 576–577. https://doi.org/10.1016/j.jamda.2020.03.025

Champagne, S. (2020, August). Without Texas nursing home visitations, isolation takes it toll. *The Texas Tribune*.

Chang, E. S., Kannoth, S., Levy, S., Wang, S. Y., Lee, J. E., & Levy, B. R. (2020). Global reach of ageism on older persons' health: A systematic review. *PLoS ONE, 15*(1), e0220857. https://doi.org/10.1371/journal.pone.0220857

Chen, Y. R. R., & Schulz, P. J. (2016). The effect of information communication technology interventions on reducing social isolation in the elderly: A systematic review. *Journal of Medical Internet Research, 18*(1), e18. https://doi.org/10.2196/jmir.4596

Chidambaram, P. (2020, April). *State reporting of cases and deaths due to COVID-19 in long-term care facilities | KFF*. Kaiser Family Foundation (KKF).

Christophorou, C., Kleanthous, S., Georgiadis, D., Cereghetti, D. M., Andreou, P., Wings, C., . . . Samaras, G. (2016). ICT services for active ageing and independent living: Identification and assessment. *Healthcare Technology Letters, 3*(3), 159–164. https://doi.org/10.1049/htl.2016.0031

Chu, C. H., Biss, R. K., Cooper, L., Quan, A. M. L., & Matulis, H. (2021b). Exergaming Platform for Older Adults Residing in Long-Term Care Homes: User-Centered Design, Development, and Usability Study. *JMIR Serious Games, 9*(1), e22370. https://doi.org/10.2196/22370

Chu, C. H., Donato-Woodger, S., & Dainton, C. J. (2020). Competing crises: COVID-19 countermeasures and social isolation among older adults in long term care. *Journal of Advanced Nursing*, jan.14467. *76*(10).https://doi.org/10.1111/jan.14467

Chu, C. H., Wang, J., Fukui, C., Staudacher, S., A Wachholz, P., & Wu, B. (2021a). The Impact of COVID-19 on Social Isolation in Long-term Care Homes: Perspectives of Policies and Strategies from Six Countries. *Journal of Aging & Social Policy*, 1–15. https://doi.org/10.1080/08959420.2021.1924346

Colenda, C. C., Reynolds, C. F., Applegate, W. B., Sloane, P. D., Zimmerman, S., Newman, A. B., . . . Ouslander, J. G. (2020). COVID-19 pandemic and ageism: A call for humanitarian care. *The Gerontologist, 60*(6), 987–988. https://doi.org/10.1093/geront/gnaa062

Comas-Herrera, A., Zalakaín, J., Litwin, C., Hsu, A. T., Lane, N., & Fernández, J.-L. (2020). *ltccovid.org | Mortality associated with COVID-19 outbreaks in care homes Mortality associated with COVID-19 outbreaks in care homes: Early international evidence*. International Long-Term Care Policy Network.

Creech, A. (2019). Using music technology creatively to enrich later-life: A literature review. *Frontiers in Psychology, 10*, 117. https://doi.org/10.3389/fpsyg.2019.00117

Dagliati, A., Tibollo, V., Sacchi, L., Malovini, A., Limongelli, I., Gabetta, M., . . . Bellazzi, R. (2018). Big data as a driver for clinical decision support systems: A learning health systems perspective. *Frontiers in Digital Humanities, 60*(2). https://doi.org/10.3389/fdigh.2018.00008

Damodaran, L., Gilbertson, T., Olphert, W., Sandhu, J., & Craig, M. (2015). Digital inclusion-the vision, the challenges and the way forward. *International Journal on Advances in Internet Technology, 8*(3/4), 78–92. http://www.thinkmind.org/index.php?view=article&articleid=inttech_v8_n34_2015_3

Damodaran, L., Olphert, C. W., & Sandhu, J. (2014). Falling off the bandwagon? Exploring the challenges to sustained digital engagement by older people. *Gerontology, 60*(2), 163–173. https://doi.org/10.1159/000357431

Davenport, T., & Kalakota, R. (2019). The potential for artificial intelligence in healthcare. *Future Healthcare Journal, 6*(2), 94–98. https://doi.org/10.7861/futurehosp.6-2-94

Deen, M. J. (2015). Information and communications technologies for elderly ubiquitous healthcare in a smart home. *Personal and Ubiquitous Computing, 19*(3–4), 573–599. https://doi.org/10.1007/s00779-015-0856-x

Dereby, J., & Luxford, W. (2010). *Hearing loss: The otolaryngologist's guide to amplification*. Plural Publishing.

Dermody, G., Whitehead, L., Wilson, G., & Glass, C. (2020). The role of virtual reality in improving health outcomes for community-dwelling older adults: Systematic review. *Journal of Medical Internet Research, 22*(6), e17331. https://doi.org/10.2196/17331

Dowding, D., Randell, R., Gardner, P., Fitzpatrick, G., Dykes, P., Favela, J., ... Currie, L. (2015, February). Dashboards for improving patient care: Review of the literature. *International Journal of Medical Informatics, 84*(2), 87–100. Elsevier Ireland Ltd. https://doi.org/10.1016/j.ijmedinf.2014.10.001

Edelman, L. S., McConnell, E. S., Kennerly, S. M., Alderden, J., Horn, S. D., & Yap, T. L. (2020). Mitigating the effects of a pandemic: Facilitating improved nursing home care delivery through technology. *JMIR Aging, 3*(1), e20110. https://doi.org/10.2196/20110

Eghtesadi, M. (2020). breaking social isolation amidst COVID-19: A viewpoint on improving access to technology in long-term care facilities. *Journal of the American Geriatrics Society, 68*(5), 949–950. https://doi.org/10.1111/jgs.16478

European Parliamentary Research Service. (2018). *Assistive technologies for people with disabilities.* Scientific Foresight Unit (STOA).

Faghanipour, S., Monteverde, S., & Peter, E. (2020). COVID-19-related deaths in long-term care: The moral failure to care and prepare. *Nursing Ethics, 27*(5), 1171–1173. https://doi.org/10.1177/0969733020939667

Flint, A. J., Bingham, K. S., & Iaboni, A. (2020). Effect of COVID-19 on the mental health care of older people in Canada. *International Psychogeriatrics, 32*(10), 1113–1116. https://doi.org/10.1017/S1041610220000708

Gitlow, L. (2014). Technology use by older adults and barriers to using technology. *Physical and Occupational Therapy in Geriatrics, 32*(3), 271–280. https://doi.org/10.3109/02703181.2014.946640

Goh, A. M. Y., Loi, S. M., Westphal, A., & Lautenschlager, N. T. (2017). Person-centered care and engagement via technology of residents with dementia in aged care facilities. *International Psychogeriatrics, 29*(12), 2099–2103. https://doi.org/10.1017/S1041610217001375

Goldsmith, S. K., Pellmar, T. C., Kleinman, A. M., & Bunney, W. E. (2002). *Reducing suicide: A national imperative.* National Academies Press.

Gonçalves, V. P., De Almeida Neris, V. P., Seraphini, S., Dias, T. C. M., Pessin, G., Johnson, T., & Ueyama, J. (2017). Providing adaptive smartphone interfaces targeted at elderly people: An approach that takes into account diversity among the elderly. *Universal Access in the Information Society, 16*(1), 129–149. https://doi.org/10.1007/s10209-015-0429-9

Hawton, A., Green, C., Dickens, A. P., Richards, S. H., Taylor, R. S., Edwards, R., ... Campbell, J. L. (2011). The impact of social isolation on the health status and health-related quality of life of older people. *Quality of Life Research, 20*(1), 57–67. https://doi.org/10.1007/s11136-010-9717-2

Hitt, L. M., & Tambe, P. (2016). Health care information technology, work organization, and nursing home performance. *Industrial and Labor Relations Review, 69*(4), 834–859. https://doi.org/10.1177/0019793916640493

Holroyd-Leduc, J. M., & Laupacis, A. (2020, June). Continuing care and COVID-19: A Canadian tragedy that must not be allowed to happen again. *Canadian Medical Association Journal, 192*(23), E632–E633. Canadian Medical Association. https://doi.org/10.1503/cmaj.201017

Holt-Lunstad, J., Smith, T. B., & Layton, J. B. (2010). Social relationships and mortality risk: A meta-analytic review. *PLoS Medicine, 7*(7), e1000316. https://doi.org/10.1371/journal.pmed.1000316

Hung, L., Chow, B., Shadarevian, J., O'Neill, R., Berndt, A., Wallsworth, C., ... Chaudhury, H. (2020). Using touchscreen tablets to support social connections and reduce responsive behaviours among people with dementia in care settings: A scoping review. *Dementia.* 20 *(3)*,1124–1143. https://doi.org/10.1177/1471301220922745

Jung, Y., Li, K. J., Janissa, N. S., Gladys, W. L. C., & Lee, K. M. (2009). Games for a better life: Effects of playing wii games on the well-being of seniors in a long-term care facility. *Proceedings of the 6th Australasian Conference on Interactive Entertainment, IE 2009.* 1–6. https://doi.org/10.1145/1746050.1746055

La Rue, F. (2011). *Promotion and protection of all human rights, civil, political, economic, social and cultural rights, including the right to development Report of the Special Rapporteur on the promotion and protection of the right to freedom of opinion and expression.* United Nations Human Rights Council.

Lee, L. N., & Kim, M. J. (2020). A critical review of smart residential environments for older adults with a focus on pleasurable experience. *Frontiers in Psychology, 10*, 3080. https://doi.org/10.3389/fpsyg.2019.03080

Leigh-Ann, T. (2020). Technologies to address the negative effects of social isolation on older adults living in long-term care. https://cadth.ca/sites/default/files/covid-19/en0024-technologies-to-address-social-isolation-long-term-care.pdf

Long-Term Care Financing Collaborative. (2015). *Vision of a better future for people needing long-term services and supports.* Urban Institute.

MacNeil, M., Koch, M., Kuspinar, A., Juzwishin, D., Lehoux, P., & Stolee, P. (2019). Enabling health technology innovation in Canada: Barriers and facilitators in policy and regulatory processes. *Health Policy, 123*(2), 203–214. https://doi.org/10.1016/j.healthpol.2018.09.018

Marcello, M., Jonathan, S., Evangelos, K., Ian, Hall., & Alex J. T. (2020, November). "Excess mortality for care home residents during the first 23 weeks of the COVID-19 pandemic in England: a national cohort study,". BMC Medicine. *19*(71).

Mccormack, B., Borg, M., Cardiff, S., Dewing, J., Jacobs, G., Janes, N., . . . Wilson, V. (2015). Person-centredness – The "state" of the art. *International Practice Development Journal, 5*, 1–15. https://www.fons.org/library/journal/volume5-person-centredness-suppl/article1

Michalik, C., Matusik, P., Nowak, J., Chmielowska, K., Tomaszewski, K. A., Parnicka, A., . . . Grodzicki, T. (2013). Heart failure, comorbidities, and polypharmacy among elderly nursing home residents. *Polskie Archiwum Medycyny Wewnetrznej, 123*(4), 170–175. https://doi.org/10.20452/pamw.1682

Moore, K. L., Boscardin, W. J., Steinman, M. A., & Schwartz, J. B. (2014). Patterns of chronic co-morbid medical conditions in older residents of U.S. nursing homes: Differences between the sexes and across the agespan. *Journal of Nutrition, Health and Aging, 18*(4), 429–436. https://doi.org/10.1007/s12603-014-0001-y

Mortenson, W. B., Demers, L., Fuhrer, M. J., Jutai, J. W., Lenker, J., & DeRuyter, F. (2013). Effects of an assistive technology intervention on older adults with disabilities and their informal caregivers: An exploratory randomized controlled trial. *American Journal of Physical Medicine & Rehabilitation, 92*(4), 297–306. https://doi.org/10.1097/PHM.0b013e31827d65bf

Moyle, W., Jones, C., Murfield, J., Dwan, T., & Ownsworth, T. (2018). 'We don't even have Wi-Fi'. descriptive study exploring current use and availability of communication technologies in residential aged care. *Contemporary Nurse, 54*(1), 35–43. https://doi.org/10.1080/10376178.2017.1411203

O'Brien, K., Liggett, A., Ramirez-Zohfeld, V., Sunkara, P., & Lindquist, L. A. (2020). Voice-controlled intelligent personal assistants to support aging in place. *Journal of the American Geriatrics Society, 68*(1), 176–179. https://doi.org/10.1111/jgs.16217

Office for National Statistics. (2020). *Deaths involving COVID-19 in the care sector.* England and Wales.

Ontario accelerating the development of long-term care homes. (2020). Office of the Premier.

Ontario Association of Residents' Councils. (2020). *Courageously living through COVID-19 together: Residents and families*. OARC.

Ontario Long Term Care Association. (n.d.). *The role of long-term care: Ontario's long-term care homes (February 2019)*.

Orecchio-Egresitz, H. (2020, April). Half of Europe's COVID-19 deaths were in long-term care facilities - Business insider. *Business Insider*.

Pollack, A. H. & Pratt, W. (2020). Association of Health Record Visualizations With Physicians' Cognitive Load When Prioritizing Hospitalized Patients. *JAMA Netw Open, 3*(1), e1919301. doi:10.1001/jamanetworkopen.2019.19301

Powell, K. R., Alexander, G. L., Madsen, R., & Deroche, C. (2019). A national assessment of access to technology among nursing home residents: A secondary analysis. *JMIR Aging, 2*(1), e11449. https://doi.org/10.2196/11449

Radionova, N., Becker, G., Mayer-Steinacker, R., Gencer, D., Rieger, M. A., & Preiser, C. (2020). The views of physicians and nurses on the potentials of an electronic assessment system for recognizing the needs of patients in palliative care. *BMC Palliative Care, 19*(1), 1–9. https://doi.org/10.1186/s12904-020-00554-9

Ramesar, V. (2020, August). Absence of volunteers creates staffing pressures at N.S. nursing homes | CBC News. *CBCNews*.

Rostamzadeh, N., Abdullah, S. S., & Sedig, K. (2020). Data-driven activities involving electronic health records: An activity and task analysis framework for interactive visualization tools. *Multimodal Technologies and Interaction, 4*(1), 7. https://doi.org/10.3390/mti4010007

Saskatchewan Health Authority. (2019) . *Saskatchewan health authority long-term care quality assessment - CEO tours, 2019*. Regina.

Scifert, A., Cotten, S. R., & Xie, B. (2020). A double burden of exclusion? Digital and social exclusion of older adults in times of COVID-19. *The Journals of Gerontology: Series B. 76*(3), e99–e103. DOI: 10.1093/geronb/gbaa098

Seifert, A., Doh, M., & Wahl, H. W. (2017). They also do it: Internet use by older adults living in residential care facilities. *Educational Gerontology, 43*(9), 451–461. https://doi.org/10.1080/03601277.2017.1326224

Sinha, S. (2020). The post-pandemic future: We will stop warehousing older people in care homes. *Toronto Life*.

Sloane, E. B., & Silva, J. R. (2020). Artificial intelligence in medical devices and clinical decision support systems. *Clinical Engineering Handbook*, 556–568. https://doi.org/10.1016/B978-0-12-813467-2.00084-5

Stall, N. M., Jones, A., Brown, K. A., Rochon, P. A., & Costa, A. P. (2020). For-profit long-term care homes and the risk of COVID 19 outbreaks and resident deaths. *Canadian Medical Association Journal*, cmaj.201197. *192*(33), e946–e955. https://doi.org/10.1503/cmaj.201197

Tak, S. H., Beck, C., & McMahon, E. (2007). Computer and Internet access for long-term care residents: Perceived benefits and barriers. *Journal of Gerontological Nursing, 33*(5), 32–40. https://doi.org/10.3928/00989134-20070501-06

Teo, A. R., Markwardt, S., & Hinton, L. (2019). Using Skype to beat the blues: Longitudinal data from a national representative sample. *American Journal of Geriatric Psychiatry, 27*(3), 254–262. https://doi.org/10.1016/j.jagp.2018.10.014

The Conference Board of Canada, & Ontario Long Term Care Association. (2011). *Elements of an effective innovation strategy for long term care in Ontario*.

U.S. Department of Health and Human Services, & Office of Disability, A. and L.-T. C. P. (2005). *Barriers to implementing technology in residential long-term care settings*. Polisher Research Institute.

Vaportzis, E., Clausen, M. G., & Gow, A. J. (2017). Older adults perceptions of technology and barriers to interacting with tablet computers: A focus group study. *Frontiers in Psychology*, 8. https://doi.org/10.3389/fpsyg.2017.01687

Vincent, C. J., Niezen, G., O'Kane, A. A., & Stawarz, K. (2015). Can standards and regulations keep up with health technology? *JMIR MHealth and UHealth*, 3(2), e64. https://doi.org/10.2196/mhealth.3918

Vollmer Dahlke, D., & Ory, M. G. (2020). Emerging issues of intelligent assistive technology use among people with dementia and their caregivers: A U.S. Perspective. *Frontiers in Public Health*, 8. https://doi.org/10.3389/fpubh.2020.00191

White, E. M., Kosar, C. M., Feifer, R. A., Blackman, C., Gravenstein, S., Ouslander, J., & Mor, V. (2020). Variation in SARS-CoV-2 prevalence in U.S. Skilled nursing facilities. *Journal of the American Geriatrics Society*, 68(10), 2167–2173. https://doi.org/10.1111/jgs.16752

Whitman, D. (2020, August). *COVID-19 has laid bare the cracks in long-term care. 17*(3), e77.

Wildevuur, S. E., & Simonse, L. W. L. (2015). Information and communication technology-enabled person-centered care for the "big five" chronic conditions: Scoping review. *Journal of Medical Internet Research*, 17(3), e77. https://doi.org/10.2196/jmir.3687

Winstead, V., Anderson, W. A., Yost, E. A., Cotten, S. R., Warr, A., & Berkowsky, R. W. (2013). You can teach an old dog new tricks: A qualitative analysis of how residents of senior living communities may use the web to overcome spatial and social Barriers. *Journal of Applied Gerontology*, 32(5), 540–560. https://doi.org/10.1177/0733464811431824

World Health Organization. (2020). *Statement – Invest in the overlooked and unsung: Build sustainable people-centred long-term care in the wake of COVID-19.*

Yourish, K. K., Lai, R., Ivory, D., & Smith, M. (2020, May). One-third of all U.S. coronavirus deaths are nursing home residents or workers - The New York Times. *New York Times.*

Zamir, S., Hennessy, C. H., Taylor, A. H., & Jones, R. B. (2018). Video-calls to reduce loneliness and social isolation within care environments for older people: An implementation study using collaborative action research. *BMC Geriatrics*, 18(1). https://doi.org/10.1186/s12877-018-0746-y

Zanwar, P., Heyn, P. C., Mcgrew, G., & Raji, M. (2018). Assistive technology megatrends to support persons with Alzheimer's disease and related dementias age in habitat: Challenges for usability, engineering and public policy. *Proceedings of ACM Human-Habitat for Health Conference*, 1–9. https://doi.org/10.1145/3279963.3279971

Zhang, X. M., Dou, Q. L., Zhang, W. W., Wang, C. H., Xie, X. H., Yang, Y. Z., & Zeng, Y. C. (2019). Frailty as a predictor of all-cause mortality among older nursing home residents: A systematic review and meta-analysis. *Journal of the American Medical Directors Association*, 20(6), 657–663.e4. https://doi.org/10.1016/j.jamda.2018.11.018

Redesigning Memory Care in the COVID-19 Era: Interdisciplinary Spatial Design Interventions to Minimize Social Isolation in Older Adults

Farhana Ferdous (iD)

ABSTRACT

Older adults living in memory care facilities are vulnerable to more than just COVID-19; they are especially harmed from social distancing guidelines, as social isolation and loneliness have important medical consequences in this population. COVID-19 has changed the way we perceive the built environment, and almost all public spaces are now adopting new design strategies to create safe indoor and outdoor environments. Eight interdisciplinary, evidence-based spatial design interventions and action plans are explored in this article with the aim of redesigning future memory care facilities to combat social isolation and loneliness in older adults during this unprecedented time and beyond.

Introduction

Time and memory are two aspects of the human life upon which spatial design is largely predicated. When it comes to addressing people with special needs, spatial design cannot be based only upon expert intuition but instead requires intimate knowledge and evidence-based approaches. The coronavirus disease 2019 (COVID-19) pandemic has devastated nursing homes, long-term care facilities (LTCFs) and memory care facilities (MCFs) across the United States (U.S.) and is particularly lethal to older adults with underlying health conditions or with cognitive impairment. As of completing this narrative commentary, more than 100,000 residents and workers at nursing homes and LTCFs have died from COVID-19, accounting for more than 38% of the deaths in the U.S. (Yourish et al., 2020). The Centers for Disease Control and Prevention (CDC) reported that 8 out of 10 deaths in the U.S. have been in adults 65 years or older. To reduce deaths and cases, assisted living facilities, LTCFs and MCFs have had to implement drastic measures to reduce disease transmission, namely those in accordance with CDC social distancing recommendations

(CDC, 2020a) such as personal hygiene, wearing masks, self-quarantine and social distancing.

The social spaces in LTCFs are recognized as places of social interaction among residents, family members and caregivers. At least half of the older adults in LTCFs live with cognitive impairment such as Alzheimer's disease and related dementias (ADRD) (CDC, 2020a). Therefore, this study included the older adults who may or may not require specialized care for cognitive impairment and often live in specialized memory care units within MCFs. Paradoxically, due to COVID-19, older adults, including individuals living with or without ADRD, may be harmed from social distancing guidelines more than they are helped: it has been established that older adults living in LTCFs and MCFs experience increased social isolation and loneliness (David, 2020; Shrira et al., 2020; Wu, 2020), and this has purportedly been worsened by social distancing guidelines (Cudjoe & Kotwal, 2020; Eghtesadi, 2020; Wu, 2020). Suddenly, the built environment now has the responsibility of combating the great momentum of the current pandemic. Architects, interior designers and other design professionals have a unique opportunity to reevaluate many ideas, including how to efficiently design the built environment while also effectively incorporating the new safety guidelines.

The relationship between the physical environment and the prevalence of social interaction has been a core topic of inquiry within environmental gerontology (Boer et al., 2018; Kang, 2012), where social interaction is considered an essential therapeutic intervention for older adults with or without ADRD. Loneliness due to social isolation is considered to be a public health threat, and the elderly are especially vulnerable to the risks associated with social isolation and loneliness, which include faster cognitive decline (Evans et al., 2019; Read et al., 2020; Yang et al., 2020), hypertension, cardiovascular and cerebrovascular disease (Holt-Lunstad & Smith, 2016; Xia & Li, 2018), and premature death in the range of 29% to 32% increased likelihood of mortality (Holt-Lunstad et al., 2015). Many targeted interventions within the fields of geriatrics and public health policy have been brought forth and are in the early stages of study where safety guidelines have been prioritized (Behrens, 2020). However, interdisciplinary approaches that emphasize spatial design guidelines and policies while also minimizing social isolation in older adults are arguably lacking. Therefore, the aim of this article is to discuss evidence-based spatial design guidelines, interdisciplinary interventions and action plans for redesigning MCFs to improve social isolation and loneliness in older adults with or without ADRD experienced during the COVID-19 pandemic.

Interdisciplinary spatial design interventions

COVID-19 has changed the way we perceive the built environment. The home or personalized indoor environment is considered the safest place, and almost all public spaces are now adopting new design strategies to create safe indoor and outdoor environments. The framework of this article has been developed by reviewing relevant evidence from multiple disciplines, such as medicine, health science, social science, evidence-based architecture, and interior design to understand what is currently in place. This article then synthesizes and organizes evidence into eight actionable themes based on interdisciplinary spatial design concepts and provides a framework for redesigning MCFs so that we may begin to think outside of the box and identify novel, creative interventions to complement those that already exist (Table 1).

Outdoor space and activities

Outdoor activities have been encouraged over indoor activities by government officials during the pandemic (CDC, 2020b; Design, 2020), and the outdoors have thus become a sanctuary for most people. Adding accessible outdoor space in the form of therapeutic gardens, courtyards, outdoor patios or simple walkways can allow access to fresh air, minimize boredom, and involve MCF residents in outdoor activities while allowing for social distancing.

Incorporating various levels of outdoor space can promote an active lifestyle through gardening, group activities, solitary activities, recreational activities and even dining, which can often easily be moved outdoors as long as there is space available, and may pose a great benefit to residents living in MCFs.

Different types of outdoor spaces with special features such as healing gardens, water bodies, fish ponds, and accessible walking paths are already recommended for older adults living in MCFs (Ferdous, 2019). The balcony has been touted as a "design hero" during the pandemic (Design, 2020), allowing social interaction from a distance and personal access to fresh air and sunlight. Another great way to encourage time spent outdoors is to allow "drive-up" visits from family members and friends; designing an outdoor socializing area to allow social interactions between residents and their visitors creates the opportunity to spend time outdoors and de-densifies the indoor common areas of the facility.

De-densification and de-centralization

The term de-densification (McFarlane, 20 Mar McFarlane, 2020) is traditionally used within the urban design and planning discipline, but de-densification can easily be implemented at the facility level. Geboy has suggested decentralizing the dining area by setting only four chairs to a table (Geboy, 2009), and this may serve as an adequate solution for maintaining communal dining while also following social distancing requirements. To maintain a lower population in the workplace, staff members could spend alternating weeks working remotely on administrative tasks for the care facility or on certain

Table 1. Framework for interdisciplinary spatial design interventions.

Interdisciplinary Spatial Design Interventions

Outdoor Space and Activities	De-densification and De-centralization	Personalized Interior and Furniture Layout	Indoor Air Quality	Make Better Use of Technology	Small-Scale Community Space	Person-Centered Approach	Spatial Design and Layout
1. Active Lifestyle 2. Fresh Air and Sunlight 3. Drive-Up Visits	1. Staggered Shift 2. Virtual Tours	1. Biophilic Design 2. Stimulating Environment 3. Furniture Use/Arrangement 4. Concept of "Hygge"	1. Air Filtration System 2. Use of Elevators 3. Air Humidity	1. Social Media and Virtual Reality 2. Telehealth Technology 3. Touchless Mechanisms	1. Keeping it Small 2. Use of Common Areas 3. Meal Services	1. Resident Advocate 2. Role of Staff 3. Therapeutic Touch	1. Negative-Pressure Isolation Rooms 2. Visitor Protocols 3. Meetings and Conferences

tasks for the residents through video chat depending on residents' needs. Staggered arrival and end times for shifts may be helpful for reducing traffic in lobbies and common areas of the MCFs during shift changes. Many care facilities are now offering virtual tours to new families. Facilities can also limit non-medical personnel by organizing virtual live entertainment for the residents. If in-person community vendors and their services are absolutely necessary to minimize boredom or loneliness for residents in this unprecedented situation, vendors could arrange shows and services for small, staggered groups of residents outdoors or arrange services so that residents can enjoy from the windows of their individual rooms.

Personalized interior and furniture layout

The immediate response to the pandemic for many MCFs was to confine residents to their rooms (Edelman et al., 2020). This is not an ideal solution, but it may continue to be necessary in communities with especially high COVID-19 case numbers. In that case, interior design may be put to good use so that residents can enjoy their private rooms a little more. A great way to improve the indoor environment is to bring plant life indoors or implement a biophilic design concept. Biophilia, or mimicking natural systems through design, is linked to decreased stress, enhanced creativity, and accelerated recovery from illness (Chmielewski, 2017; Stanke, 2014). Biophilia is fairly pleasing to most people, may even be therapeutic (Minton & Batten, 2016), and can be widely implemented in common areas and even residents' personal rooms, but other aspects of design and décor must be personalized for residents. Creating a personalized, stimulating environment in the residents' rooms or adjacent balconies is another best practice to consider. Caregivers can work with residents to establish a craft corner or a reading nook; redecorate their rooms; bring in seed starters to celebrate spring; or procure a small fish tank for animal lovers. In fact, observing fish has been shown to improve self-reported measures of mood and relaxation (Gee et al., 2019).

Furniture in common areas could be placed six feet apart to maintain social distancing guidelines. Multiple-seat couches and sofas could be replaced with single-seat furniture or could be labeled or used by only specific users during this pandemic. The facility could request that family members bring the residents' own furniture to the facility, and this cost-effective, person-centered strategy will minimize the spread of viruses. Even design elements, such as floor tile patterns or marks on the floor that are six feet apart, may be useful in serving as guides for placement of common area furniture. Furniture on wheels can allow residents and staff to arrange the space with a personal touch and maintain the person-centered aspect.

The mind-set of "*hygge*," a Danish concept that roughly translates to coziness and/or togetherness in English and is thought to contribute to high levels of happiness in the population (Wiking, 2017), has been popularized in American culture over the last several years. *Hygge* is much more than interior design, but some elements of *hygge*, including warm blankets, soft lighting, potted plants, nature-based and minimalistic décor, souvenirs, and photographs (Linnet, 2011), may be applied to the interior design of residents' rooms in a creative way to help memory care residents enjoy their personal space.

Indoor air quality

Great strides have been made in technology to improve indoor air quality, but implementation of these strategies is still not widespread in care facilities. Retrofitting existing buildings with a special focus on indoor air quality should be prioritized in the COVID-19 era. Measures can include high-quality air filters and ultraviolet lights to help purify indoor air for a safer indoor environment (Morawska & Milton, 2020; Mousavi et al., 2020). These measures could be considered for both design of future care facilities and for current MCFs via retrofitting where financially feasible. High efficiency air filtration and ultraviolet light could be used in MCFs to minimize air transmission of the virus in the building. Air flow dynamics are a part of mechanical architectural design and can be better implemented in improving indoor air quality by altering ventilation infrastructure; another less expensive option is to install more ceiling fans (Design, 2020).

Elevators notoriously hold air particles for a longer time due to poor air circulation, and they also typically require touching of buttons for operation, providing two different modes of transmitting viral particles. Escalators may provide an open-air, touchless option for traveling between floors; some other countries, namely Japan, have even developed wheelchair accessible escalators (Japan, 2020). When elevators are the only option, as in the case of taller buildings, button panels can be replaced with larger buttons to make it easier to use an elbow or cane to push the button (Design, 2020), and ultraviolet-based filters or air circulators can be installed to improve air quality (García De Abajo et al., 2020). Air humidity of above 50% has been shown to harbor the lowest amount of airborne viral particle transmission in animals (García De Abajo et al., 2020), and regulating indoor humidity and temperature is a feasible intervention that warrants further study.

Make better use of technology

Technology seems to be the go-to strategy for overcoming social isolation during the pandemic, and not just for older adults. It is important to remember that older adults' abilities and motivations for using technology vary widely and should be assessed rather than assumed (Eghtesadi, 2020), and accommodations should be made where necessary. Video chat-based platforms (e.g., Zoom, Facetime, Skype), use of social media, and virtual reality technology (Banskota et al., 2020; Berg-Weger & Morley, 2020; Eghtesadi, 2020; Padala et al., 2020) could be used as effective intervention strategies or therapies for mitigating COVID-19-related loneliness in the elderly who have reduced sensory ability, reduced mobility, and/or impaired cognition. *"Telemedicine,"* *"Telehealth"* or *"Telephone Outreach"* saves travel time for both the patient and the provider and may allow patients to receive a wider range of services without having to travel to a healthcare facility (Goodman-Casanova et al., 2020; Husebo & Storm, 2014; Van Den Berg et al., 2012; Van Dyck et al., 2020; Zubatsky et al., 2020).

Touchless technology can be made more prevalent at every level of the care facility. All doors, electrical switches, bathroom faucets and dispensers, soap and towel dispensers, and other hand-held touchable devices should be replaced with touchless sensing mechanisms (e.g., eye/hand movement, or voice detection systems) when possible. Foot pedals can also be used to operate doors, trash can lids, or even electrical switches. For surfaces that require touch, copper has been shown to have anti-microbial properties (Colin et al., 2018).

Small-scale community space

Previous research in MCFs showed that greater visibility and accessibility of common areas are actually associated with low-level compared to high-level (i.e. more meaningful) social interaction (Ferdous & Moore, 2015). This may be taken to mean that high-level social interaction occurs in more small-scale, home-like settings (Adlbrecht et al., 2020; Boer et al., 2018), and this conveniently parallels the need to reduce large group gatherings. Smaller gatherings of residents can be encouraged during meal times, group activities, and social hours by either physically spacing out or staggering activity times. This can also be applied to the design of floor plans by redesigning smaller common areas intended for use by 4–5 residents rather than larger common areas for use by all residents (Boer et al., 2018; Frankowski et al., 2011).

Instead of outright limiting social and communal gathering to keep residents safe, community activities such as meetings, grooming, and memory-care or fitness activities can be spread out across the facility in activity rooms and also in other common areas (such as bistros, living rooms, dining rooms, activity rooms, courtyards or outdoor patios) while maintaining social distancing guidelines. These activities can help MCF residents to maintain an active lifestyle and mitigate loneliness. Communal dining can still be enjoyed while maintaining social distancing and hygiene guidelines by extending the spacing between tables, adding additional meal service shifts for staff and switching to single-use table linens, condiments, menus, and service ware.

Person-centered approach

In the context of older adults, person-centered care can involve many domains, including holistic or whole-person care, respect, value, choice, dignity, self-determination, and purposeful living (Kogan et al., 2016). These concepts must be considered when determining how well safety guidelines for reducing disease transmission address the needs of the intended beneficiary (in this case, residents and staff members of MCFs).

A designated staff member at each facility could be assigned as the resident advocate. It might be someone who can take the time to listen to each resident and find out what will make each of them feel most valued, dignified, comfortable and cared for during this time. This advocate can then inform decisions for interior design, furniture layout and personalized activities, subsequently conserving facility resources for things that are most important to the residents. Staff members may also deserve a stake in these decisions, as they tend to know the residents most closely and also benefit from improvements to resident care. Of note, it especially behooves stakeholders of MCFs to invest in this aspect of care for residents and staff members, as downstream effects may include reduced staff turnover and improved staff satisfaction and performance (Koren, 2010).

The human aspect, implicit to spatial design, can be catered to in MCFs during the current and future pandemics. Face masks, which have become a necessary precaution, can be fun to wear; administrators can consider implementing themed mask days or promoting creative expressions of both residents (if they are physically able) and staff by encouraging use of brightly colored masks. The benefit of therapeutic touch, exemplified by caregivers physically helping the resident to wash their own hands, cannot be overstated (Hawranik & Deatrich, 2008; Woods & Dimond, 2002).

Spatial design and layout

Architecture and spatial design can play a significant role in redesigning future MCFs by maintaining social distancing guidelines, incorporating technology and following the occupancy and safety requirements for its users. To accommodate de-densification and social distancing guidelines, future MCFs could rethink, re-organize, retrofit, or redesign floor plans and alter building plans by incorporating the following spatial design strategies.

Incorporating negative-pressure isolation rooms (Miller et al., 2017, 2020) within each care facility could be a great way to control COVID-19 transmission. Negative-pressure isolation rooms are used to prevent the spread of airborne infectious disease from an infected patient to others in hospitals (Herrick, 2017). Sometimes memory care is embedded within nursing homes, assisted living facilities or LTCFs; isolating each specialized unit within the care facility with dedicated entry/exit points instead of a single main lobby might be a great design strategy to follow in future. Staggering and setting appointments for visiting hours to reduce traffic in the lobby or central areas could be an immediate solution for facilities. Care facilities could also install individual glass cubicles for visitation near the lobby where family members can visit the residents and even enjoy meals together. Meeting spaces can be redesigned so that seats are placed according to social distancing guidelines. If space limitation is an issue, community or staff meetings could take place in the existing conference rooms at reduced capacity and allow others to join virtually. If weather permits, meetings could also take place outside, and designers could accommodate this aspect when designing future care facilities.

Discussion

The long-term care system in the United States has never been flawless, but it has been neglected for decades (Werner et al., 2020). Even prior to COVID-19, the quality of care facilities has long been a critical issue that now requires immediate attention. The COVID-19 pandemic exposed the fragile and critical condition of the United States' long-term care system, and now it is time to reimagine the role of all care homes including MCFs in supporting older adults with or without ADRD. Lack of financial stability, inadequate resources, insufficiently monitored institutions, and understaffing of the existing long-term care system demands more subsidies and a newer model for delivering satisfactory, affordable care for vulnerable older adults with memory impairment who can no longer care for themselves at home.

Slowing the spread of the novel coronavirus requires immediate adjustments on how we use and inhabit existing spaces. Some advocates estimate that it will take up to 15 USD billion in federal funds for LTCFs to survive the COVID-19 pandemic (Goldstein et al., 2020). According to the Coronavirus Aid, Relief, and Economic Security (CARES) Act, Medicare-certified LTCFs with six or more certified beds will receive a baseline payment of 50,000 USD followed by additional performance-based distributions to address the critical needs and challenges directly linked to this pandemic such as increased testing, staffing, personal protective equipment needs and technological support (HHS, 2020b).

In reusing, repurposing, retrofitting and redesigning the existing MCFs to serve the urgent demands of the pandemic (e.g., "social distancing"), architects and designers are now facing new kinds of challenges. To begin with, the physical design and existing model of MCFs must be revised to accommodate the need for social isolation, physical distancing, staff protection, and safety and satisfaction of residents with or without ADRD during this unprecedented time when infectious diseases are flourishing. Although most of the interventions mentioned in this article are affordable, cost-effective, immediate and sustainable spatial design solutions, those interventions that are more cost-intensive may warrant use of additional relief funds. These interventions may include improving indoor air quality, replacing furniture, changing the spatial design layout, and incorporating touchless technology and will help to achieve longer-term benefits even after the COVID-19 era.

Additional funding may allow for the above-mentioned spatial design interventions; however, this is not the only solution to support the physical, mental, and social wellbeing of our older community while they battle the pandemic. Instead, we need a comprehensive, sustainable, affordable strategy; a collaborative approach; effective regulations; and advancement in policy at the institutional and administrative levels to support the long-term care system in the United States. In June of 2019, the Department of Health and Human Services (HHS) developed a contemporary, collaborative approach to improve the quality performance of U.S. healthcare providers called the "Health Quality Roadmap" (HHS, 2020a). Although COVID-19 has pushed back the project timeline, once implemented, this roadmap will enhance the effectiveness and efficiency of the U.S. healthcare system across federal programs and will create an opportunity for successful collaborative public-private partnerships (HHS, 2020a). To accommodate the mental wellbeing and psycho-social needs of older adults with or without ADRD, the most important aspects to consider in this novel situation are: 1) adapting and retrofitting existing LTCFs through interdisciplinary spatial design interventions and 2) redeveloping a newer model by revisiting the existing model of the U.S. long-term care system.

Conclusion

Rethinking the spatial design of care facilities in order to prepare for any future contagious respiratory pathogens is one of the prime concerns across the globe now. The objective of this article was to discuss evidence-based, interdisciplinary spatial design concepts, interventions, and action plans for redesigning future MCFs to minimize social isolation in older adults with or without ADRD. There is a strong need for evidence-based design solutions to accommodate the personal, social, and psychological needs of the residents, staff, caregivers, and family members as they are proportionately related to physiological and psychological health and well-being. Older adults living in MCFs will benefit greatly from a thoughtful revision of the incorporation of social distancing guidelines to reduce disease transmission. As of today, smaller-scale, family-style facilities with small numbers of residents, plenty of outdoor spaces, and modified interior layouts that prioritize social distancing, de-densification, and purified indoor air quality could be considered the most effective solutions for combatting the virus. The above interdisciplinary spatial design interventions and strategies may inspire not only MCFs but also nursing home and LTCF administrators, caregivers, family members of residents, policymakers, health care design professionals and researchers across many disciplines. We may very well be at the frontier of a new era of architecture, one that is again inspired by a public health crisis (Megahed & Ghoneim, 2020).

Key points

Older adults living in memory care facilities may be harmed from COVID-19 social distancing guidelines due to increased social isolation and loneliness.

Interdisciplinary approaches that emphasize spatial design guidelines and policies to minimize social isolation in older adults are arguably lacking.

Spatial design principles can inform public health policy and facility-level protocols with creative, evidence-based interventions.

Eight actionable, interdisciplinary spatial design themes are explored here that could be useful in redesigning memory care facilities and making future policy decisions.

Disclosure statement

No potential conflict of interest was reported by the author(s).

ORCID

Farhana Ferdous (iD) http://orcid.org/0000-0003-1622-2516

References

Adlbrecht, L., Bartholomeyczik, S., Hildebrandt, C., & Mayer, H. (2020). Social interactions of persons with dementia living in special care units in long-term care: A mixed-methods systematic review. *Dementia, 20*(3), 967–984. https://doi.org/10.1177/1471301220919937

Banskota, S., Healy, M., & Goldberg, E. M. (2020, April 14). 15 Smartphone Apps for Older Adults to Use While in Isolation During the COVID-19 Pandemic. *Western Journal of Emergency Medicine, 21*(3), 514–525. https://doi.org/10.5811/westjem.2020.4.47372

Behrens, L. L. (2020, June 4). "We are Alone in This Battle": A Framework for a Coordinated Response to COVID-19 in Nursing Homes. *Journal of aging & social policy, 32*(4–5), 316–322. https://doi.org/10.1080/08959420.2020.1773190

Berg-Weger, M., & Morley, J. E. (2020). Loneliness and Social Isolation in Older Adults during the COVID-19 Pandemic: Implications for Gerontological Social Work. *The journal of nutrition, health & aging, 24*(5), 456–458. https://doi.org/10.1007/s12603-020-1366-8

Boer, B. D., Beerens, H. C., Katterbach, M. A., Viduka, M., Willemse, B. M., & Verbeek, H. (2018). The Physical Environment of Nursing Homes for People with Dementia: Traditional Nursing Homes, Small-Scale Living Facilities, and Green Care Farms. *Healthcare, 6*(4), 137. https://doi.org/10.3390/healthcare6040137

CDC. (2020a). *Centers for Disease Control and Prevention: COVID-19 and Older Adults.* Retrieved November 09, 2020, from https://www.cdc.gov/coronavirus/2019-ncov/need-extra-precautions/older-adults.html

CDC. (2020b). *Personal and Social Activities*. Retrieved September 11, 2020, from https://www.cdc.gov/coronavirus/2019-ncov/daily-life-coping/personal-social-activities.html

Chmielewski, E. (2017). *Designing for memory care, senior-living facilities. Health Facilities Management Magazine.* https://www.hfmmagazine.com/articles/2730-designing-for-memory-care

Colin, M., Klingelschmitt, F., Charpentier, E., Josse, J., Kanagaratnam, L., De Champs, C., & Gangloff, S. C. (2018). Copper Alloy Touch Surfaces in Healthcare Facilities: An Effective Solution to Prevent Bacterial Spreading. *Materials (Basel)*, *11*(12), 2479. https://doi.org/10.3390/ma11122479

Cudjoe, T. K. M., & Kotwal, A. A. (2020, June). "Social Distancing" Amid a Crisis in Social Isolation and Loneliness. *Journal of the American Geriatrics Society*, *68*(6), E27–E29. https://doi.org/10.1111/jgs.16527

David, E. (2020, 14 April). The unspoken COVID-19 toll on the elderly: Loneliness. *abc News*. https://abcnews.go.com/Health/unspoken-covid-19-toll-elderly-loneliness/story?id=69958717

Design, M. (2020). *How do we design for safe interaction, not social isolation?* Designing Senior Housing for Safe Interaction. The Role of Architecture in Fighting COVID-19.*Mass Design Group.* https://massdesigngroup.org/sites/default/files/multiple-file/2020-07/Designing%20Senior%20Housing%20for%20Safe%20Interaction.pdf

Edelman, L. S., McConnell, E. S., Kennerly, S. M., Alderden, J., Horn, S. D., & Yap, T. L. (2020, May 26). Mitigating the Effects of a Pandemic: Facilitating Improved Nursing Home Care Delivery Through Technology. *JMIR Aging*, *3*(1), e20110. https://doi.org/10.2196/20110

Eghtesadi, M. (2020, May). Breaking Social Isolation Amidst COVID-19: A Viewpoint on Improving Access to Technology in Long-Term Care Facilities. *Journal of the American Geriatrics Society*, *68*(5), 949–950. https://doi.org/10.1111/jgs.16478

Evans, I. E. M., Martyr, A., Collins, R., Brayne, C., & Clare, L. (2019). Social Isolation and Cognitive Function in Later Life: A Systematic Review and Meta-Analysis. *Journal of Alzheimer's Disease*, *70*(s1), S119–S144. https://doi.org/10.3233/JAD-180501

Ferdous, F. (2019, September 13). Positive Social Interaction by Spatial Design: A Systematic Review of Empirical Literature in Memory Care Facilities for People Experiencing Dementia. *Journal of aging and health*, *32*(9), 898264319870090. https://doi.org/10.1177/0898264319870090

Ferdous, F., & Moore, K. D. (2015, March). Field observations into the environmental soul: Spatial configuration and social life for people experiencing dementia. *American Journal of Alzheimer's Disease & Other Dementiasr*, *30*(2), 209–218. https://doi.org/10.1177/1533317514545378

Frankowski, A. C., Roth, E. G., Eckert, J. K., & Harris-Wallace, B. (2011). The Dining Room as Locus of Ritual in Assisted Living. *Generations*, *35*(3), 41–46. https://pubmed.ncbi.nlm.nih.gov/25663740/

García De Abajo, F. J., Hernández, R. J., Kaminer, I., Meyerhans, A., Rosell-Llompart, J., & Sanchez-Elsner, T. (2020, July 28). Back to Normal: An Old Physics Route to Reduce SARS-CoV-2 Transmission in Indoor Spaces. *ACS Nano*, *14*(7), 7704–7713. https://doi.org/10.1021/acsnano.0c04596

Geboy, L. (2009). Linking Person-Centered Care and the Physical Environment: 10 Design Principles for Elder and Dementia Care Staff. *Alzheimer's Care Today*, *10*(4), 228–231. https://doi.org/10.1097/ACQ.0b013e3181bef153

Gee, N. R., Reed, T., Whiting, A., Friedmann, E., Snellgrove, D., & Ka., S. (2019). Observing Live Fish Improves Perceptions of Mood, Relaxation and Anxiety, But Does Not Consistently Alter Heart Rate or Heart Rate Variability. *International Journal of*

Environmental Research and Public Health, 16(17), 3113. https://doi.org/10.3390/ijerph16173113

Goldstein, M., Gebeloff, R., & Silver-Greenberg, J. (April 21, 2020). *Pandemic's costs stagger the nursing home industry.* New York Times. Retrieved December 7, 2020, from https://www.nytimes.com/2020/04/21/business/coronavirus-nursing-home-finances.html?auth=login-google

Goodman-Casanova, J. M., Dura-Perez, E., Guzman-Parra, J., Cuesta-Vargas, A., & Mayoral-Cleries, F. (2020, May 22). Telehealth Home Support During COVID-19 Confinement for Community-Dwelling Older Adults With Mild Cognitive Impairment or Mild Dementia: Survey Study. *Journal of Medical Internet Research, 22*(5), e19434. https://doi.org/10.2196/19434

Hawranik, P., & Deatrich, J. P. (2008). Therapeutic Touch and Agitation in Individuals With Alzheimer's Disease. *Western Journal of Nursing Research, 30*(4), 417–434. https://doi.org/10.1177/0193945907305126

Herrick, M. (2017). *Planning and maintaining hospital air isolation rooms. ASHE Health Facilities Management Magazine.* https://www.hfmmagazine.com/articles/2671-planning-and-maintaining-hospital-air-isolationrooms#:~:text=Negative%20isolation%20rooms.,to%20others%20in%20the%20hospital

HHS. (May 18, 2020a). *National Health Quality Roadmap.* Retrieved December 7, 2020, from https://www.hhs.gov/about/leadership/eric-d-hargan/quality-roadmap/index.html

HHS. (May 22, 2020b). *HHS Announces Nearly $4.9 Billion Distribution to Nursing Facilities Impacted by COVID-19.* https://www.hhs.gov/about/news/2020/05/22/hhs-announces-nearly-4.9-billion-distribution-to-nursing-facilities-impacted-by-covid19.html

Holt-Lunstad, J., & Smith, T. B. (2016, July 1). Loneliness and social isolation as risk factors for CVD: Implications for evidence-based patient care and scientific inquiry. *Heart, 102*(13), 987–989. https://doi.org/10.1136/heartjnl-2015-309242

Holt-Lunstad, J., Smith, T. B., Baker, M., & Harris, T. (2015). Loneliness and social isolation as risk factors for mortality: A meta-analytic review. *Perspectives on Psychological Science, 10* (2), 227–237. https://doi.org/10.1177/1745691614568352

Husebo, A. M., & Storm, M. (2014). Virtual visits in home health care for older adults. *The Scientific World Journal, 2014*, 689873. https://doi.org/10.1155/2014/689873

Japan, A. (2020). *No Elevator, No Problem.Accessible Japan.* Retrieved September 15, 2020, from https://www.accessible-japan.com/no-elevator-no-problem/#:~:text=Wheelchair%20Accessible%20Escalators&text=They%20are%20usually%20operated%20by,special%20arca%20of%20the%20steps .

Kang, H. (2012). Correlates of social engagement in nursing home residents with dementia. *Asian Nursing Research, 6*(2), 75–81. https://doi.org/10.1016/j.anr.2012.05.006

Kogan, A. C., Wilber, K., & Mosqueda, L. (2016). Person-Centered Care for Older Adults with Chronic Conditions and Functional Impairment: A Systematic Literature Review. *Journal of the American Geriatrics Society, 64*(1), 1–7. https://doi.org/10.1111/jgs.13873

Koren, M. J. (2010). Person-centered care for nursing home residents: The culture-change movement. *Health affairs(Millwood), 29*(2), 312–317. https://doi.org/10.1377/hlthaff.2009.0966

Linnet, J. T. (2011). Money Can't Buy Me Hygge Danish Middle-Class Consumption, Egalitarianism, and the Sanctity of Inner Space. *Social Analysis, 55*(2), 21–44. https://doi.org/10.3167/sa.2011.550202

McFarlane, C. (2020, March 20). De/re-densification: A relational geography of urban density. *City, 24*(1–2), 314–324. https://doi.org/10.1080/13604813.2020.1739911

Megahed, N. A., & Ghoneim, E. M. (2020, October 1). Antivirus-built environment: Lessons learned from Covid-19 pandemic. *Sustainable Cities and Society, 61,* 102350. https://doi.org/10.1016/j.scs.2020.102350

Miller, S. L., Clements, N., Elliott, S. A., Subhash, S. S., Eagan, A., & Radonovich, L. J. (2017, June 1). Implementing a negative-pressure isolation ward for a surge in airborne infectious patients. *American journal of infection control, 45*(6), 652–659. https://doi.org/10.1016/j.ajic.2017.01.029

Miller, S. L., Mukherjee, D., Wilson, J., Clements, N., & Steiner, C. (2020, October 3). Implementing a negative pressure isolation space within a skilled nursing facility to control SARS-CoV-2 transmission. *American journal of infection control, 49*(4). https://doi.org/10.1016/j.ajic.2020.09.014

Minton, C., & Batten, L. (2016). Rethinking the intensive care environment: Considering nature in nursing practice. *Journal of Clinical Nursing, 25*(1–2), 269–277. https://doi.org/10.1111/jocn.13069

Morawska, L., & Milton, D. K. (2020, July 6). It is Time to Address Airborne Transmission of COVID-19. *Clinical infectious diseases, 71*(9), 2311–2313. https://doi.org/10.1093/cid/ciaa939

Mousavi, E. S., Kananizadeh, N., Martinello, R. A., & Sherman, J. D. (2020, September 11). COVID-19 Outbreak and Hospital Air Quality: A Systematic Review of Evidence on Air Filtration and Recirculation. *Environmental science & technology, 55*(7), 4134-4147. https://doi.org/10.1021/acs.est.0c03247

Padala, S. P., Jendro, A. M., & Orr, L. C. (2020, June). Facetime to reduce behavioral problems in a nursing home resident with Alzheimer's dementia during COVID-19. *Psychiatry Research, 288,* 113028. https://doi.org/10.1016/j.psychres.2020.113028

Read, S., Comas-Herrera, A., & Grundy, E. (2020, January 14). Social Isolation and Memory Decline in Later-life. *The Journals of Gerontology: Series B, 75*(2), 367–376. https://doi.org/10.1093/geronb/gbz152

Shrira, A., Hoffman, Y., Bodner, E., & Palgi, Y. (2020, May 27). COVID-19-Related Loneliness and Psychiatric Symptoms Among Older Adults: The Buffering Role of Subjective Age. *The American Journal of Geriatric Psychiatry, 28*(11), 1200–1204. https://doi.org/10.1016/j.jagp.2020.05.018

Stanke, S. (2014). *Connecting to Nature in Interior Dementia Care Environments,* Master of Arts in Sustainable Design. https://islandora.mcad.edu/islandora/object/MASD%3A33/datastream/OBJ/view

Van Den Berg, N., Schumann, M., Kraft, K., & Hoffmann, W. (2012, October). Telemedicine and telecare for older patients–a systematic review. *Maturitas, 73*(2), 94–114. https://doi.org/10.1016/j.maturitas.2012.06.010

Van Dyck, L. I., Wilkins, K. M., Ouellet, J., Ouellet, G. M., & Conroy, M. L. (2020, June 5). Combating Heightened Social Isolation of Nursing Home Elders: The Telephone Outreach in the COVID-19 Outbreak Program. *The American Journal of Geriatric Psychiatry, 28*(9), 989–992. https://doi.org/10.1016/j.jagp.2020.05.026

Werner, R. M., Hoffman, A. K., & Coe, N. B. (2020, September 3). Long-Term Care Policy after Covid-19 - Solving the Nursing Home Crisis. *New England Journal of Medicine, 383*(10), 903–905. https://doi.org/10.1056/NEJMp2014811

Wiking, M. (2017). *The Little Book of Hygge: Danish Secrets to Happy Living.* William Morrow.

Woods, D. L., & Dimond, M. (2002). The Effect of Therapeutic Touch on Agitated Behavior and Cortisol in Persons with Alzheimer's Disease. *Biological Research For Nursing, 4*(2), 104–114. https://doi.org/10.1177/1099800402238331

Wu, B. (2020). Social isolation and loneliness among older adults in the context of COVID-19: A global challenge. *Global Health Research and Policy*, *5*(1), 27. https://doi.org/10.1186/s41256-020-00154-3

Xia, N., & Li, H. (2018). Loneliness, Social Isolation, and Cardiovascular Health. *Antioxidants & redox signaling*, *28*(9), 837–851. https://doi.org/10.1089/ars.2017.7312

Yang, R., Wang, H., Edelman, L. S., Tracy, E. L., Demiris, G., Sward, K. A., & Donaldson, G. W. (2020). Loneliness as a mediator of the impact of social isolation on cognitive functioning of Chinese older adults. *Age and Ageing*, *49*(4), 599–604. https://doi.org/10.1093/ageing/afaa020

Yourish, K., Rebecca Lai, K. I. D., & Smith, M. (2020, December 4). More Than 100,000 U.S. Coronavirus Deaths Are Linked to Nursing Homes. *NY Times*. https://www.nytimes.com/interactive/2020/us/coronavirus-nursing-homes.html

Zubatsky, M., Berg-Weger, M., & Morley, J. (2020, May 11). Using telehealth groups to combat loneliness in older adults through COVID-19. *Journal of the American Geriatrics Society*, *68*(8), 1678–1679. https://doi.org/10.1111/jgs.16553

Index

Note: Figures are indicated by italics. Tables are indicated by bold.

absorptive transnational elder care 187–8
active aging 63, 75, 76; counter infections of 69–70
adaptive transnational elder care 185–7
advance care planning (ACP) 200, 207–8; high interpersonal barriers 200–1; high sociostructural barriers 201; limiting the practitioners' capacities 202; as structured process for chronic illness 201–2
advanced care planning (ACP) 12
age: at 70, 67–9; categorization 65, 69–72; discrimination 68, 69, 73; limit 67–8, 72–3; rejection of 76; restriction 65, 66, 68, 69, 71–7
age-based recommendations 63–5, 67, 70–5
ageism/aging 6, 10, 92, 241–2; and implications on mental well-being 235–6; parallel outbreak of 34; in place 35, 37
Alajlani, M. 223
Alzheimer's disease and related dementias (ADRD) 264, 271, 272
Andersson, J. 76
anxiety 75–6, 88, 89, 91, 92, 103
anxiety in Northern California 24, 26, 29, 30; correlation between isolation and 26, **27**, 29; limitations and future research for 29–30
Armitage, R. 37
Aronson, L. 34
artificial intelligence (AI) 252
Australia, telemedicine reimbursement 223
avoidance coping 46

Batsis, J. A. 222
Bayesian Information Criterion (BIC) 24, 26
biological age 67, 69, 74
biophilia 267
biopolitics 62, 65, 75
biopower 62, 65, 69
bitterness 88
Black, Indigenous, or other Persons of Color (BIPOC) residents 121, 126
"BoomerRemover" hashtag 34
borderline situation 76
borderline situations 76

Brazilian Health Regulatory Agency 165, 167
Brazil, LTC homes in 164, 167; interdisciplinary leadership groups 170; prohibition of visitors 165
brokering agencies 179, 180, 182–4, 187, 188, 190, 191
Brooke, J. 241
Brooks, A. K. 241
Bureau of Health and Welfare for the Elderly 150–1, 155

Canada, LTC homes in 164, 248; ban of visitors 166; ban of volunteers 167; eliminating movement of staff 166–7; Resident Support Aides (RSAs) 169; visitor restrictions 167
care gap 188
caregivers 103–5, 110; demographic characteristics of **104**; isolation 106; visitation restrictions/strategies 100, **104**, 104–8
care recipient 99–100, 103; inhumane care to 106–7; isolation 106; lack of oversight due to short staffing 107–8; rapid decline, mental and physical state of 106, 108, 109
care retirement community (CCRC) 121
caring for psychological health 54
Carr, D. 110
Centers for Medicare and Medicaid Services (CMS) datasets 118, 119
Certification and Survey Provider Enhanced Reporting (CASPER) system 119, 121
Chaudoir, S. R. 48
China, LTC homes in 164; elimination of visitors 165; interdisciplinary leadership groups 170; preventing the staffs from leaving 167
chronological age 67, 69, 74, 75
Clarke, M. 223
class 201
clinical decision-making support systems (CDS) 252–3
Cohen, S. 48
communal dining 167, 269
communal gathering 269

communication to mitigate social isolation residents 170
community-dwelling older adults: coping strategies 90–1, 93, 94; mixed experiences 84–5, 87–8, 91; negative experiences 84–5, 88–9; positive experiences 84–7, 89–90, 92; resilience 91, 94; thematic map 84–5, 89, *90*, 92
community safety 37
community value 37, 39
complex symptom management 209
compliance: with age-based recommendations 66, 71; and resistance 75, 77–8
confirmatory factor analysis (CFA) 23–4, 26, 27, 49–50; fit indices for 26, **28**
contagion 235
Coronavirus Aid, Relief, and Economic Security (CARES) Act 271
COVID-19 pandemic: challenge for medical services by 220–1; deaths 4–6, 110, 148–50, **149**; impact on long-term care systems 10–12; personal experiences with 9–10; role of end-of-life care in 12; technologies and innovations for 12–13
COVID-19 pandemic: telemedicine for 221–5
cross-border: medical practices 220; mobility 180; older adults 218, 220, 224; social policy for Hong Kong's older adults in China 218–20

data: analysis 84–5, 102–3, 185; collection 102; visualization 252
de-centralization 265, 267; de-densification 265, 270
de-densification 265, 270
dementia 249, 251–3
demographic data analysis 84
Department of Health and Human Services (HHS) 272
depression 88, 89, 91, 92, 103, 234
descriptive statistics 24, **25**
de-stigmatization 53–4
disappointment 88
Disease Control and Prevention (CDC) 263
distress 236
durable power of attorney for health care (DPAHC) 200, 208–9

economic disparities 8
Ehni, H. -J. 74
electronic medical records (EMRs) 252
elevators 268
emotional resilience 234
emotional support 231, 232, 234, 236–43
end-of-life care 12
escalators 268
Ethical Guidelines on the Practice of Telemedicine in 2019 223
ethnicity 201
Ethnographic Content Analysis 64

"failure to plan" 163
family caregivers *see* caregivers

family-resident interaction 169
fear of disclosure 45, 53, 54; analytic strategy 50; measure 48; regression analyses 51–2
Federation of Trade Unions (FTU) 221, 224
female caregivers 179
Ferdous, F. 13
financial security and safety 36
Folkman, S. 46
formal care setting (FCS) 101, 109–11; *see also* visitation restrictions; experiences with 104–5
formal care setting (FCS) residents *see* care recipient
formal care workers 179
for-profit LTCFs 153, 155–7
Foucault, Michel: biopolitics 62, 75; biopower 62; governmentality 62, 63
Fujian Scheme 219
furniture layout 267

gastroenteritis 156
Geboy, L. 265
German-Polish mobility 191
Germany 179; absorptive transnational care 187; adaptive transnational care 186–7; brokering agencies 184; restricted mobility 181–2, 186; transformative transnational care 188–9; transnational care system 180, 190–1
Gitlow, L. 251
global recession 7
Golant, S. M. 37
good convergent and discriminant validity 49
governmentality 62, 63, 69
Greenberg, N. 241
grief 110
Guangdong-Hong Kong-Macao Greater Bay Area 219–20
Guangdong Scheme 219

Hackenbroich, J. 190
health care system 202
"Health Quality Roadmap" 272
health resources 38
high efficiency air filtration 268
higher-intensity emotional support 239
HIV-status disclosure 46
Hokenjo 152
Holt-Lunstad, J. 108
home-based care 177–8
Hong Kong 217
Hong Kong's older adults in mainland China 217–18; challenge for medical services by COVID-19 220–1; chronic diseases 221; cross-border social policy for 218–20; telemedicine for COVID-19 pandemic 221–5
hospitalization 5
hours per resident day (HPRD) 120
hygge 267–8

identity-place relationship 37, 39
indoor air quality 268

inequalities 201, 254; racial and
    socioeconomic 12
influenza 22, 44, 151, 152, 156
informal care 179–80, 189
informal care givers 179
inhumane care to care recipient 106–7
innovations 12–13
inpatient palliative care 210–11
intelligent assistive technologies (IATs) 253–4
intentional concealment of epicenter travel 53
interdisciplinary leadership groups 170
interdisciplinary spatial design interventions
    264–5, **266**, 272
interior design 267–8
internet access 250–1
interpersonal barriers to ACP 200–1
Irwin, R. 66
isolation *see* social isolation
Israel: COVID-19 pandemic impact on
    older adults' mental well-being 233–4;
    deterioration in older adults' physical and
    mental health 233–4; emotional resilience of
    older adults 234; impact of the lockdown 234;
    loneliness of older adults 233–4
Israel Gerontological Society 236, 237, 240,
    241, 243
Italy: COVID-19 outbreak 134; long-term care
    policies 138; National Health System (NHS)
    of 141–3

Jackson, D. 241
Japan, COVID-19 in 11; features and pandemic
    response 155–7; institutional response 157;
    long-term care facilities (LTCFs) (*see*
    long-term care facilities (LTCFs), Japan);
    Long-Term Care Insurance 152; LTCF
    system 152–5; mortality 150; number of
    deaths 148, **149**; small death toll 148–50;
    social welfare corporations 153; swift decision
    to lockdown LTCFs 150–2
Japan, LTC homes in 164; ban of
    volunteers 167; seasonal lockdowns 166;
    visitor restrictions 167

Kenny, D. A. 50
Kruk, M. E. 190, 191
Kuwahara, K. 38

labor force participation 7, 8
lack of oversight due to short staffing 107–8
Langabeer, J. R. 222
Lazarus, R. S. 46
Leiber, S. 180
Leiblfinger, M. 186
leisure technologies 253
lockdowns 150–2, 156, 231, 234, 235, 238, 250,
    253, 255
Lombardy, nursing homes in 135; coverage
    rate of residential beds 137–8, *138*, **139**;
    decentralization by regional governments 140;
    financial unsustainability 142; funding
    mechanism in 141; institutional context

137–42; lack of personal protective
    equipment 136; long-term health care
    services 140; medium-to-high intensity
    health services 140; mortality rate 11, 135–6,
    136, 143; national lockdown of 136; number
    of hospitalized patients in *140*, 142; policy
    strategy 136, 137; poor development of long-
    term care policy 137; poor development of
    residential care 138; public funding 142, 143;
    recent trends 142–3; reduction of staff 142;
    share of residential beds *141*; size of 141
loneliness 6, 9, 54, 81–2, 163, 200, 231, 232–3,
    251, 264
loneliness in Northern California 21, 24, 26;
    correlation between isolation, anxiety and
    26, **27**; feelings of 26, 29–30; and isolation 28–
    9; limitations and future research for 29–30;
    prevalence of 21–2, 26, 29
loner advantage 87, 93
long-distance caregivers 103
long-term care facilities (LTCFs) 5–6, 263, 271–
    2; social spaces in 264
long-term care facilities (LTCFs), Japan 148–
    50, 157–8; disease prevention and control
    150–2, 155–6; features and pandemic
    response 155–7; five categories of **154**;
    for-profit facilities 153, 155–7; lockdown
    decision 150–2; nonprofit facilities 153;
    regulatory framework 153, **154**; system 152–5
long-term care (LTC) homes 162–3, 247;
    barriers and challenges in technology
    implementation 254–5; Canada 248; clinical
    decision-making support systems (CDS) 252–
    3; COVID-19 policies 164; eliminating
    movement of staff and volunteers 166–7;
    elimination of visitors 165–6; intelligent
    assistive technologies (IATs) 253–4;
    international perspective of 164; internet
    access 250–1; policies and countermeasures
    in 164–8; restricting resident activities
    and interactions 167–8; social
    isolation of residents 164–71; social
    technologies 253; software and peripheral
    accessories 251–2; staffing issues 168–9;
    structural deficiencies 248; technology access
    to 248–55; Wi-Fi access 250–1
long-term care insurance (LTCI) 152–3, 155
Long-Term Care Insurance in 2000, Japan 152
long-term care systems 10–12
low-intensity emotional support 239
lung tissue, 72 years old 70
Lutz, H. 180

McGoogan, J. M. 220
machine learning 252
Masi, C. M. 233
mediation mechanism 46–7, 53
memory care facilities (MCFs) 263, 264, 271–
    2; better use of technology 268–9; de-
    centralization 265, 267; furniture layout 267;
    indoor air quality 268; interdisciplinary
    spatial design interventions 264–5, **266**, 272;

outdoor space and activities 265; personalized interior 267–8; person-centered care 270; small-scale community space 269

mental health: hotlines 239; services 38

Ministry for Social Equality's hotline 237

Ministry of Health, Labor and Welfare (MHLW) 150–1, 153, 155, 156

mixed experiences 84–5, 87–8, 91; *see also* negative experiences; positive experiences

monitoring the residents 168

Morrow-Howell, N. 241

mortality rate: nursing homes in Lombardy 135–6, *136*, 143; Tokyo 150

multimorbidity 206; palliative care for patients with 207–12

National Council on Aging (NCOA) 36, 38

National Health System (NHS) of Italy 141–3

negative experiences 84–5, 88–9

negative-pressure isolation rooms 270

neighborhood changes and moving 38, 39

neighborhood-feeling 37, 38

Nellums, L. B. 37

neoliberal governmentality 62, 63, 69, 75

non-profit LTCFs 153

nonprofit organizations 153, 155

North America, LTC homes in 167; ban of volunteers 167; ban on visitors 166

North Atlantic Treaty Organization (NATO) 222

Northern California: anxiety in (*see* anxiety in Northern California); loneliness in (*see* loneliness in Northern California); social isolation in (*see* social isolation in Northern California)

Nursing Home Improvement and Accountability Act 7–8

nursing homes 11; challenges 130; facilities 129–30; in Lombardy (*see* Lombardy, nursing homes in); nature and structure of 130; Ohio (*see* Ohio nursing homes, impact of COVID-19 on); policies 130; poor and high-quality 129; reimbursement system 130

Ohio Department of Health (ODH) data 118–19, 122

Ohio nursing homes, impact of COVID-19 on 117–18; analytic approach 122; cases 119–22, 126; expansion in intensity among 123; facility structure 121, 122, 126, 129; financial resources measure 121; higher staffing levels 126; high number of cases among facilities with a case 126, **127–8**; licensed beds 119, 120, 122, 129, 131; licensed practical nurses 126; nursing staff and quality measures 120–2; occupancy 121, 126; overall 5-star ratings 126, **128**, 128–9; payer-mix 121, 126; prevalence 117–18, 123, **123**, 129; quality 126, 129; regression analyses 120–2; resident case-mix 126; rurality 121, 126; summary statistics and

factors 123, **124–5**, 126; test positive case 122–3, 126; virus case information 131

Old Age Allowance (OAA) 219

Old Age Living Allowance (OALA) 219

older adults: COVID-19 pandemic impact on the mental well-being of 233–4; economic effects and 7–8; health effects and 5–6; isolation 232–3; loneliness 232–3; in memory care facilities 13; psychological health care 54; racial and ethnic disparities and 8; relationship to place matters 35; social effects and 6–7

Older Americans Act 39

online social support 241

Ouslander, J. G. 241

outdated building design 248

outdoor space and activities 265

outpatient palliative care 210; *see also* inpatient palliative care

"overly restrictive reactive policies" 163

Palenga-Möllenbeck, E. 180

palliative care 12; advance care planning 207–8; complex symptom management 209; description 207; expanding and integrated roles 210–11; goals of 207–8; inpatient 210–11; outpatient 210; for patients with multimorbidity 207–12; settings 202; supporting caregivers 209; surrogate decision-making 208; teams 209–12; telemedicine 210

"parallel outbreak of ageism" 34

Payroll-Based Journaling (PBJ) data 119

perceived stress measure 48

personal experiences 9–10

personalized interior 267–8

personal safety 37

person-centered care (PCC) 110, 248–55, 270

Person-Place Fit Measure for Older Adults 9

person-place fit measure for older adults (PPFM-OA) 36–9

physical distancing 167

Pilot Residential Care Services Scheme 219, 224

place 35; attachment 37, 39

PLHIV (people living with HIV) 46

Poland 179; absorptive transnational care 187; adaptive transnational care 186; brokering agencies 183, 186; caregivers 186; COVID-19 cases 182; restricted mobility 181–2, 186, 189; transformative transnational care 188–90; transnational care system 180, 190–1

policy implications 39

policy/practice for safer visitation 109–10

positive experiences 84–7, 89–90, 92

primary/basic needs and necessities 36–7, 39

psychological first aid 54

qualitative analysis 102

qualitative data analysis 84

quality of care 187–8

quarantine 47, 48, 53, 54

Quinn, D. M. 48

racial and ethnic minority older adults 8
racial inequality 201
rapid decline 233; of care recipient's mental and
    physical state 106, 108, 109
Razian, S. 48
regression analyses 50–2, **52**, 120–2, 126, 128
resident-resident interaction 169
Resident Support Aides (RSAs) 169
resilience 178, 186, 234; transnational elder care
    system 180–2, 188, 190, 191
restricted mobility 181–6, 188, 189
Rose, Nicolas 62

sadness 105
safe resident interactions 169
Scheizer, K. 24
self-quarantining 200
sending agencies 182–3, 188, 190
Shinzo Abe 151
short staffing 107–8
Shrira, A. 234
Skilled Workers Immigration Act 191
small-scale community space 269
social avoidance 45, 46, 53, 54; analytic
    strategy 50–1; measure 48; regression
    analyses 51–2; scale 51
social connectedness 250
social distancing 22, 167, 200, 231, 235;
    guidelines 264, 265, 267, 269, 270, 272
social gathering 269
social interaction 264
social isolation 6, 9, 12, 37, 81–2, 108,
    109, 163, 171, 200, 231–3, 251, 264; *see
    also* loneliness; of caregivers 106; of care
    recipient 106; in long-term care homes 11;
    for LTC home residents 164–8; of LTC
    staffs 167; strategies for mitigating the
    residents of 168–71
social isolation in Northern California 21,
    24, 26; correlation between anxiety, loneliness
    and 26, **27**; feelings of 26, 29–30; limitations
    and future research for 29–30; loneliness
    and 28; prevalence of 21–2, 26, 29
social media 53, 54
social networks 37
social technologies 253
social welfare corporations , Japan 153
Social Welfare for the Elderly, Article 30 of the
    Act on 156
socioeconomic inequality 201
sociostructural barriers to ACP 201
software and peripheral accessories 251–2
solidarity 66–7, 76
spatial design and layout 270–1
staff-resident interaction 169
staff's clinical decision making, technology
    for 252–3
stay-at-home order 22, 23, 26, 28–30, 231
Steinman, M. A. 241
stigmatization 43–5, 47, 53, 54; analytic
    strategy 50–1; measure 48; regression
    analyses 51–2; scale 51; and stress 45–6

stress 53, 54; analytic strategy 50; mediating
    role of 46–7; perceived, measure 48;
    regression analyses 51–2; stigmatization
    and 45–6
structural equation modeling (SEM) 50–1
successful aging 61, 63, 74
surrogate decision-making 208–9
Sweden, age restriction in 65
Swedish culture 66, 75
Swedish response to COVID-19 pandemic 65–
    6, 74, 75
Switzerland, LTC homes in 164,
    167, 170; ban of volunteers 167; safe resident
    interactions 169; social distancing 167;
    visitor restrictions 166
system resilience 178, 186, 190, 191

technology 12–13; access to LTC homes
    248–55; better use of 268–9; to mitigate social
    isolation residents 170
Tegnell, A. 60, 66
telemedicine/telehealth 210, 218, 249, 269;
    barriers against wide implementation
    of 224; cost savings for patients. 222; cross-
    border 224–5; future of 221–5; Hong Kong's
    older adults in mainland China 221–5;
    legislation 222; providing the clinical
    services at a distance 221–2; reimbursement
    for 222–3; training 224; video conferencing
    system 223
telephone-based emotional care program 13
telephone outreach 269
telephone relationships 238, 239
telephone-support initiative 241–2; additional
    benefits of 240–1; establishing the 236–7;
    goal of 237; program development 237;
    program implementation 238; type of
    support 239–40; unique features of 238–9
thematic analysis 84
thematic map 84–5, 89, *90*, 92
Tokyo 150
touchless technology 269
transformative transnational elder
    care 188–90
transnational home-based elder care
    179–81; absorptive capacity 187–8;
    adaptive capacity 185–7; legal regulations
    and policy 190; quality of care 187–8;
    resilience 180–2, 188, 190; transformative
    capacity 188–90
transnational mobility 186, 191
travel restrictions 181–6, 188, 189
trust 66, 75

ultraviolet light 268
unemployment 7, 8
United States (US): COVID-19 cases and
    deaths 4; long-term care system 271–2
United States (US), LTC homes in 164; ban of
    volunteers 167; elimination of visitors 165;
    visitor restrictions 166, 167

vaccination 4, 6
vaccines 3–4
Vaportzis, E. 251
video conferencing 223, 249
visitation restrictions 100, 104, 108, 109, 167, 249; feelings regarding reduction of **105**, 105–8; mitigating the negative impacts of 168–9; policy/practice 109–10; thematic analysis 105–8

visitors: elimination 165–6; limitations 208, 211; restrictions 167
volunteers 167; emotional support to older adults 236–42

Wahl, H. -W. 74
Wi-Fi access 250–1
Wuhan 22, 165, 167
Wu, Z. 220

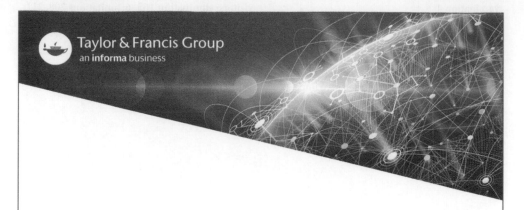
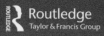
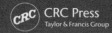